PROGRESS IN CARDIAC ARRHYTHMIA RESEARCH

PROGRESS IN CARDIAC ARRHYTHMIA RESEARCH

IRA R. TARKOWICZ
EDITOR

Nova Biomedical Books
New York

Library of Congress Cataloging-in-Publication Data

Progress in cardiac arrythmia research / Ira R. Tarkowicz (editor).
p. ; cm.
Includes bibliographical references and index.
ISBN-13: 978-1-60021-796-8 (hardcover)
ISBN-10: 1-60021-796-6 (hardcover)
1. Arrhythmia. I. Tarkowicz, Ira R.
[DNLM: 1. Arrhythmia. WG 330 P9632 2007]
RC685.A65P77 2007
616.1'28--dc22 2007021895

Published by Nova Science Publishers, Inc. ✦ New York

Contents

Preface

Cardiac arrhythmia is a term that denotes a disturbance of the heart rhythm. Cardiac arrhythmias can range in severity from entirely benign to immediately life-threatening. A cardiac arrhythmia, also called cardiac dysrhythmia, is a disturbance in the regular rhythm of the heartbeat. Several forms of cardiac arrhythmia are life-threatening and a medical emergency.Cardiac arrhythmias sometimes are classified according to their origin as either ventricular arrhythmias (originating in the ventricles) or supraventricular arrhythmias (originating in heart areas above the ventricles, typically the atria). They also can be classified according to their effect on the heart rate, with bradycardia indicating a heart rate of less than 60 beats per minute and tachycardia indicating a heart rate of more than 100 beats per minute. This new book presents important research in the field from around the globe.

The chances for successful restoration of spontaneous circulation (ROSC) in cardiac arrest follwing ventricular fibrillation (VF) deteriorate rapidly with time. Improved myocardial reperfusion, e.g. by way of cardiopulmonary resuscitation (CPR), may improve the prospect for successful defibrillation. In addition, electrocardiographic (ECG) waveform analysis can help determine the optimal timing for defibrillation and thus prevent unnecessary damage caused to the myocardium by unsuccessful electric shocks. Computer-assisted ECG analysis with removal of CPR-associated noise and artifacts allows the outcome of defibrillation to be predicted without causing potentially detrimental interruptions in CPR. The likelihood that defibrillation in patients with sustained VF will be successful can be further improved by administering thrombolytics during CPR. While dissolution of coronary artery thrombosis resolves the underlying cause of myocardial infarction in the majority of patients, improved microcirculatory reperfusion and alteration of the electrical activity of the fibrillation process may increase the likelihood of restoring spontaneous circulation during resuscitation. An increase in fibrillation frequency, fibrillation amplitude or in amplitude spectrum area (AMSA) as calculated from electrocardiography (ECG) signals indicates that thrombolytic therapy is improving ventricular fibrillation status, thus improving the chances for successful defibrillation.

As presented in Chapter 1, contemporary preclinical *in vitro* and *in vivo* methods have been imperfect in predicting drug-induced Torsades de Pointes (TdP) arrhythmia in humans. A better understanding of additional relevant factors in the genesis of drug-induced TdP besides the relationships between *h*ERG inhibition, action potential duration, and QT interval is necessary and supports the evolution of new methods to assess the cardiovascular safety of new drug candidates in the future.

New, sophisticated *in vitro* techniques, such as arterially perfused ventricular wedge preparations or isolated perfused hearts, potentially offer a better understanding of torsadogenic mechanisms and a refinement of drug testing. Of particular interest are the dispersion of repolarization and the refractoriness of different cell types across the ventricular wall, triangulation of the action potential, reverse use dependence and instability of the action potential duration. *In vivo* models in conscious and anesthetized non-rodents are currently refined by establishing the relevance of parameters such as beat-to-beat-variability and T-wave morphology as derived from the *in vitro* proarrhythmia indices. Animal models of proarrhythmia are to date not recommended for routine evaluation, since the models are insufficiently established to provide any certainty of detecting relevant effects. This holds true for *in vitro* and *in vivo* techniques.

Pharmacodynamic interactions with combinations of torsadogenic compounds at the level of the hERG channel on the plasma membrane and interactions with other channel proteins is another area to be considered. Little is known about channel/receptor cross talk, although considerable evidence exists that cardiac G protein-coupled receptors can modulate *h*ERG channel function. More investigations are necessary to further evaluate the role of altered gene expression, mutations and polymorphisms in drug-induced TdP. Down-regulation of hERG channels under pathophysiological conditions contributes significantly to the enhanced liability of the repolarization process. A recently discovered mechanism of drug-induced torsadogenesis is the reduced expression of hERG channel protein on the plasma membrane due to a trafficking defect.

Pharmacokinetic and metabolism data of NCE are crucial for calculating the risk of a torsadogenic potential in man. Consideration of intracardiac accumulation via effects on active transport mechanisms that facilitate access of the drug to the "active site" may help in delineating any pharmacokinetic-pharmacodyamic relationships and potential pharmacokinetic drug-drug interactions that may occur beyond the hepatic cytochrome P450 level.

In silico methods possess the potential to improve the prediction of torsadogenic risk. For early risk assessment of new drug candidates, virtual screening procedures to predict hERG block would become a promising tool. The role of *in silico* modeling of TdP arrhythmia is likely to become increasingly important, however, the pathogenesis of arrhythmias is complex and vast amounts of data need to be considered. At present *in silico* methods cannot replace existing preclinical models.

Chapter 2 discusses the role of antagonists of the renin-angiotensin system in the prevention of atrial fibrillation.

Background: Atrial fibrillation (AF) is the most frequently encountered arrhythmia in clinical practice and is associated with increased mortality and morbidity. Its incidence has grown due to the increasing prevalence of risk factors for AF development, which include age, diabetes, hypertension, heart failure (HF), valvular and ischemic heart diseases. Retrospective studies and small prospective trials have suggested a preventive effect of antagonists of the renin-angiotensin system (RAS), including angiotensin-converting enzyme (ACE) inhibitors and angiotensin-II receptor blockers (ARB), on AF occurence.

Method and Results: The authors performed a systematic literature search on the role of RAS antagonists in the prevention of AF. They looked in particular at the pathophysiology of AF, including the concepts of atrial ionic and anatomical changes induced by AF, called electrical and structural remodelling. The authors reviewed the published data on the potential beneficial effect of RAS inhibitors on AF occurrence in various experimental and clinical settings.

Conclusions: Inhibition of the renin-angiotensin system seems to prevent AF occurrence in patients with associated disease such as heart failure, hypertension and population with few co-morbidities but persistent AF. The role of these agents in the routine management of AF remains to be determined.

As explained in Chapter 3, the Ro-ribonucleoproteins (52- and 60-kDa) are the main intracellular targets of the anti-Ro/SSA-antibodies, frequently detected in autoimmune rheumatic diseases, particularly Sjögren's syndrome, and systemic lupus erythematosus, but occasionally also in asymptomatic individuals. Passive trans-placental passage of anti-Ro/SSA-antibodies from mother to foetus is associated with a peculiar syndrome named *neonatal lupus*, where the congenital heart block (CHB) represents the most severe clinical feature. In fact, CHB is responsible of significant mortality (about 20%) and morbidity, with over 60% of surviving affected children requiring pace-maker. In anti-Ro/SSA-positive mothers, the risk of giving birth to a newborn with CHB is around 1-2 %, with a recurrence risk in a subsequent child of 10-16%.

On this basis, great scientific interest arose about the pathogenetic mechanisms underlying CHB development, aimed at identifying possible therapeutic targets. In the inflammatory theory, the occurrence of apoptosis during the development of foetal heart represents the pivotal factor in the beginning of the pathogenetic cascade, thus resulting in translocation of Ro/SSA-antigens to cell surface where they are bound by maternal autoantibodies. The subsequent phagocytosis of opsonized cells by tissue macrophages induces the secretion of pro-inflammatory and pro-fibrotic cytokines producing cardiac damage and irreversible scarring. Other authors proposed an electrophysiological theory, in which anti-Ro/SSA-antibodies block specific ion channels critically involved in the function of the atrio-ventricular (AV) node. In fact, it has been demonstrated that purified anti-Ro/SSA antibodies induce AV-block in isolated human foetal heart and inhibit inward calcium fluxes through L-type calcium-channels in human heart ventriculocytes.

More recently, other cardiac rhythm disturbances different from CHB have been reported in children born from anti-Ro/SSA-positive mothers, among which sinus bradycardia and corrected QT (QTc)-interval prolongation. The pathogenetic mechanisms of such abnormalities are also largely unknown, even if experimental data suggest an electrophysiological interference on both T- and L-type calcium-channels in the genesis of sinus bradycardia

Although anti-Ro/SSA-antibodies have been traditionally considered dangerous only for the foetal heart, recent studies demonstrated the presence of QTc prolongation at the electrocardiogram also in anti-Ro/SSA-positive adults affected with connective tissue diseases (CTD), as a possible sign of cardiac damage. This feature may be of particular clinical relevance, being the QTc prolongation an established risk factor for life-threatening arrhythmias and sudden death in the general population. On this basis, studies aimed at defining the incidence of complex ventricular arrhythmias and their relationship with the QTc prolongation in anti-Ro/SSA-positive CTD patients are presently in progress.

Chapter 4 discusses the development and Evaluation of a high-Fidelity Simulator prototype for electrophysiology.

Background: Advances in clinical electrophysiology should go hand in hand with training of young physicians, so that their theoretical knowledge is complemented by practicing of manual skills. Generally in medicine, training is based on the master-apprentice model. Although the use of simulators for medical training has been already reported, no prior experience on development and use of simulators for electrophysiologic procedures is available.

Methods: Development of an electrophysiology simulator has been planned starting from the Procedicus VIST, previously realized for simulation and training in endovascular procedures. This hybrid simulator consists of a computer connected to an interface unit (the virtual patient), in which catheters or devices are inserted and manipulated in virtual vessels. Catheters are real in their proximal part and simulated in their distal part. Implementation of this system for electrophysiology includes: 1) integration with computed tomography of a normal heart; 2) increase of the number of vascular accesses to place the catheters necessary for an electrophysiology study and consequent adaptation of the simulation software; 3) developing of different modules that simulate electrophysiology procedures with highest priority given to development of the basic catheter placement and trans-septal catheterization modules. Early evaluation of the prototype by a panel of international experts was planned to get necessary feedback on simulation quality. Evaluators are required to attribute a score to the different characteristics of the simulation in a 1-5 scale (5 highest).

Results: In the prototype, catheter placement in the coronary sinus and His bundle area and recording of the intracavitary signals from these sites is possible. A complete trans-septal catheterization procedure can be simulated realistically, including complications. For each procedure a report is automatically generated by the system, which provides essential data to evaluate objectively the trainee performance. For each of the characteristics of the trans-septal simulation evaluated by the international panel, the mean score was > 4.0, ranging from 4.0 to 4.4; > 90% of the evaluators agreed that this simulator could be useful for training purposes. Development of other modules to simulate arrhythmia ablation and three-dimensional mapping procedures has been already planned.

Conclusions: Simulation of electrophysiologic procedures is feasible in a realistic and high fidelity prototype. So far, complete simulation has been obtained for basic catheter placement and trans-septal catheterization. The quality of the simulation has been considered satisfactory by an international panel of electrophysiologists. The clinical impact of virtual training will be assessed in prospective randomized studies.

As explained in Chapter 5, atrial fibrillation (AF) is the most common cardiac arrhythmia in the adult population and is associated with increased cardiovascular morbidity and mortality, and stroke. Currently available antiarrhythmic drugs are moderately effective in restoring normal sinus rhythm in patients with AF. However, excessive delay of ventricular repolarization (excessive QT prolongation) by these agents may be associated with increased risk for proarrhythmia (early afterdepolarization leading to *torsades de pointes* arrhythmia). Therefore, selective blockers of cardiac ion channels that are exclusively present in the atria are highly desirable, as it is expected to be devoid of any ventricular proarrhythmia.

NIP-142 and the hydrochloride salt (NIP-141) are novel benzopyrane derivatives which block potassium, calcium and sodium channels and shows atrial selective action potential duration prolonging profile. These compounds preferentially block the ultrarapid delayed rectifier potassium current (I_{Kur}) and the acetylcholine-activated potassium current (I_{KACh}). Because I_{Kur} and I_{KACh} have been shown to be expressed more abundantly in atrial than in ventricular myocyte, the atiral specific repolarization prolonging effects of NIP141 and NIP-142 are thought to be due to the blocking of these potassium currents. In canine models, NIP-

142 was shown to terminate the microreentry type of AF induced by vagal nerve stimulation and the macroreentry type of atrial flutter induced by an intercaval crush. These effects of NIP-142 have been thought to be due to the prolongation of atrial effective refractory period (ERP), because this compound prolonged atrial ERP without affecting intraatrial and interatrial conduction time in these models. The ERP prolongation by NIP-142 was greater in the atrium than in the ventricle. NIP-142 also terminated the focal activity type of AF induced by aconitine. In addition, NIP-141 restored the atrial ERP shortening and the loss of rate adaptation induced by short-term rapid atrial pacing in anesthetized dogs. Although clinical trials are required to provide evidence of efficacy and safety, the novel mixed channel blocker NIP-141/142 would be a useful drug for treatment of several type of AF with a low risk of proarrhythmia.

QRS detection is the crucial first step in every automatic ECG analysis. Subsequent ECG processing, e.g. automatic arrhythmia classification, relies on an accurate QRS detection performance. Much work has been carried out in automatic QRS complex detection, using various methods ranging from filtering and threshold methods, through wavelet methods, to neural networks, and others. Performance is generally good, but each method has situations where it fails. In particular, cardiac arrhythmias continue to present challenges to automatic ECG detection algorithms due to the irregular rhythms and waveforms. In Chapter 6 the authors describe and evaluate an approach to improve QRS detection performance by automatically combining different detection algorithms, here the Pan-Tompkins and wavelet method. The goal is to benefit from the strengths of both algorithms. A key point of the algorithm is to balance the contribution of the individual methods by introducing appropriate parameters. These parameters are estimated in a data-driven way. The authors provide experimental results on the Massachusetts Institute of Technology-Beth Israel Hospital (MIT-BIH) Arrhythmia Database. It is shown that our combination approach improves overall QRS detection results compared to both individual methods. A set of examples is provided to illustrate the results of our combination algorithm. Furthermore, they address the performance of our method specifically during arrhythmic episodes of the patients. They also discuss patient individual optimizations of the combination parameters for further performance improvements.

The fast (I_{Kr}) and the slow (I_{Ks}) components of the delayed rectifier potassium current are important targets for class III antiarrhythmic drugs that exert their antiarrhythmic potential by prolongation of repolarization. In the present study, the authors analyzed the effects of blocking I_{Kr} and I_{Ks} on action potential repolarization in isolated perfused rabbit heart. Dofetilide (10^{-8} to 10^{-5} M) was used as I_{Kr} blocker, and chromanol 293B (293B) (10^{-7} to $3x10^{-5}$ M) to block I_{Ks}. Epicardial monophasic action potentials were recorded by means of contact electrodes and the action potential duration (APD) was measured at 20% (APD_{20}), 50% (APD_{50}) and 90% (APD_{90}) repolarization.

Dofetilide exhibited a dose-dependent prolongation of APD_{90}, and, to a lesser extent of APD_{50} at all cycle lengths (1000, 750, 600, 500, 400, and 333 ms) with an IC_{50} of 4.7 nM (APD_{90}). Under basal conditions, the application of 293B resulted in a mild APD prolongation which was significant only for APD_{20} (20.7 ± 12.2%, $p<0.05$ at a cycle length of 500 ms, IC_{50}: 7.0 μM). APD_{90} was not prolongated at concentrations up to $3x10^{-5}$ M.

It is shown in Chapter 7, that the delay in repolarization observed with dofetilide displayed a clear reverse rate- dependence whereas the effects of 293B were similar at all frequencies tested.

Under β-adrenergic stimulation with isoproterenol (10^{-8}M, 15 min), dofetilide exerted only a small, temporal prolongation of APD_{90} (14.1 ± 12.6%, $p<0.05$), while a much more pronounced effect was observed with 293B over the complete registration period (34.7 ± 17.9%, $p<0.05$). Both substances exhibited no significant effect on APD_{50} and APD_{20} under β-adrenergic stimulation.

Conclusions: Dofetilide showed a potent and dose-dependent APD prolongation which was associated with a reverse rate-dependence, while 293B effect was rate-independent and less pronounced under basal conditions.

With an increase in adrenergic tone, the effect of I_{Ks} block increased substantially and the APD prolongation was stronger compared to I_{Kr} block. These properties of I_{Ks} block make this channel an interesting target for novel antiarrhythmic agents with a potentially advantageous profile over currently available drugs.

Cardiac arrhythmias are commonly observed in the intensive care unit (ICU) setting. These arrhythmias may result in life threatening events, hence requiring good knowledge of management strategies including urgent transcutaneous pacing. The types of arrhythmias which may be encountered in the ICU can be broadly divided into bradyarrhythmias and tachyarrhythmias. They could vary from "innocent" premature atrial contractions to ventricular tachycardia or complete atrio-ventricular block. It is of note that patients with an underlying disorder are more prone to develop life threatening arrhythmias than healthy subjects. However, there are certain subgroups of previously healthy critical care patients, such as patients with severe brain injury due to trauma, who exhibit a number of changes in heart rate and cardiovascular control. Furthermore, many factors may impair pacemaker automa-ticity or myocardial impulse conduction in critical care patients such as drugs, electrolyte and pH disturbances, myocardial ischaemia, anaesthesia, sepsis, shock, hypoxia, insertion of central venous catheters, trauma and head injury. Also, of great interest is the recent delineation of at least four different hereditary syndromes characterised by myocardial ion channel abnormalities. Clinically these syndromes manifest as a prolonged QT interval on surface electrocardiogram (ECG), associated with sudden death in some affected individuals. Other myocardial ion channel abnormalities such as the Brugada syndrome have been also reported in the ICU setting.

The purpose of Chapter 8 is to provide a comprehensive update of the diagnosis, physiopathology and therapeutic strategies of cardiac arrhythmias in the ICU setting. In this review, the authors also discuss the occurrence of cardiac arrhythmias in unique subpopulations of critical care patients as well as management guidelines for potentially lethal arrhythmias.

As explained in Chapter 9, in the United States 350 000 people die annually of SCD which does not spare any age, gender, or socioeconomic group. The major cause of SCD is CAD, but a small percentage is due to cardiac diseases other then CAD. The main substrate of the latter are cardiac arrhythmias, mainly caused by ARVD/C, Long QT sy and WPW sy in this otherwise healthy population. A special problem exists in professional sports and dieing during sport activities, in spite of regular thorough examinations.

The most mysterious among aforementioned is arrhythogenic right ventricular dysplasia and/or cardiomyopathy (21 clinical genotype types) which unfortunately, apparently, has no clinical warning sign at the early stage, sometimes having SCD for the first and only presenting dramatic event. The arrhythmias leading to SCD may be identified by electrophysiological testing, and significant percentage of patients can have polymorphic VT or VF as the only inducible arrhythmia, which seems to be the exact scenario for the fatal outcome in the whole group of patients. So what might be the underlying cause and could it be prevented?

ARVD/C is a genetically inherited condition with autosomal-dominant pattern of inheritance (as most common), as consequence of single gene mutations which lead to complex patterns of altered localization of desmosomal proteins. These mutations may change cytosolic pools of cell-cell junction proteins which lead to desmosome disorganization and gap junction distortion. Latter is explanation for loss of contact between cardiomyocites and earlier start of apoptosis.

Pathological hallmark of ARVD/C is the atrophy of myocites with fatty or fibro-fatty infiltration of the right ventricle. Typical clinical picture encompasses arrhythmias with left bundle branch block morphology and ventricular tachyarrhythmias, while less frequent presentation are signs of right heart failure (fatigue and shortness of breath). The disease may be localized or widespread, with biventricular involvement in some cases.

Valid WHO criteria during last 12 years failed to detect disease at its early stage and recommended diagnostic methods were shown to have low sensitivity for the majority of patients even in its overt phase (because of lack of scoring system). Investigation of this population is further complicated by disease rarity and lack of large databases. New research published data give priority to vectorcardiography and ultrasound.

The possible explanation for this lies in the existence of specific place in the heart exposed to most physical forces during cardiac cycle. Nevertheless, this place is *locus minoris rezistentiae* during contraction and relaxation of the heart. It is presently the focus of an ongoing clinical study regarding two aforementioned methods in detecting early stage of ARVD/C. It is also registered by WIPO as SOPHIE methodology (suggesting wisdom to detect). Soon enough the authors can expect this technique to be incorporated in newly medical equipment (for stratification of risk for SCD).

Expert Commentaries

In: Progress in Cardiac Arrhythmia Research
Editor: Ira R. Tarkowicz, pp. 3-9
ISBN: 1-60021-796-6

Population-Based Developments in Genetic Screening for long QT Syndrome

Stephen M. Modell
From the Department of Health Management and Policy, University of Michigan School of Public Health, USA

Introduction

The majority of cases of sudden cardiac death (SCD) are due to disturbances in cardiac rhythm, with tachyarrhythmias (ventricular fibrillation or tachycardia), bradyarrhythmias, and asystole being the most common mechanisms. While more than half of the deaths are due to ischemia and myocardial infarction associated with age, arrhythmic cardiac deaths also occur in otherwise healthy individuals of all ages, representing a significant proportion of those dying of cardiovascular causes [1]. In instances where no structural heart disease exists, inherited arrhythmia syndromes are usually responsible.

The inherited arrhythmia syndromes consist of a heterogeneous group of conditions including primary ventricular tachycardia and primary ventricular fibrillation, Wolf-Parkinson-White syndrome, Brugada syndrome, and the long QT family of syndromes (LQTS) [2]. Long QT syndrome (LQTS) refers to a group of "channelopathies" – disorders that affect cardiac potassium and sodium ion channels. The "family" concept of syndromes has been applied to the expanding set of congenital LQTS genotypes, currently LQT1-10, which exhibit converging mechanisms leading to QT prolongation and slowed ventricular repolarization [3-5]. Resultant early after depolarizations can lead to a polymorphic form of ventricular tachycardia known as *torsade de pointes*, resulting in syncope, sudden cardiac death, or near-death. In this commentary I will review the population relevance of this potentially fatal arrhythmic disease family, a variety of ongoing genetic screening approaches, and future public health-oriented directions.

Population Relevance of LQTS Genetic Variants

The public health importance of LQTS is highlighted by the fact that it may be responsible for as many as 3,000 unexpected deaths in children and young adults annually in the U.S. [6]. In children and young athletes, long QT syndrome and hypertrophic cardiomyopathy represent the two main causes of SCD. In the absence of treatment, 6 to 13% of affected individuals succumb to cardiac arrest or sudden cardiac death (SCD) before the age of 40 years [7,8]. Demographic characteristics among patient groups, such as sex, age at first event, and mean age first seen in clinic for the event, tend to vary by genotype. The frequency of cardiac events (syncope, aborted cardiac arrest and sudden death) tends to be higher in individuals with LQT2 (rapidly deactivating potassium channel) mutations than in those with LQT1 (slowly deactivating potassium channel) or LQT3 (sodium channel) mutations. However, a higher percentage of lethal events by age 40 is associated with the LQT3 genotype [8]. Certain families may display a more pronounced phenotype than others, with a high frequency of syncope and sudden death, especially in the young.

Two forms of familial inheritance exist for the panoply of LQTS mutations. The most common familial form, Romano-Ward syndrome (RWS), displays the cardiac electrocardiographic abnormalities typical of LQTS and normal hearing. It is inherited in autosomal dominant fashion, with an estimated prevalence of 1 gene carrier in 7,000 persons in the general U.S. population [6]. The second familial form, Jervell and Lange-Nielsen syndrome (JLNS), is associated with homozygous KCNQ1 (LQT1) and KCNE1 (LQT5) mutations. JLNS carries a more severe phenotype than RWS, with marked QT prolongation and a high incidence of sudden death (inherited in autosomal dominant fashion) and bilateral sensorineural deafness (autosomal recessive inheritance). On the other, it has a distinctly lower population prevalence, with one study in the United Kingdom estimating 1.6 to 6 cases per million [9].

Phenotypes of individuals with compound heterozygote genotypes containing two different alleles lie midway, in terms of degree of QT prolongation, frequency and severity of cardiac events, between those of RWS (1 functional mutation), and those connected with JLNS and other LQTS homozygous mutations. Relatives of individuals with 2 variant gene copies display variable phenotype. The frequency of fatal cardiac arrest in relatives is less than that of probands, but greater than zero. The higher-than-expected proportion of compound heterozygotes in some recent studies is an additional piece of evidence suggesting the prevalence of LQTS gene carriers in the general population may be much higher than generally accepted [10].

LQTS is also gaining increasing attention from a broader population perspective as its prevalence across the globe and in diverse racial-ethnic groups has come to be recognized. The expanse of LQTS human-subject related articles cited in major LQTS article collections such as the European Society of Cardiology Working Group on Arrhythmias LQTS gene database [11] and the international Human Genome Organisation (HUGO) database [12] is truly global in extent, connecting countries as distanced as the USA and Canada, France and Britain, Australia and New Zealand, Israel and the Arabic countries, and Asia from China to Thailand [13].

Among the most frequently cited mutations in each of their genotype categories, KCNQ1 mutations G314S, A341V, A344A [14]; HERG mutations A561V, A614V [14]; SCN5A

(LQT3) mutation R1623Q [15]; and KCNE1 mutation D76N [16] have been found across geographically and culturally disparate continents – Europe, the Americas, Asia, and the Middle East. Within this set, KCNQ1 A341V (reported in USA, Netherlands, France, and Japan); A344A (USA, Denmark, England, France, Japan); and HERG A561V (USA, Italy, Japan) mutations are thought to be mutational hotspots, coding regions especially prone to harboring various mutations.

Cases and families bearing the same mutation may be separated by considerable distance, e.g., the HERG A614V missense mutation, a reported hotspot detected in Japanese families and multiple unrelated families of European descent, and the HERG S818L missense mutation detected in unrelated families from Belgium and Ireland. In many instances these recurrent genetic events are considered sporadic [17]. However, the JLNS R518X mutation found on 2 different haplotypes in Norwegian families of Swedish and Scottish ancestry suggest the possibility of a founder effect [9]. Four alleles studied in the Finnish population – KCNQ1 G589D and IVS7-2A->G (KCNQ1-FinA and B, respectively), and HERG L552S and R176W (HERG-FinA and B, respectively) – represent founder mutations enriched by the historic isolation of that country [18].

Over the last 5 years investigative teams have also launched systematic racial-ethnic studies of LQTS genetic variants. Ackerman et al., in looking at genetic repository samples from 744 healthy individuals representing the 4 major U.S. racial-ethnic groups, discovered that 86% of the cardiac potassium channel genetic variants were ethnicity specific [19]. For example, the KCNQ1 G643S polymorphism was identified at higher rates in African-American and Asian participants (heterozygous frequencies of 5.9% and 6.0%, respectively) than in Caucasians and Latinos (0% and 1.1%). The heterozygous frequency for HERG P448R was appreciably higher in Asian- Americans (16.4%) than the other groups (next highest: African-Americans – 0.3%). HERG A915V was identified only in Asian participants (4.5%). Six of the potassium channel allelic variants that were identified with higher frequency in specific racial-ethnic categories – the LQT5 KCNE1 V109I and LQT6 KCNE2 Q9E polymorphisms in African-Americans; HERG N33T, R176W, P347S, and P917L in Caucasians – have been reported in the literature as potentially pathogenic. In follow-up studies of sodium channel variants in 829 healthy individuals, 3 of the variants identified that show similar specificities – SCN5A S1102Y in African-Americans; R1193Q in the Japanese; and V1951L in Latinos – have also been reported as potentially pathogenic [20]. This area of investigation is evolving. Future efforts will likely involve functional characterization of variants showing racial-ethnic predilection, and confirmation in population-based studies [19].

Directions in Genetic Screening

Genetic screening for LQTS occurs in the neonatal, family, and population-level contexts. Testing for LQTS in newborns typically takes place with referral for ECG abnormalities, while workup can involve either ECG alone, or in combination with mutation testing. Preliminary data from a prospective study assessing QTc (the rate-corrected QT interval) in 50,000 consecutive neonates has shown that newborn population screening for LQTS is possible, though overall feasibility is uncharted [21].

While bodies such as the European Society of Cardiology have advocated neonatal ECG inspection as a step towards arrhythmia-related SIDS prevention [22], consensus in this area is not yet established. Newborn screening for SIDS-related metabolic conditions such as the fatty acid oxidation disorders (MCAD, LCAD, and VLCAD) is progressing more rapidly on an institutionalized level. In a study by Schwartz et al. showing a high proportion of infants with QTc > 440 ms (msec) among SIDS fatalities [23], 2.5% of the newborns with QTc > 440 ms did not suffer from SIDS, and would be considered false-positives. One hundred infants would need to be placed on beta-blockers to save 2 lives [24]. Strategies such as repeat screening for particular QTc thresholds have been suggested, but the cost of purchasing monitoring devices for vast numbers of infants must also be born in mind.

Clinicians and epidemiologists envision an early warning system for at-risk families. A warning system based on decedent information could be used to alert surviving family members and relatives having little or no knowledge of arrhythmic death in the family, reflecting public health's assurance role [25]. Several teams have successfully used PCR and direct sequencing to perform "molecular autopsy" of paraffin block and post-mortem tissue samples of deceased individuals, resulting in the detection of LQT1, 2, and 3 mutations and alerting of relatives [26-28]. Were warning systems to become established, policymakers would need to balance health privacy laws with needed care for at-risk families.

Population screening for LQTS is now occurring on an international level. In China, ECG screening using ST-T-wave patterns to determine genotype is regularly performed on new entries into the national LQTS registry [29]. The presence of the Statens Serum Institute in Denmark has facilitated inclusion of LQTS patients into a mutations-based national long QT registry [30]. The recent commercial marketing of short turn-around time (~ 6 weeks) long QT syndrome genetic diagnostic testing [31], and increasing availability of testing through university-affiliated laboratories in several countries, could in the not so distant future establish genetic testing as a clinical tool alongside more commonly used electrocardiographic means.

Genetic screening of particular subgroups showing susceptibility to LQTS could also be a part of future programs. In their study of the SCN5A S1102Y polymorphism which appears with increased frequency in individuals of African descent, Splawski et al. concluded that the greatest risk lies in the effect of concomitant factors – medications, hypokalemia, and structural heart disease – on the polymorphism [32]. The authors note the increased prevalence of the variant in African-Americans and suggest testing as part of future preventive strategies in those at risk. Here again, the drive to move testing for LQTS to the population level should be accompanied by appropriate analysis of the social and ethical issues involved, especially if particular groups are singled-out for increased monitoring.

Conclusion – The Role of Public Health

In addressing prevention strategies for particular groups, Splawski et al. choose to focus on the value of avoiding particular medications, maintaining normal potassium levels, and beta-blocker therapy [32]. Public health action would be equally effective, however, in maintaining and promoting institutional mechanisms such as cardiac arrhythmia and LQTS registries and monitoring systems that could be used to alert at-risk families. Public health also has a significant educational role to play. Lay persons are often unaware of the more common causes of sudden cardiac death, as well as ways to minimize risk such as the avoidance of particular competitive sports and strenuous activities in individuals with detected LQT1 and 2 mutations, for example [33]. Education of professionals is especially important given assessed shortcomings in the ability of medical residents and practitioners in the field to accurately read ECGs and calculate QT intervals [34], and lack of knowledge among physicians of drugs that can prolong the QT interval and lead to arrhythmia [35].

On a more fundamental level, investigation of the genetic epidemiology of mutations and polymorphisms in international populations, and comparison of affected and control populations in different countries and kindreds, will continue to expand the list of known variants and understanding of their functional effects. Long QT syndrome depicts the continuum between basic research, clinical application, and population-wide dissemination of interventions in the vaster universe of cardiac arrhythmias.

References

[1] Spooner PM, Albert C, Benjamin EJ, Boineau R, Elston RC, George AL, Jr., Jouven X, Kuller LH, MacCluer JW, Marban E, Muller JE, Schwartz PJ, Siscovick DS, Tracy RP, Zareba W, Zipes DP. Sudden cardiac death, genes, and arrhythmogenesis: consideration of new population and mechanistic approaches from a National Heart, Lung, and Blood Institute workshop, Part I. *Circulation* 2001;103:2361-2364.

[2] Roberts R. Genomics and cardiac arrhythmias. *J Am Coll Cardiol* 2006;47:9-21.

[3] Shah M, Akar FG, Tomaselli GF. Molecular basis of arrhythmias. *Circulation* 2005;112:2517-2529.

[4] Splawski I, Timothy KW, Sharpe LM, Decher N, Kumar P, Bloise R, Napolitano C, Schwartz PJ, Joseph RM, Condouris K, Tager-Flusberg H, Priori SG, Sanguinetti MC, Keating MT. $Ca_v1.2$ calcium channel dysfunction causes a multisystem disorder including arrhythmia and autism. *Cell* 2004;119:19 31.

[5] Roden DM, Spooner PM. Inherited long QT syndromes: a paradigm for understanding arrhythmogenesis. J *Cardiovasc Electrophysiol* 1999;10:1664-1683.

[6] Vincent GM. Long QT syndrome. *Cardiol Clin* 2000;18:309-325.

[7] Priori SG, Schwartz PJ, Napolitano C, Bliose R, Ronchetti E, Grillo M, Vicentini A, Spazzolini C, Nastoli J, Bottelli G, Folli R, Cappelletti D. Risk stratification in the long-QT syndrome. *N Engl J Med* 2003;348:1866-1874.

[8] Zareba W, Moss AJ, Schwartz PJ, Vincent GM, Robinson JL, Priori SG, Benhorin J, Locati EH, Towbin JA, Keating MT, Lehmann MH, Hall WJ. Influence of genotype on the clinical course of the long-QT syndrome. International Long-QT Syndrome Registry Research Group. *N Engl J Med* 1998;339:960-965.

[9] Tranebjaerg L, Bathen J, Tyson J, Bitner-Glindzicz M. Jervell and Lange-Nielsen syndrome: a Norwegian perspective. *Am J Med Genet* 1999;89:137-146.

[10] Schwartz PJ, Priori SG, Napolitano C. How really rare are rare diseases?: the intriguing case of independent compound mutations in the long QT syndrome. *J Cardiovasc Electrophysiol* 2003;14:1120-1121.

[11] European Society of Cardiology Working Group on Arrhythmias (WGA). Gene Connection for the Heart: Long QT Syndrome. 2007. Available at: http://pc4.fsm.it:81/cardmoc/main.htm. Last accessed: 2/27/07.

[12]Human Genome Organisation (HUGO). 2003. Long QT Syndrome Database. Available at: http://www.ssi.dk/graphics/html/lqtsdb/lqtsdb.htm. Last accessed: 2/27/07.

[13]Modell SM, Lehmann MH. The long QT syndrome family of cardiac ion channelopathies: A HuGE review. *Genet Med* 2006;8:143-155.

[14]Tester DJ, Will ML, Haglund CM, Ackerman MJ. Compendium of cardiac channel mutations in 541 consecutive unrelated patients referred for long QT syndrome genetic testing. *Heart Rhythm* 2005;2:507-517.

[15]Splawski I, Shen J, Timothy KW, Lehmann MH, Priori S, Robinson JL, Moss AJ, Schwartz PJ, Towbin JA, Vincent GM, Keating MT. Spectrum of mutations in long-QT syndrome genes. *KVLQT1, HERG, SCN5A, KCNE1*, and *KCNE2*. *Circulation* 2000;102:1178-1185.

[16]Schulze-Bahr E, Wang Q, Wedekind H, Haverkamp W, Chen Q, Sun Y, Rubie C, Hordt M, Towbin JA, Borggrefe M, Assmann G, Qu X, Somberg JC, Breithardt G, Oberti C, Funke H. *KCNE1* mutations cause Jervell and Lange-Nielsen syndrome. *Nat Genet* 1997;17:267-268.

[17]Miller TE, Estrella E, Myerburg RJ, de Viera JG, Moreno N, Rusconi P, Ahearn ME, Baumbach L, Kurlansky P, Wolff G, Bishopric NH. Recurrent third-trimester fetal loss and maternal mosaicism for long-QT syndrome. *Circulation* 2004;109:3029-3034.

[18]Fodstad H, Swan H, Laitinen P, Piippo K, Paavonen K, Viitasalo M, Toivonen L, Kontula K. Four potassium channel mutations account for 73% of the genetic spectrum underlying long-QT syndrome (LQTS) and provide evidence for a strong founder effect in Finland. *Ann Med* 2004;36 Suppl 1:53-63.

[19]Ackerman MJ, Tester DJ, Jones GS, Will ML, Burrow CR, Curran ME. Ethnic differences in cardiac potassium channel variants: implications for genetic susceptibility to sudden cardiac death and genetic testing for congenital long QT syndrome. *Mayo Clin Proc* 2003;78:1479-1487.

[20]Ackerman MJ, Splawski I, Makielski JC, Tester DJ, Will ML, Timothy KW, Keating MT, Jones G, Chadha M, Burrow CR, Stephens JC, Xu C, Judson R, Curran ME. Spectrum and prevalence of cardiac sodium channel variants among black, white, Asian, and Hispanic individuals: implications for arrhythmogenic susceptibility and Brugada/long QT syndrome genetic testing. *Heart Rhythm* 2004;1:600-607.

[21]Stramba-Badiale M, Goulene K, Bosi G, Bini R, Priori SG, Bloise R, Crotti L, Salice P, Fesslova V, Mannarino S, Latini G, Giorgetti R, Arsizio AO, Arsizio B, Schwartz PJ. The role of neonatal electrocardiography in the early identification of genetic arrhythmogenic disorders and congenital cardiovascular diseases: prospective data from 21,000 infants. (Abstract) *Circulation* 2004;110 Suppl III:III-407.

[22]Schwartz PJ, Garson A, Jr., Paul T, Stramba-Badiele M, Vetter VL, Villain E, Wren C. Guidelines for the interpretation of the neonatal electrocardiogram. *Eur Heart J* 2002;23:1329-1344.

[23]Schwartz PJ, Stramba-Badiale M, Segantini A, Austoni P, Bosi G, Giorgetti R, Grancini F, Marni ED, Perticone F, Rosti D, Salice P. Prolongation of the QT interval and the sudden infant death syndrome. *N Engl J Med* 1998;338:1709-1714.

[24]Van Langen IM, Hofman N, Tan HL, Wilde AA. Family and population strategies for screening and counseling of inherited cardiac arrhythmias. *Ann Med* 2004;36 Suppl 1:116-124.

[25]Beskow LM, Khoury MJ, Baker TG, Thrasher JF. The Integration of Genomics into Public Health Research, Policy and Practice in the United States. *Community Genet* 2001;4:2-11.

[26]Wang DW, Desai RR, Crotti L, Arnestad M, Insolia R, Pedrazzini M, Ferrandi C, Vege A, Rognum T, Schwartz PJ, George AL, Jr. Cardiac sodium channel dysfunction in sudden infant death syndrome. Circulation 2007;115:368-376.

[27]Chugh SS, Senashova O, Watts A, Tran PT, Zhou Z, Gong Q, Titus JL, Hayflick SJ. Postmortem molecular screening in unexplained sudden death. *J Am Coll Cardiol* 2004;43:1625-1629.

[28]Ackerman MJ, Tester DJ, Driscoll DJ. Molecular autopsy of sudden unexplained death in the young. *Am J Forensic Med Pathol* 2001;22:105-111.

[29]Li C, Hu D, Qin X, Li Y, Li P, Liu W, Li Z, Li L, Wang L. Clinical features and management of congenital long QT syndrome: a report on 54 patients from a national registry. *Heart Vessels* 2004;19:38-42.

[30]Kanters JK, Bloch Thomsen PE, Toft E, Christiansen M. Clinical characteristics in long QT syndrome from the Danish Long QT Registry. *Heart Rhythm* 2005;2(5 Suppl 9);S311.

[31]Genaissance Pharmaceuticals. FAMILION: a genetic test for cardiac ion channel mutations. 2004. Available at: http://www.familion.com/physicans/home.html. Last accessed: 2/27/07.

[32]Splawski I, Timothy KW, Tateyama M, Clancy CE, Malhotra A, Beggs AH, Cappuccio FP, Sagnella GA, Kass RS, Keating MT. Variant of SCN5A sodium channel implicated in risk of cardiac arrhythmia. *Science* 2002;297:1333-1336.

[33]Maron BJ, Chaitman BR, Ackerman MJ, de Luna AB, Corrado D, Crosson JE, Deal BJ, Driscoll DJ, Estes M, 3rd, Araujo CG, Liang DH, Mitten MJ, Myerburg RJ, Pelliccia A, Thompson PD, Towbin JA, Van Camp SP, for the Working Groups of the American Heart Association Committee on Exercise, Cardiac Rehabilitation, and Prevention; Councils on Clinical Cardiology and Cardiovascular Disease in the Young. Recommendations for physical activity and recreational sports participation for young patients with genetic cardiovascular diseases. *Circulation* 2004;109:2807-2816.

[34]Viskin S, Rosovski U, Sands AJ, Chen E, Kistler PM, Kalman JM, Rodriguez Chavez L, Cruz F FE, Centurion OA, Fujiki A, Maury P, Chen X, Krahn A, Roithinger F, Zhang L, Vincent GM, Zeltser D. Inaccurate electrocardiographic interpretation of long QT: the majority of physicians cannot recognize a long QT when they see one. *Health Rhythm* 2005;2:569-574.

[35]Shaoul R, Shahory R, Tamir A, Jaffe M. Comparison between pediatricians and family practitioners in the use of the prokinetic cisapride for gastroesophageal reflux disease in children. *Pediatrics* 2002;109:1118-1123.

In: Progress in Cardiac Arrhythmia Research
Editor: Ira R. Tarkowicz, pp. 11-16
ISBN: 1-60021-796-6

Thrombolytic Therapy in Patients with Ventricular Fibrillation

W. Lederer and A. Amann
Department of Anaesthesiology and Critical Care Medicine, Innsbruck Medical UniversityA-6020 Innsbruck, Austria

Abstract

The chances for successful restoration of spontaneous circulation (ROSC) in cardiac arrest follwing ventricular fibrillation (VF) deteriorate rapidly with time. Improved myocardial reperfusion, e.g. by way of cardiopulmonary resuscitation (CPR), may improve the prospect for successful defibrillation. In addition, electrocardiographic (ECG) waveform analysis can help determine the optimal timing for defibrillation and thus prevent unnecessary damage caused to the myocardium by unsuccessful electric shocks. Computer-assisted ECG analysis with removal of CPR-associated noise and artifacts allows the outcome of defibrillation to be predicted without causing potentially detrimental interruptions in CPR. The likelihood that defibrillation in patients with sustained VF will be successful can be further improved by administering thrombolytics during CPR. While dissolution of coronary artery thrombosis resolves the underlying cause of myocardial infarction in the majority of patients, improved microcirculatory reperfusion and alteration of the electrical activity of the fibrillation process may increase the likelihood of restoring spontaneous circulation during resuscitation. An increase in fibrillation frequency, fibrillation amplitude or in amplitude spectrum area (AMSA) as calculated from electrocardiography (ECG) signals indicates that thrombolytic therapy is improving ventricular fibrillation status, thus improving the chances for successful defibrillation.

Keywords: AMSA; cardiovascular diseases; electric countershock; fibrinolysis; myocardial ischemia; reperfusion; ROSC.

Introduction

Since the first scientific investigations of the efficacy of basic life support (BLS) in the late fifties, the fundamentals of cardiopulmonary resuscitation (CPR) and its outcome have not changed substantially [1]. Time is still the most important single factor determining survival, in particular the arrest-to-CPR interval and the arrest-to-defibrillation interval in ventricular fibrillation (VF) [2]. When circulatory arrest is recognized early and basic life support is started immediately the hospital discharge rate of out-of-hospital cardiac arrest (OOH-CA) survivors is almost double [3]. VF is presumably the most common cardiac rhythm after OOH-CA. Homberg et al. reported 43% VF in the first ECG on arrival of the Emergency Medical System (EMS), suggesting a high initial incidence of VF among OOH-CA patients and a slow rate of transformation to a non-shockable rhythm [4].

For VF and pulseless ventricular tachycardia immediate electrical defibrillation is the internationally recommended treatment [5]. With increasing delay to defibrillation, the survival rate declines rapidly from approximately 50% immediately after CA to 5% at 15 minutes. Survival of more than one month was reported in 1.6% of patients with non-shockable rhythms, e.g. asystole and pulseless electrical activity, and in 9.5% of patients with VF [4]. It is presumed that each minute of delay diminishes the chances for successful defibrillation by 7% to 10 % [6]. Wik et al., however, reported that patients with VF and ambulance response intervals of more than 5 minutes had better outcomes when CPR was initiated before attempting defibrillation [7]. In their investigation Wik et al. reported return of spontaneous circulation (ROSC) in 58% of patients with CPR prior to defibrillation vs. 38% in the control group. This effect is even more remarkable when considering that BLS can rarely produce a cardiac output exceeding 25 % of what is considered adequate under normal conditions [8]. Controversy still surrounds the effects of vasopressors on myocardial reperfusion and coronary perfusion pressure (CPP) during advanced cardiac life support (ACLS) in OOH-CA [9,10]. There are, however, patients who do not respond to prolonged CPR, administration of vasopressors or repeated defibrillation attempts. In cases of sustained VF, administration of thrombolytic agents, e.g. recombinant tissue plasminogen activator (rt-PA), may increase the likelyhood of successful defibrillation, again by improving reperfusion of the myocardium. In a retrospective study conducted in patients with OOH-CA due to sustained VF we more frequently observed termination of VF when rt-PA, 50 mg alteplase (Actilyse®, Boehringer Ingelheim), was administered in addition to conventional CPR [11]. Patients with sustained VF, defined as three or more unsuccessful defibrillation attempts, had a significantly better outlook for ROSC and for surviving the first 24 hours if they received thrombolytic treatment (81.0% vs. 64.9% in controls; $p=0.029$). Results of our data evaluation indicate that administration of rt-PA facilitates successful defibrillation in patients who do not respond to repeated defibrillation attempts. Successful resuscitation, however, depends on a number of variables and there are several limitations on these findings, e.g. patients were not randomly assigned to one of the two groups and administration of rt-PA was optional and at the discretion of the emergency physician. Böttiger et al. reported ROSC in about 70% of prospectively assessed, rt-PA treated patients with OOH-CA [12]. Böttiger et al argued that the underlying cause of OOH-CA would be resolved by lysis with rt-PA. Furthermore, dissolution of a causative thrombus in acute myocardial infarction (AMI), as shown by coronary artery patency, is associated with rescue of myocardial tissue. Unfortunately, we still lack the data to prove that this effect occurs in CA survivors [13]. Successful recanalization is achievable in up to 80% of patients, but will not occur before 60 to 90 minutes following administration of a thrombolytic drug [14]. Under the conditions of extended hypotension, as typical for CPR, complete recanalization of blood vessels will be even further delayed. Therefore, we postulate that the increased probability of ROSC following thrombolysis must be due to a different mode of action [15].

During CPR ischemia/hypoxia is prolonged and causes formation of microthrombi that further impair organ perfusion [16,17]. While endogenous fibrinolysis is delayed and inadequate, extrinsic activation of plasminogen by rt-PA effectively counteracts coagulation and exerts positive effects on microcirculatory reperfusion [18]. We attribute the early effects of thrombolysis to the improved microperfusion resulting from dissolution of microthrombi and decrease in blood viscosity, e.g. by splitting circulating fibrinogen and enhanced collateral reperfusion. This is particularly relevant to perfusion of the heart and brain, and might also explain the exceptionally high rate of hospital discharge and the good neurological outcome despite prolonged resuscitation procedures that have been observed when thrombolytics were administered during and after CPR [19,20].

Achleitner et al. showed in a porcine model that improved perfusion of the myocardium is associated with increased mean VF frequency that correlated positively with the coronary perfusion pressure and the mean arterial pressure [21]. Mean fibrillation frequencies exceeding 5 Hz increase the chances for successful defibrillation [22]. In the surface ECG frequencies of VF are centered around 5Hz ± 3Hz (range: 1-15 Hz). The mean frequency – i.e., the mean of all frequencies occurring in the ECG – and the amplitude of VF in ECG can be used to predict defibrillation outcome [23, 24]. Initially, both amplitude and frequency of VF signals are relatively high, but quickly deteriorate with duration of cardiac arrest. The higher the mean VF frequency, the higher the likelihood of spontaneous sinus rhythm after defibrillation [24].

Mechanically, the impairment of cellular ion pumps and the irregular opening of ion channels give rise to an irregular sequence of polarization and depolarization, resulting in a massive influx of calcium into myocardial cells within a few minutes of VF onset [25]. It is possible that there is interaction between fibrinolysis, fibrillation and Ca^{2+}overload. Ca^{2+} overload can damage mitochondria during ischemia and reperfusion [26] and may consequently impair maintenance of membrane potential at reperfusion [27]. Moreover, high extracellular Ca^{2+} load increases Vf activity [28] and enhances fibrinolysis [29]. We assume that the impairment of ion pumps and the consequent Ca^{2+}overload in myocardial cells progress during sustained VF [15,30]. Further investigations of the impact of thrombolysis on the electrical activity during VF are needed

ECG waveform analysis can help determine the optimal timing of defibrillation and prevent unnecessary damage caused to the myocardium by unsuccessful electric shocks [31,32]. Computer-assisted ECG analysis with removal of CPR-associated noise and artifacts allows the outcome of defibrillation to be predicted without causing potentially detrimental interruptions in CPR [31,33]. However, selection of an appropriate predictor for successful defibrillation requests a highly sophisticated algorithm. Analysis of VF-ECG in animal experiments revealed a positive predictive value equivalent to that of CPP [21]. Furthermore, amplitude spectrum area (AMSA) was reported to have better predictive power for defibrillation success than does mean amplitude, mean frequency or even CPP. The negative predictive value was as high as 96% [23].

In a small subgroup analysis of a prospective study we investigated changes in AMSA in patients with sustained VF, who received either rt-PA variant, tenecteplase 0.5 mg/kg/BW (Metalyse®, Boehringer Ingelheim), in addition to standard CPR or were given standard treatment only [34]. A Welsh-Allyn defibrillator equipped for data acquisition was used to store and subsequently analyze fibrillation ECG data. Time of administration of thrombolytic therapy and ROSC onset were drawn from treatment protocols. Mean VF frequency, mean VF amplitude and AMSA were determined and their respective values before and after thrombolytic administration compared. The power spectrum of the ECG (square of the windowed Fourier transformation) was computed. Patients with sustained VF who received thrombolytic treatment more frequently showed an increase in AMSA. Presumably, administration of thrombolytics was successful in terminating sustained VF in cardiac arrest patients by improving myocardial reperfusion and altering the electrical activity of the fibrillation process, as was expressed by changes in AMSA. Thus, the effect of thrombolytics on myocardial fibrillation status with an increase in defibrillation success could promote a new strategy for emergency medical care in CPR.

Conclusion

Improved myocardial reperfusion, e.g. by way of CPR, can improve the chances for defibrillation success. In addition, ECG waveform analysis can help determine the optimal timing of defibrillation and prevent unnecessary damage caused to the myocardium by unsuccessful electric shocks. Further trials are needed to investigate whether increased ROSC frequency is associated with improved VF electrical activity and outcome.

References

[1] Kouwenhoven WB, Jude JR, Knickerbocker GG. Closed-chest cardiac massage. *JAMA* 1960;173:1064-1067.

[2] Valenzuela TD, Roe DJ, Cretin S, Spaite DW, Larsen MP. Estimating effectiveness of cardiac arrest interventions: a logistic regression survival model. *Circulation.* 1997;96(10):3308-3313.

[3] Cummins RO, Eisenberg MS. Prehospital cardiopulmonary resuscitation: is it effective? *JAMA* 1985;253:2408-2412.

[4] Holmberg M, Holmberg S, Herlitz J. Incidence, duration and survival of ventricular fibrillation in out-of-hospital cardiac arrest patients in Sweden. *Resuscitation.* 2000 Mar;44(1):7-17.

[5] International Liaison Committee on Resuscitation (ILCOR). Part 4: Advanced life support. *Resuscitation.* 2005;67:213-247.

[6] Larsen MP, Eisenberg MS, Cummins RO, Hallstrom AP. Predicting survival from out-of-hospital cardiac arrest: a graphic model. *Ann Emerg Med* 1993;22:1652-1658.

[7] Wik L, Hansen TB, Fylling F, Steen T, Vaagenes P, Auestad BH, Steen PA. Delaying defibrillation to give basic cardiopulmonary resuscitation to patients with out-of-hospital ventricular fibrillation: a randomized trial. *JAMA* 2003;289(11):1389-1395.

[8] Chamberlain D.: Wonders, Disappointments, and Hopes in Resuscitation. Scandinavian CPR Congress (2001)

[9] Wenzel V, Krismer AC, Arntz HR, Sitter H, Stadlbauer KH, Lindner KH. European Resuscitation Council Vasopressor during Cardiopulmonary Resuscitation Study Group. A comparison of vasopressin and epinephrine for out-of-hospital cardiopulmonary resuscitation. *N Engl J Med* 2004;350(2):105-113.

[10]Nolan JP, De Latorre FJ, Steen PA, Chamberlain DA, Bossaert LL. Advanced life support drugs: do they really work? *Curr Opin Crit Care*. 2002(3):212-218.

[11]Lederer W, Lichtenberger C, Kroesen G, Baubin M. Thrombolytic therapy in sustained ventricular fibrillation. *Acta Anaesthesiologica Scand* 2001;45(8):1054

[12]Bottiger BW, Bode C, Kern S, Gries A, Gust R, Glatzer R, Bauer H, Motsch J, Martin E. Efficacy and safety of thrombolytic therapy after initially unsuccessful cardiopulmonary resuscitation: a prospective clinical trial. *Lancet* 2001;357(9268):1583-1585.

[13]Ober MC, Ober C, Hagau A, Mot S, Iancu A, Literat S, Capalneanu R. Prodromal angina reduces infarcted mass less in interventionally reperfused than in thrombolysed myocardial infarction. *Rom J Intern Med*. 2004;42(3):533-543.

[14]Bode C, Nordt TK, Peter K, Smalling RW, Runge MS, Kubler W. Patency trials with reteplase (r-PA): what do they tell us? *Am J Cardiol*. 1996;78(12A): 16-19.

[15]Lederer W, Schlimp CJ, Niederklapfer T, Amann A. Altered electrical activity of fibrillation process following thrombolytic therapy in out-of-hospital cardiac arrest patients with sustained ventricular fibrillation. *Med Hypotheses* 2006; 67(2):333-335.

[16]Gando S, Kameue T, Nanzaki S, Nakanishi Y. Massive fibrin formation with consecutive impairment of fibrinolysis in patients with out-of-hospital cardiac arrest. *Thrombosis and haemostasis* 1997;77:2 78-82.

[17]Fischer M, Böttiger BW, Popov-Cenic S, Hossmann KA. Thrombolysis using plasminogen activator and heparin reduces cerebral no-reflow after resuscitation from cardiac arrest: an experimental study in the cat. *Intensive Care Med* 1996;22:1214-1223.

[18]Böttiger BW, Motsch J, Bohrer H, Boker T, Aulmann M, Nawroth PP, Martin E. Activation of blood coagulation after cardiac arrest is not balanced adequately by activation of endogenous fibrinolysis. *Circulation* 1995;92:2572-2578.

[19]Schreiber W, Gabriel D, Sterz F, Muellner M, Kuerkciyan I, Holzer M, Laggner AN. Thrombolytic therapy after cardiac arrest and its effect on neurological outcome. *Resuscitation* 2002;52(1):63-69.

[20]Voipio V, Kuisma M, Alaspaa A, Manttari M, Rosenberg P. Thrombolytic treatment of acute myocardial infarction after out-of-hospital cardiac arrest. *Resuscitation* 2001;49(3):251-258.

[21]Achleitner U, Wenzel V, Strohmenger HU, Lindner KH, Baubin MA, Krismer AC, Mayr VD, Amann A. The beneficial effect of basic life support on ventricular fibrillation mean frequency and coronary perfusion pressure. *Resuscitation*. 2001;51(2):151-158.

[22]Strohmenger HU, Hemmer W, Lindner KH, Schickling J, Brown CG. Median fibrillation frequency in cardiac surgery: influence of temperature and guide to countershock therapy. *Chest*. 1997;111(6):1560-1564.

[23]Povoas HP, Bisera J. Electrocardiographic waveform analysis for predicting the success of defibrillation. *Crit Care med* 2000;28(11):210-211.

[24]Noc M, Weil MH, Tang W, Sun S, Pernat A, Bisera J. Electrocardiographic prediction of the success of cardiac resuscitation. *Crit Care Med*. 1999;(4):708-714.

[25]Zaugg C. Current Concepts on Ventricular Fibrillation: A Vicious Circle of Cardiomyocyte Calcium Overload in the Initiation, Maintenance, and Termination of Ventricular Fibrillation. *Indian Pacing and Electrophysiology Journal* 2004;4(2):85-92.

[26]Radhakrishnan J, Wang S, Ayoub IM, Kolarova JD, Levine RF, Gazmuri RJ. Circulating Levels of Cytochrome C after Resuscitation from Cardiac Arrest: A Marker of Mitochondrial Injury and Predictor of Survival. *Am J Physiol Heart Circ Physiol.* 2006; Epub

[27]Garcia-Rivas Gde J, Carvajal K, Correa F, Zazueta C. Ru360, a specific mitochondrial calcium uptake inhibitor, improves cardiac post-ischaemic functional recovery in rats in vivo. *Br J Pharmacol.* 2006;149(7):829-837.

[28]Wang X, Tsuji K, Lee SR, Ning M, Furie KL, Buchan AM, Lo EH. Mechanisms of hemorrhagic transformation after tissue plasminogen activator reperfusion therapy for ischemic stroke. *Stroke*. 2004;35:2726-2730.

[29]Kojima Y, Urano T, Kojima K, Serizawa K, Takada Y, Takada A. The significant enhancement of fibrinolysis by calcium ion in a cell free system: the shortening of euglobulin clot lysis time by calcium ion. *Thromb Haemost.* 1994;72(1):113-118.

[30]Heyman SN, Hanna Z, Nassar T, Shina A, Akkawi S, Goldfarb M, Rosen S, Higazi AA. The fibrinolytic system attenuates vascular tone: effects of tissue plasminogen activator (tPA) and aminocaproic acid on renal microcirculation. *Br J Pharmacol.* 2004;141(6):971-978.

[31]Kracher G, Werther T, Klotz A, Feichtinger H, Gilly H, Baubin M, Amann A (2007). CPR Artefact Removal in ECG Signals Using Gabor Multipliers. *preprint.*

[32]Lederer W, Rheinberger K, Lischke V, Amann A. [Analysis of ventricular fibrillation signals for the evaluation of defibrillation success in the treatment of ventricular fibrillation] *Anasthesiol Intensivmed Notfallmed Schmerzther.* 2003;38(12):787-794.

[33]Rheinberger K, Steinberger T, Baubin M, Klotz A Amann A (2007). Removal of CPR artifacts from the ventricular fibrillation ECG by adaptive regression on lagged reference signals. *preprint.*

[34]Lederer W, Schlimp CJ, Ritter EM, Niederklapfer T, Baubin MA, Amann A. Influence of tenecteplase on amplitude spectrum area in out-of-hospital cardiac-arrest patients with sustained ventricular fibrillation. *preprint.*

Research and Review Studies

In: Progress in Cardiac Arrhythmia Research
Editor: Ira R. Tarkowicz, pp. 19-65
ISBN: 1-60021-796-6

Chapter 1

Drug-Induced Torsadogenesis: Evolving Trends and New Technologies

Peter Hoffmann, Berengere Dumotier, Robert Pearlstein and Barbara Warner
Preclinical Safety, Novartis Pharma AG, MUT-2881.205, CH-4002, Basel, Switzerland

Abstract

Contemporary preclinical *in vitro* and *in vivo* methods have been imperfect in predicting drug-induced Torsades de Pointes (TdP) arrhythmia in humans. A better understanding of additional relevant factors in the genesis of drug-induced TdP besides the relationships between *h*ERG inhibition, action potential duration, and QT interval is necessary and supports the evolution of new methods to assess the cardiovascular safety of new drug candidates in the future.

New, sophisticated *in vitro* techniques, such as arterially perfused ventricular wedge preparations or isolated perfused hearts, potentially offer a better understanding of torsadogenic mechanisms and a refinement of drug testing. Of particular interest are the dispersion of repolarization and the refractoriness of different cell types across the ventricular wall, triangulation of the action potential, reverse use dependence and instability of the action potential duration. *In vivo* models in conscious and anesthetized non-rodents are currently refined by establishing the relevance of parameters such as beat-to-beat-variability and T-wave morphology as derived from the *in vitro* proarrhythmia indices. Animal models of proarrhythmia are to date not recommended for routine evaluation, since the models are insufficiently established to provide any certainty of detecting relevant effects. This holds true for *in vitro* and *in vivo* techniques.

Pharmacodynamic interactions with combinations of torsadogenic compounds at the level of the hERG channel on the plasma membrane and interactions with other channel proteins is another area to be considered. Little is known about channel/receptor cross talk, although considerable evidence exists that cardiac G protein-coupled receptors can modulate *h*ERG channel function. More investigations are necessary to further evaluate the role of altered gene expression, mutations and polymorphisms in drug-induced TdP. Down-regulation of hERG channels under pathophysiological conditions contributes significantly to the enhanced liability of the repolarization process. A recently discovered mechanism of drug-induced

torsadogenesis is the reduced expression of hERG channel protein on the plasma membrane due to a trafficking defect.
Pharmacokinetic and metabolism data of NCE are crucial for calculating the risk of a torsadogenic potential in man. Consideration of intracardiac accumulation via effects on active transport mechanisms that facilitate access of the drug to the "active site" may help in delineating any pharmacokinetic-pharmacodyamic relationships and potential pharmacokinetic drug-drug interactions that may occur beyond the hepatic cytochrome P450 level.
In silico methods possess the potential to improve the prediction of torsadogenic risk. For early risk assessment of new drug candidates, virtual screening procedures to predict hERG block would become a promising tool. The role of *in silico* modeling of TdP arrhythmia is likely to become increasingly important, however, the pathogenesis of arrhythmias is complex and vast amounts of data need to be considered. At present *in silico* methods cannot replace existing preclinical models.

Keywords: Torsades de pointes, QT interval, Mechanisms, Pre-clinical models, Emerging trends.

Introduction

Potential for drug-induced cardiac arrhythmia has increasingly resulted in non-approval, relabellings, warnings, and withdrawals of some drugs from the market (Redfern et al. 2003; Belardinelli et al. 2003) and the termination of many compounds in pharmaceutical industry pipelines. Drug-induced polymorphic ventricular tachyarrhythmia, known as torsades de pointes (TdP), is at the center of interest. It is a rare but potentially life threatening arrhythmia leading to syncope or, even more rarely, to ventricular fibrillation and sudden cardiac death, and it is typically not seen in clinical trials prior to registration of a new drug. For terfenadine, recognition of this rare event required extensive use (> 10 million prescriptions per 24 million patient years) and detailed monitoring from 1985 until 1998 before the drug was finally recalled because of 125 terfenadine-related deaths in the US alone in patients with seasonal hay fever (Rangno 1997).

Putting TdP into perspective, the reporting rate for drug-induced ventricular fibrillation not related to TdP, e.g., due to sodium channel inhibition, is much higher and has lower probability of survival (Shah & Hondeghem, 2005). Inhibition of cardiac sodium channels appears much more dangerous, but effects are easily monitorable with the surface ECG and will be easily detected pre-clinically and during clinical development.

The current conceptualization of TdP, which determines health authorities' requirements and pharmaceutical industry practice is as follows (Figure 1). TdP has been linked to delayed cardiac repolarization, as manifested by a prolongation of the QT interval on the electrocardiogram (ECG). QT interval prolongation is so frequently associated with TdP that prolongation of the QT interval became a surrogate marker for the potential of a drug to induce TdP. Since almost all compounds that produce TdP in man also inhibit the rapid form of the delayed rectifier potassium current $I_{Kr,}$ whose alpha subunit is encoded by the hERG gene, the blockade of this channel and derived electrophysiological consequences on the cellular (action potential duration, APD) and organ level (QT interval) became the primary parameters to predict drug-induced torsadogenesis.

This concept of drug-induced torsadogenesis by hERG channel inhibition appears to be supported by the congenital long QT syndrome as manifested by a mutation of hERG gene (LQT2) (Roden and Kuperschmidt 1999; Moss 2003). But not all patients with a hERG mutation show a clear QT interval prolongation. In addition, mutations in other genes for cardiac ion channels (KCNQ1 for I_{Ks} = slow form of the delayed rectifier potassium current, or SCN5A for the Na^+ channel) can also lead to TdP. Thus, the comparison of drug-induced and congenital long QT syndrome indicates that there may be other factors than hERG channel inhibition and QT prolongation that are involved in drug-induced torsadogenesis.

A recent survey of pharmaceutical industry practice (Hammond et al. 2001), articles of opinion leaders in the area (Gralinski 2000; Haverkamp et al. 2000), and guidelines from regulatory authorities (European Agency for the Evaluation of Medical Products, CPMP/986/96, 1997; ICH S7B guideline Oct 2005) describe a core battery of three preclinical assays typically used to predict torsadogenic potential in man. These include (1) an *in vitro* assay investigating the inhibitory potential of a compound on I_{Kr} (mandatory assay); (2) an *in vitro* repolarization assay that evaluates changes in the APD in an integrated electrophysiological system (such as Purkinje fiber or papillary muscle); and (3) an *in vivo* assay evaluating changes in the QT interval of the ECG (mandatory assay). The use of three assays is reasoned by the fact that no one assay is totally predictive for torsadogenesis in man. The use of models displaying different integrated information (cell, tissue, organ) is necessary.

The assumption of the central role of hERG channel inhibition as the mechanism of drug-induced TdP also led to the idea that screening of new chemical entities for hERG inhibitory activity early in the drug development process may eliminate termination of compounds in later preclinical or clinical development stages (Netzer et al. 2003). Early screening during lead identification/lead optimization implies the ability to test large numbers of compounds in a short period of time with minimal effort in terms of materials and costs. Several approaches are being used to measure drug effects on the hERG channel indirectly or directly. In binding assays, the replacement of a radioactively labeled channel antagonist (e.g., [^{3}H]-dofetilide) by the compound under investigation is measured, assuming the same binding site for both drugs. Other assays have been developed. Rubidium flux assays rely on the high permeability of Rb^+ through voltage sensitive K^+ channels. Fluorescence assays make use of voltage–sensitive dyes, which measure the membrane potential of a living cell. Every assay showed advantages but also limitations related to reduced sensitivity and selectivity. Furthermore, all these tests suffer from measuring the effects on the hERG channel indirectly and are therefore prone to artifacts. Thus, the patch clamp technique is still regarded as the gold standard. But the manual handling of the patch clamp systems is very time consuming and can therefore not be used in early drug development stages. Recently, several companies have increased the throughput by automating electrophysiological experiments.

By using the above methodology in drug development, significant advances have been made in the ability to test for drug effects on the I_{Kr} current, APD and the QT interval over the last years, and the risk of drug-induced changes in cardiac repolarization and TdP in man has been considerably reduced but not eliminated.

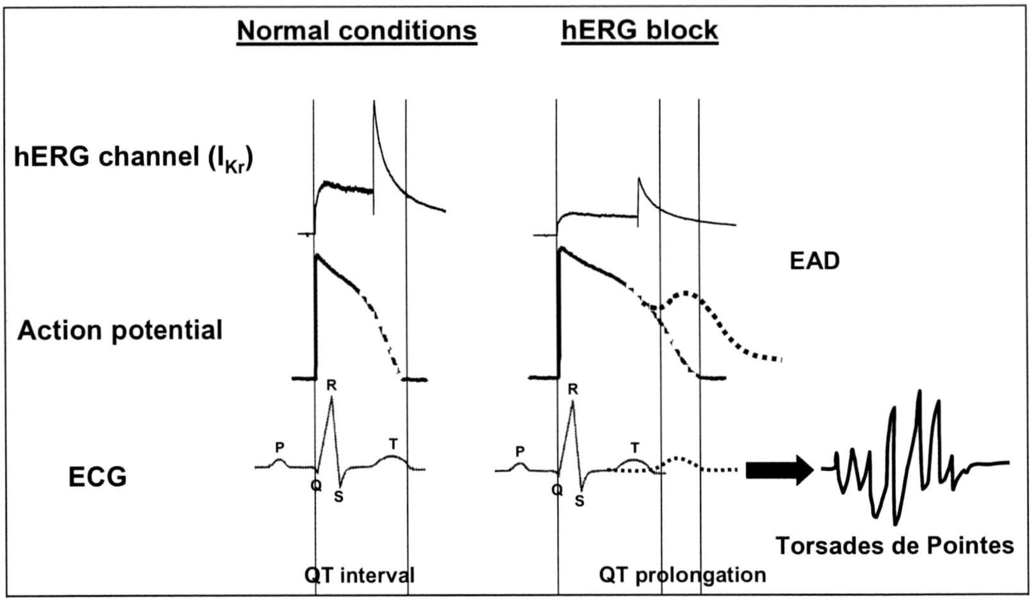

Figure 1. Summary of the traditional concept of drug-induced torsadogenesis. According to this view, hERG channel inhibition delays the repolarization which leads to a prolongation of the action potential duration. Under these conditions early afterdepolarizations (EAD) are provoked. EADs are abnormal cellular depolarizations occurring before repolarization is completed. They are likely carried by increases in intracellular Ca^{2+}. EADs may give rise to premature APs or even trains of APs that may lead to torsades de pointes.

The S7B guideline was finalized in October 2005 and proposed a preclinical core battery with the hERG assay and an *in vivo* QT assay. The problem was that the predictive value of these assays for clinical QT effects was unknown. Early indications were that the preclinical data are quite predictive of the clinical outcome. Experiments had been initiated that aimed at retrospectively test the predictive value of the preclinical tests by using compounds with known QT prolonging properties in the clinic. Two series of experiments were performed, one in the US and one in Japan that used similar preclinical assays (hERG assay, *in vitro* APD assay and *in vivo* QT assay). Taken together, results of these studies support the potential for an overall good level of predictivity for clinical effects on QT. These experiments were performed in well-chosen laboratories with well-standardized protocols.

A recent analysis by the FDA, however, concluded that the predictive value of preclinical tests for clinical QT outcome is insufficient. On the contrary, leading companies in the QT field claim that their preclinical in-house models predict QT effects in humans very well using well-defined criteria in an integrated risk assessment. At Novartis, an internal review was performed to compare preclinical data with available results from 6 "thorough QT studies" in humans. These compounds are under development for six different indications (cancer, infection, psychosis, allergy, autonomic dysfunction) with different mechanisms of action. Criteria for data evaluation were:

Clinical (only "thorough QT studies" in healthy volunteers)
- *study type:* 1 multiple dose studies, 4 single dose study
- *dose:* <0.6 to 3 times therapeutic target dose

positive study: mean increase in QTc > 5 ms

Preclinical

hERG:

expression system: mammalian cell

positive study: TI ≤ 30

APD assay

Purkinje fiber (sheep, dog), papillary muscle (guinea pig) or isolated heart (rabbit)

positive study: TI ≤ 30

In vivo whole animal:

5 dogs (4 conscious, 1 anesthetized)

1 monkey (conscious)

positive study: TI ≤ 30

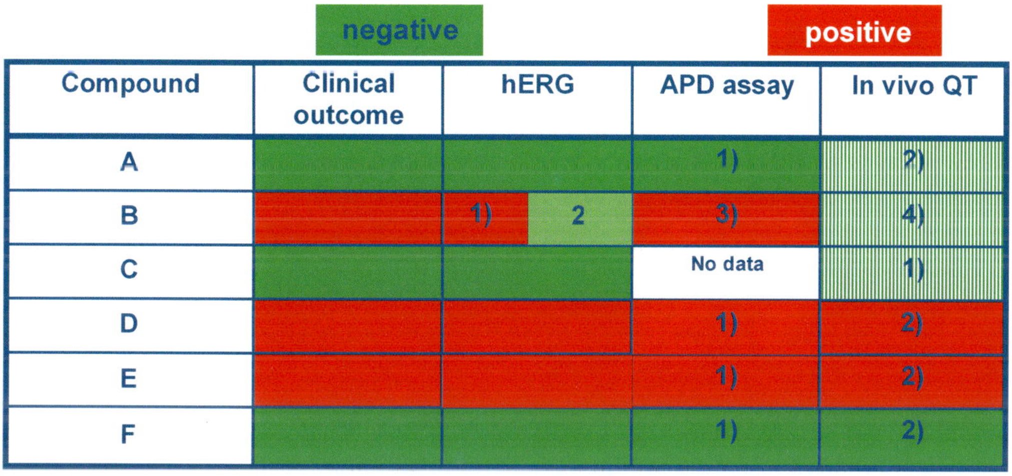

Figure 2. Predictive values of individual preclinical tests for QT effects in humans. A: 1) results from sheep Purkinje fiber and isolated rabbit heart 2) max dose in telemetered dogs resulted i n TI = 7; B: 1) based on phase 2 data 2) based on phase 3 data 3) dog Purkinje fiber 4) max dose in telemetered dogs resulted in TI=1-5; C: 1) max dose resulted in TI = 10 in telemetered dogs; D: 1) guinea pig papillary muscle 2) anesthetized dogs; E: 1) Isolated rabbit heart 2) telemetry monkey; F: 1) Rabbit Purkinje fiber indicated mixed cardiac ion channel inhibition (K, Na, Ca) 2) anesthetized dogs.

The therapeutic Index (TI) was calculated with the therapeutic free plasma concentration as denominator. The most recent definition of the therapeutic dose during the development of the drugs was used to calculate this value, i.e., not necessarily the value that may have been considered valid at the time when the preclinical tests were performed. The numerators were IC50-values for the hERG assay, highest concentration without effect on APD for the APD assay, and free Cmax at the no-effect-level for the *in vivo* QT assay, respectively. The results are summarized in Figure 2. Using TI ≤ 30 as a criterion for a positive outcome, the individual preclinical assays predicted the clinical outcome in most cases correctly and an integrated safety assessment for the six molecules correctly predicted compounds with repolarization issues. The individual tests never produced false positive results. False negative data were obtained for an antipsychotic (substance B). This is partially due to the difficulties in defining the therapeutic plasma concentration during the preclinical phase of drug development. Preclinical disease models, in particular for antipsychotic drugs, often poorly predict therapeutic pharmacologically active doses in humans. The final definition of the therapeutic dose and plasma concentrations occurs in phase 2 studies or even later. It was evident that uncertainties in defining the therapeutic plasma concentration during early drug development are the main obstacles for applying the concept of a TI $\leq$ 30. In the case of compound B, a lower therapeutic dose was assumed during the phase 2 studies and with the lower doses the TI for the hERG assay was > 30.

In *in vivo* assays with conscious, telemetered non-rodents treated with low multiples of the therapeutic doses (often << 30-fold therapeutic doses) often produce signs of toxicity. Since these animals are typically re-used in other studies, investigators are understandably hesitant to dose higher. Dose limitations are frequently observed for compounds with central nervous system indications that often produce peripheral effects on the cardiovascular system and with oncology indications. Cancer drugs usually have a low TI. An alternative for overcoming problems with conscious telemetered non-rodents is using anesthetized animals.

Different opinions exist currently amongst regulatory agencies in the acceptance of the relevance of preclinical data. There is still no agreement on the extent to which preclinical data can exclude a clinical risk, and regulatory authorities in some regions will require clinical evaluation of a new drug in a "thorough QT-study" during clinical Phase I for almost all new drugs independent of the outcome of the preclinical investigations including cases of negative hERG data.

Certain risk factors for the development of TdP in man have been identified and include female gender, hypokalemia, heart diseases, marked elevations of plasma drug concentrations following iv administration or inhibition of metabolism, and baseline QT prolongation (Roden 2004). Despite the identification of such risk factors, the development of TdP and, even more importantly, the outcome of the arrhythmic event remain unpredictable in an individual subject. This highly variable response to drug therapy suggests that additional as yet undefined factors may be involved in the pathogenesis of TdP arrhythmia.

Limitations of Current Test Methods for Torsadogenic Potential (Figure 3)

hERG Assay: Blockade of the hERG Channel is not Synonymous with Clinical TdP Risk

Indeed, "false positive" and "false negative" results for TdP prediction in man are documented. Compounds showing inhibitory potential in the hERG assay may not be torsadogenic for the human heart. Verapamil and clozapine are examples that potently block the hERG channel, but both compounds lack torsadogenic potential in man. This may be attributed to their properties to reduce, in the same concentration range, the Na^{+} and the Ca^{++} currents, respectively, which theoretically opposes the repolarization delay (Cavero and Crumb 2001; Warner and Hoffmann 2002). From industry as well as regulatory perspectives it is of concern that the hERG assay generates a high rate of equivocal or "false positive" results if performed according to the draft guidelines S7B, e.g., testing of substances at concentrations up to the limit of solubility. It has become clear that 75 – 86 % of NCE tested in the pharmaceutical industry during early phases of drug development show hERG inhibitory activity (Shah 2005). Provided that the concentration is high enough, it seems that almost any compound will inhibit the hERG channel *in vitro*. One only has to torture nature long enough - in its desperation it will give you an answer. Screening of all drugs in the pharmacopoeia would probably unearth some potent hERG blockers that have never been associated with QT interval prolongation or TdP in man. "False positive" outcomes in the hERG assay appear logical when considering that the action potential is the integral of several sequentially activated channels and ion transporters. It means, though, that more electrophysiological data must be generated to understand compensating or mitigating effects such as inhibition of I_{Na} or I_{Ca}. Concerning "false negatives" with the hERG assay, nifedipine, amiodarone, diphenhydramine, and arsenic trioxide are examples that cause TdP in man but have no or very low inhibitory potential for the hERG channel (Redfern et al. 2003).

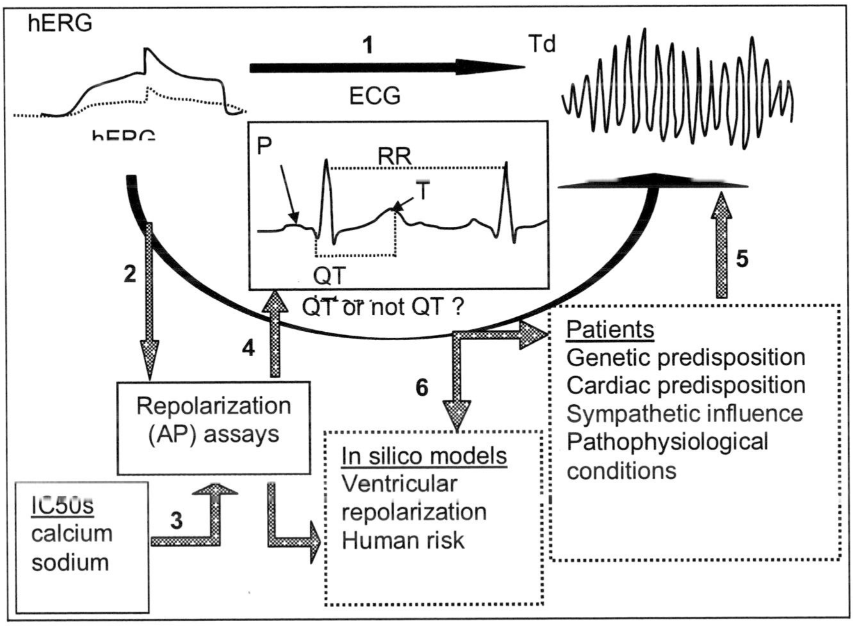

Figure 3. General overview of potential relationship between the reduction of the current generated by the human ether-à-gogo-related gene (hERG) and occurrence of Torsade de Pointes (TdP) in patients. 1: absence of direct correlation between the potency of hERG blockade and TdP incidence in patients; 2: absence of direct correlation between potency of hERG blockade and the duration of ventricular repolarization measured in action potentials (AP); 3: additional inhibition of sodium and/or calcium inward currents evaluated by their respective IC50-values can mitigate the effects of hERG blockade on the duration of ventricular repolarization; 4: modification of AP duration may not translate into an increase in the ventricular repolarization measured at the whole heart level by the QT interval on a body surface electrocardiogram (ECG); 5: patients may carry genetic and cardiac predispositions which may strongly modify drug effects in the myocardium; 6: computerized models appear to constitute a very valuable approach integrating any component from gene to integrated human physiology potentially interfering with normal cardiac functions and pathological conditions. (Dumotier and Georgieva 2007, reproduced with permission of the authors).

APD Assay: Inhibition of the hERG Channel Does not always Translate into APD Prolongation

Martin et al. (2004) investigated the APD prolonging potential of ten hERG blockers in the canine Purkinje fiber model. Only four compounds demonstrated convincing monotone concentration-dependent APD prolongation. Comparable levels of hERG block did not result in the same APD prolongation due to different electrophysiological drug profiles (ability to reduce other ion currents than hERG). Indeed, bell-shaped concentration response relationships are seen frequently and further complicate the interpretation of the data with this model. Investigations in an isolated rabbit heart model with 5079 hERG blockers revealed that hERG blockade was associated with APD prolongation only in 76 % of the compounds, but shortening of APD with hERG blockers was also seen (Hondeghem 2005). It is still difficult to determine an APD prolonging effect of terfenadine in canine and porcine Purkinje fiber preparations (Gintant et al. 2001). On the contrary, ebastin prolongs APD in the isolated rabbit heart but is not torsadogenic in man (Valentin et al. 2004). In a systematic validation approach of the International Life Science Institute, results with canine Purkinje fibers indicated a poor correlation between APD prolongation and torsadogenic risk in man (International Life Science Institute (ILSI) workshop "Cardiovascular Risk Assessment", Washington June 3 – 4, 2003). Considering the data generated preclinically and using different animal models, it is increasingly questioned whether prolongation of APD per se can be used as a reliable predictor of TdP arrhythmia in man. Hondeghem et al. (2001) investigated the correlation between APD prolongation and TdP proarrhythmia using 702 compounds in 1071 isolated rabbit heart preparations. In general, their findings supported the concept that APD prolongation is associated with proarrhythmia. Some compounds, however, prolonged APD and were anti-arrhythmic. This clearly indicates that proarrhythmic events beyond a sole APD prolongation are needed to favor the development of TdP.

QT Interval: Accumulating Evidence Suggests that Only a Weak Correlation Exists between QT Prolongation and TdP in Humans

Prolongation of the QT interval in telemetered dogs and primates has a high predictive value for QT interval prolongation in humans. But accumulating evidence suggests that only a weak correlation exists between QT prolongation and TdP in humans. For seven antipsychotics this was recently reviewed by Warner and Hoffmann (2002) as summarized in Figure 4. It is estimated that the therapeutic free plasma concentration of these antipsychotics would result in approximately 10 – 20 % inhibition of the hERG channel. This, however, translates into very different increases in the QTc (frequency corrected QT) interval in the target population. Additionally, the magnitude of QTc prolongation does not correlate with the torsadogenic risk in humans. Specifically, haloperidol causes an increase in mean QTc of only 5 to 7 ms, but TdP in humans are frequently observed at therapeutic dose. By contrast, ziprasidone prolongs QTc to a greater extent than haloperidol, risperidone and olanzapine but so far, ziprasidone has not been associated with TdP and sudden death in the clinic (Taylor, 2003). Sertindole, on the other hand, prolongs QTc to the same extent as ziprasidone but is torsadogenic in humans. For the potent hERG blocker clozapine, no effects on QT_C were observed during clinical trials in phase I – III and no reliable data are available postmarketing that could clearly demonstrate a potential QT prolonging effect (Warner and Hoffmann 2002). Erythromycin is another example. It markedly prolongs the QT interval at therapeutic doses (35 ms). Cases of TdP, though, are very rare, and there were almost always additional predisposing factors (Redfern et al. 2003). Sildenafil and vardenafil are weak hERG blockers relative to their clinical exposure and were not found to prolong QT interval in preclinical models. However, these compounds show a QT prolongation up to 10 ms in man (see below).

In conclusion, these examples show that hERG inhibition, APD prolongation and prolongation of the QT interval are not reliable indicators of torsadogenic potential in man. New arrhythmogenic markers are clearly needed. They should not only identify the potential of a new drug to cause TdP, but ideally they should also enable us to identify patients at risk for proarrhythmia. We need to understand the mechanisms from genes to the effects on individual channels, to interactions with other cellular processes, to the ECG (Noble 2001). New approaches are emerging which can help in better understanding these mechanisms.

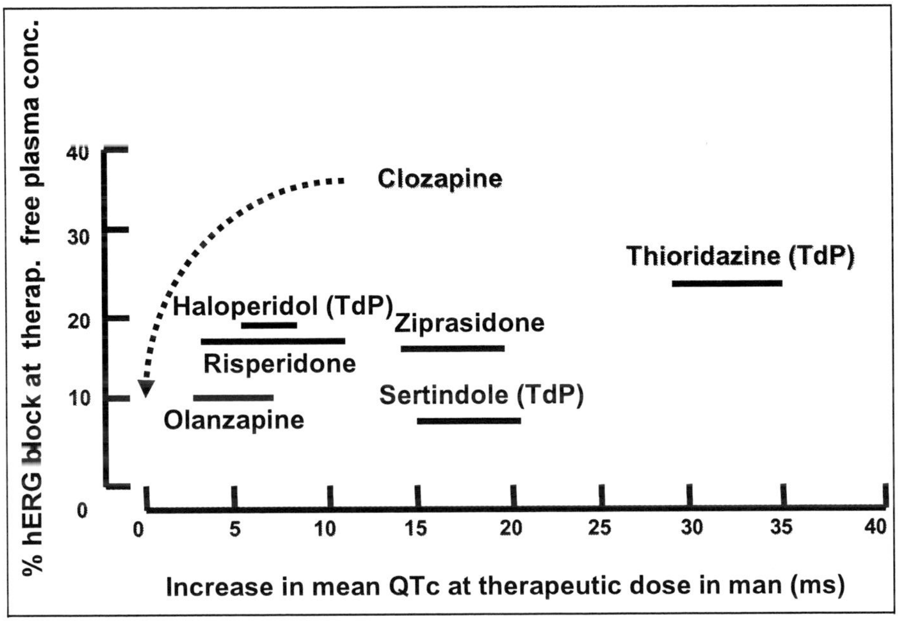

Figure 4. hERG block at therapeutic free plasma concentrations for seven antipsychotics is plotted vs mean change of QTc interval at therapeutic doses. TdP means that compounds are torsadogenic in humans at therapeutic doses (graph according to data from Warner and Hoffmann 2002).

Impact on the Development of New Drugs

Health authorities currently scrutinize all hERG blockers that delay repolarization to cause QT prolongation. Since a direct link between QT prolongation and TdP arrhythmia does not exist we are faced with the inability to distinguish between safe and potentially torsadogenic hERG blockers and APD/QT prolongers. Pharmaceutical companies must now assess the potential torsadogenic risk of new drugs using a number of preclinical assays and clinical trials. Pfizer initiated about 50 "thorough QT-studies" in 2002 (Fermini and Fossa

2003). Such a study for a single compound with a preclinical QT signal approximates nearly US $1 million. Thus, in the current environment the upfront costs required to address the issue of torsadogenesis become very significant. Once it is clear that a compound under development has a QT prolonging potential at therapeutically relevant exposure in man, a company must evaluate the approvability and labeling implications.

Given these hurdles it is conceivable that some molecules with great therapeutic potential will be terminated. In the current scientific and regulatory environment, one can question whether companies would pursue the development of drugs like clozapine and fluoxetine, which were introduced into the market 1969 and 1987, respectively. These compounds have been utilized by tens of millions of patients and revolutionized the treatment of schizophrenia and depression, with low incidence of arrhythmogenic liability (Fermini and Fossa 2003; Warner and Hoffmann 2002). Both compounds are, however, potent hERG blockers, and it is unlikely that these molecules would have survived the rigorous test batteries and decision criteria currently applied during early drug development. Is the drug development paralyzed, preventing some drugs with substantial health benefits from reaching the market?

On the following pages, preclinical methods beyond those currently used as the core battery of torsadogenicity testing will be reviewed with special emphasis on evolving new scientific approaches. The methods will be critically evaluated considering their potential to refine how cardiovascular safety of new drug candidates can be assessed in the future. The relevance and the predictive value of these methods have, however, yet to be made clear.

In Vitro Models

Several in vitro studies simulating pathophysiological conditions have been published. Many of those dealing with basic ionic mechanisms of delayed repolarization were performed in isolated cells, whereas studies investigating the electrophysiologic aspects of a torsadogenic effect mainly used isolated tissues or whole heart preparations.

Isolated cells: The current standard hERG screen using stably transfected cells (HEK or CHO) does not include proarrhythmic risk factors. Pathological conditions may alter electrophysiology and thereby influence the propensity of a compound to produce TdP; some attempts have been made to address this problem. Cavero et al. (2000) proposed adapting the hERG assay to conditions known to amplify adverse effects on cardiac repolarization such as low K^+ concentration, low rate of stimulation imitating bradycardia, bath solutions mimicking cardiac ischemia, and concurrent use of multiple drugs that can prolong repolarization to investigate pharmacodynamic interactions. Measurement of ion currents and APD in primary cultures of disaggregated cardiomyocytes including human preparations are as yet infrequently performed. Proteolytic dispersion and storage conditions appear to damage channels or alter channel expression and cause high variation of electrophysiologic parameters. Unsuccessful attempts were undertaken to create a cardiomyocyte cell line that proliferates in culture while maintaining a differentiated phenotype. VistaGen Therapeutics (2005) recently published ongoing research activities to develop an immortalized cardiomyocyte cell line from human fetal or adult cardiomyocyte precursors using a conditional immortalization technology (http://www.vistagen-inc.com/htm_pages/homepage.htm). A renewable source of standardized human cardiomyocytes could be a valuable tool for assessing drug effects on cardiac ion channels in their native environment.

Isolated tissues/hearts: *In vitro* techniques can be employed to better understand the relationship between prolongation of APD and torsadogenic risk. Eckardt et al. (2001) have developed an isolated rabbit heart model aimed at reproducing conditions that are associated clinically with an increased propensity to develop TdP arrhythmia. Bradycardia was achieved by complete AV block and a low K^+ concentration was used in the perfusate. Monophasic action potentials were simultaneously recorded from up to 8 sites evenly spread in a circular pattern around both ventricles. TdP was produced with several QT prolonging agents, and occurrence of abnormalities in repolarization phase (EADs) predicted TdP arrhythmia.

Hondeghem et al. (2001) and Hondeghem and Hoffmann (2003) investigated the correlation between APD prolongation and proarrhythmia in isolated rabbit heart preparations. In this model, the His bundle is sectioned to better control ventricular pacing by stimulating electrodes, and the monophasic action potential are recorded from the left ventricle epicardium and subendocardium (populated with some Purkinje fibers). In general, their findings supported the concept that APD prolongation is associated with pro-arrhythmia when associated with repolarization disturbances. By contrast, some compounds prolong APD but are anti-arrhythmic. For these compounds, APD prolongation was not accompanied by proarrhythmia indices referred to as triangulation of the action potential (defined as selectively slowing phase 3 repolarization to give triangular shaped action potentials), instability (defined as high variability of beat-to-beat APD), or reverse use dependence (defined by more marked effects of the compound at lower stimulation rates). Examples for triangulation and instability are illustrated in Figures 5 and 6. Spatial (intramural) and temporal (beat-to-beat) dispersion are additional proarrhythmia indices found to be highly reliable in this model. These and other experiments showed that a set of repolarization disturbances characterized by Triangulation, Reverse use dependence, Instability and Dispersion (= TRIaD), rather than simple changes in the duration of the AP, provides the proarrhythmic substrate (Hondeghem 2005). The isolated heart model described as SCREENIT allows a high throughput and is now used in several companies for early drug screening in the clinical candidate selection phase (Valentin et al. 2004). So far, over 16000 experiments have been conducted, including approximately 300 blinded tests of 70 widely used clinical drugs with both torsadogenic and non-torsadogenic properties (Valentin et al. 2004). Using the above proarrhythmia indices, there are no documented instances of torsadogenic compounds that are negative on TRIaD and, conversely, there is no TRIaD signal for compounds that are safe clinically in terms of proarrhythmia.

Recent studies from a number of laboratories have delineated three distinct cell types with different electrophysiological properties in the ventricular myocardium of a number of species: epicardial, midmyocrdial (M cells) and endocardial cells (Antzelevitch 2004 a; Belardinelli et al. 2003). Distinctive repolarization features of M cells are due in part to a lesser contribution of I_{Ks}, a larger late Na^+ current, and a larger Na^+/Ca^{2+} exchange current compared to epicardial and endocardial cells (Antzelevitch 2004 b). Under physiological conditions, M cells exhibit the longest APD in the left ventricular myocardium, which makes them especially vulnerable to agents that prolong APD (Poelzing and Rosenbaum 2005). This vulnerability is further enhanced by the fact that the electrical coupling of M cells to epicardial cells is very low in normal myocardium, supporting the establishment of an APD gradient between epicardial and M cells (Poelzing and Rosenbaum 2005). An amplification of electrical heterogeneities intrinsic to the ventricular myocardium, i.e., transmural dispersion of repolarization, combined with regional expression patterns in electrical coupling, appear to be important for the development of TdP arrhythmias. Findings like these provide increasing insight into the mechanisms of TdP and make clear why measurement of the QT interval is too crude a parameter to predict drug-induced torsadogenesis, since such subtle electrophysiological changes will not be seen in the surface ECG.

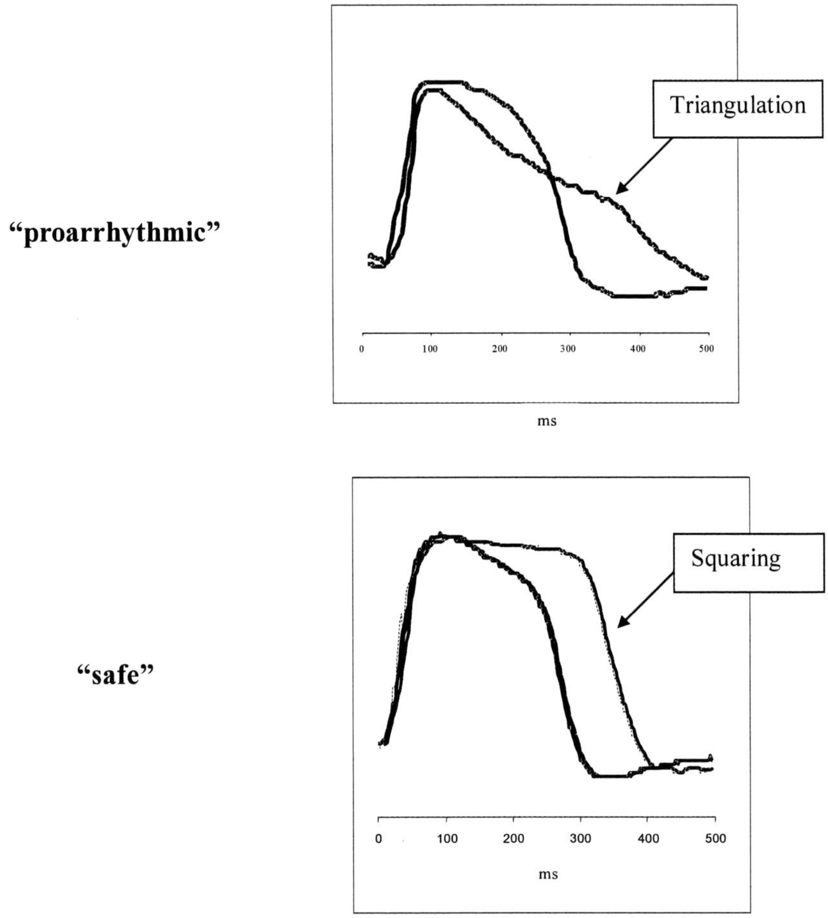

Figure 5. Examples of proarrhythmic (upper) and safe (lower) prolongation of an action potential in the isolated rabbit heart model: Triangulation vs Squaring of the action potential (Hondeghem 2005, reproduced with permission of the author).

Isolated, arterially perfused ventricular wedge preparations from dog, rabbit, and feline left ventricles were used to investigate action potentials from the epicardial, midmyocardial (M cells) and endocardial region (Aiba et al. 2005; Joshi et al. 2004). Using a canine ventricular wedge preparation, prolongation of APD after terfenadine was observed in M cells (Antzelevitch 2004 b). The rabbit ventricular wedge preparation appears even more sensitive to the genesis of early afterdepolarizations and TdP in the presence of QT prolonging agents, due to the smaller or missing I_{Ks} current in the ventricular wall of this species (Yan et al. 2001). With the rabbit model, intracellular recording provided direct evidence that early afterdepolarizations can be generated in the intact ventricular wall. Early afterdepolarizations of sufficient conduction and amplitude can propagate across the ventricular wall causing a transmural dispersion of repolarization and initiation of TdP.

Isolated arterially perfused ventricular wedge preparations have a high selectivity (90 %) and specificity (100 %) for human torsadogens (Antzelevitch 2004 b). However, being technically challenging, they are difficult methods thus the number of molecules that can be investigated is rather limited. This model may be best used for follow up mechanistic studies.

"proarrhythmic"

"safe"

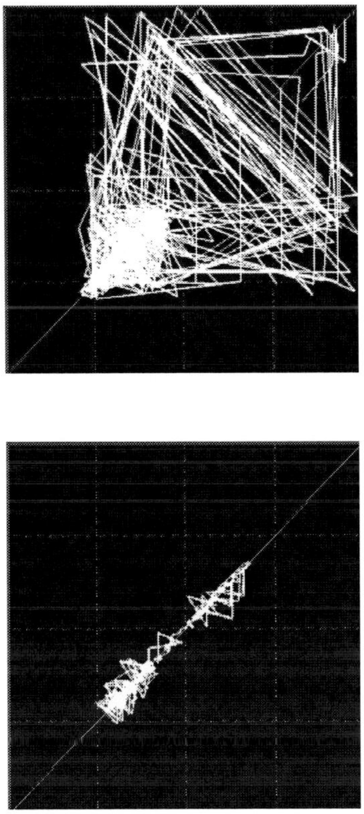

Figure 6. Poincaré plot for a proarrhythmic (upper) and safe (lower) compound in the isolated rabbit heart model. Each APD_{60} (= APD until 60 % repolarization) is plotted against the previous beat's APD_{60} and for clarity the points are connected. The axes show an interval of 800 ms. Proarrhythmic APD_{60} changes generate many points far removed from the diagonal line. (Hondeghem 2005, reproduced with permission of the author).

In Vivo Models

Direct assessment of the proarrhythmic risk of compounds that prolong QT interval in an animal TdP arrhythmia model would seem the most likely to predict human experience. However, mimicking the clinical setting where drugs elicit TdP arrhythmia is very difficult in vivo. Generally, data from conscious animals are preferable but only a few methods to examine TdP proarrhythmia in conscious animals exist. Chezalviel Guilbert et al. (1995) introduced a conscious dog model with TdP like polymorphic ventricular tachycardia, in which bradycardia and hypokalemia were combined. Bradycardia was achieved by chemically or electrically induced complete AV block, whereas hypokalemia was induced over a period of weeks using high doses of diuretics. Quinidine, sotalol, and almokalant, but not lidocaine, flecainide, or propranolol, exhibited significant proarrhythmic effects in this model. Carlsson et al. (1993) used a conscious rabbit model and found that infusion of APD prolonging antiarrhythmic agents such as almokalant, dofetilide, clofilium, or semaltilide was associated with the induction of TdP.

Nevertheless, most of the TdP arrhythmia models in use involve anesthetized animals, mainly rabbits and dogs. Voss et al. (1995) described a canine model with chronic AV block where different pacing modes were used to produce TdP. QT prolonging compounds induced TdP in this model, showing promise in discriminating the proarrhythmic effects of various hERG blocking agents. Anesthetized rabbits concomitantly treated with the α_1 adrenergic agonist methoxamine exhibited TdP-like polymorphic ventricular tachycardia in the presence of agents prolonging the repolarization process (Carlsson et al. 1993). The results indicate that the anesthetized rabbit, which like humans presents a high density of α_1 adrenergic receptors, may be a relevant model for studies of torsadogenic compounds. Other *in vivo* canine models, such as an anesthetized open-chest model with myocardial infarction, models with ventricular pacing, and cesium or neurotoxin treatment, are useful mainly for the study of the etiology of TdP and not for assessing the torsadogenic potential of new drug candidates (Eckardt et al. 1998).

There are important limitations of *in vivo* proarrhythmia models, including the high variability in the occurrence of TdP. No model shows 100% reproducibility. In addition, all the *in vivo* models utilize complex techniques, which indicate how difficult it is to induce TdP under experimental conditions. The rare occurrence of TdP arrhythmia in animal models suggests that other predisposing and, so far, unknown factors may contribute to TdP development. For example, it is still difficult to detect the torsadogenic potential of terfenadine in animal models even though terfenadine was withdrawn from the market due to TdP and sudden death in man. Due to technical complexity, lack of experience, and high effort in terms of time and costs, proarrhythmia models are rarely used and very little data are available with these methods. The role of these models in drug development appears difficult to define at this time. An ongoing ILSI initiative is planning a series of experiments to systematically investigate the predictive value of TdP arrhythmia models for torsadogenic risk in man (Methods to increase the predictive value of drug-induced torsades de pointes. Workshop planned November 2 -3, 2005, in Washington).

Experimental mouse models with congenital long QT syndrome represent a more recent approach. The mouse genome contains a hERG related gene (Merg1) expressed in the heart (Londan and Pan 1998). Mice with homozygous deletion of Merg1 die early during development and a Merg1 B-specific knock out mouse has a normal QT duration but shows abrupt episodes of sinus bradycardia (Lees-Miller et al. 2003). Models with LQT1, LQT3, LQT4 , and LQT5 syndrome have also been established (Charpentier et al. 2004). But the main disadvantage of transgenic mouse models is that repolarization in adult rodents is mainly driven by transient outward currents, whereas I_{Kr} and I_{Ks} (carried by hERG and KvLQT1 channels, respectively) play little role if any, and that it is extremely difficult to define precisely the end of the T wave of the ECG due to very high cardiac frequency in mouse. Therefore most agree that transgenic rodent models are inappropriate for the study of drug-induced TdP. In the near future, we may see transgenic rabbit models emerging). These appear to be a more promising approach.

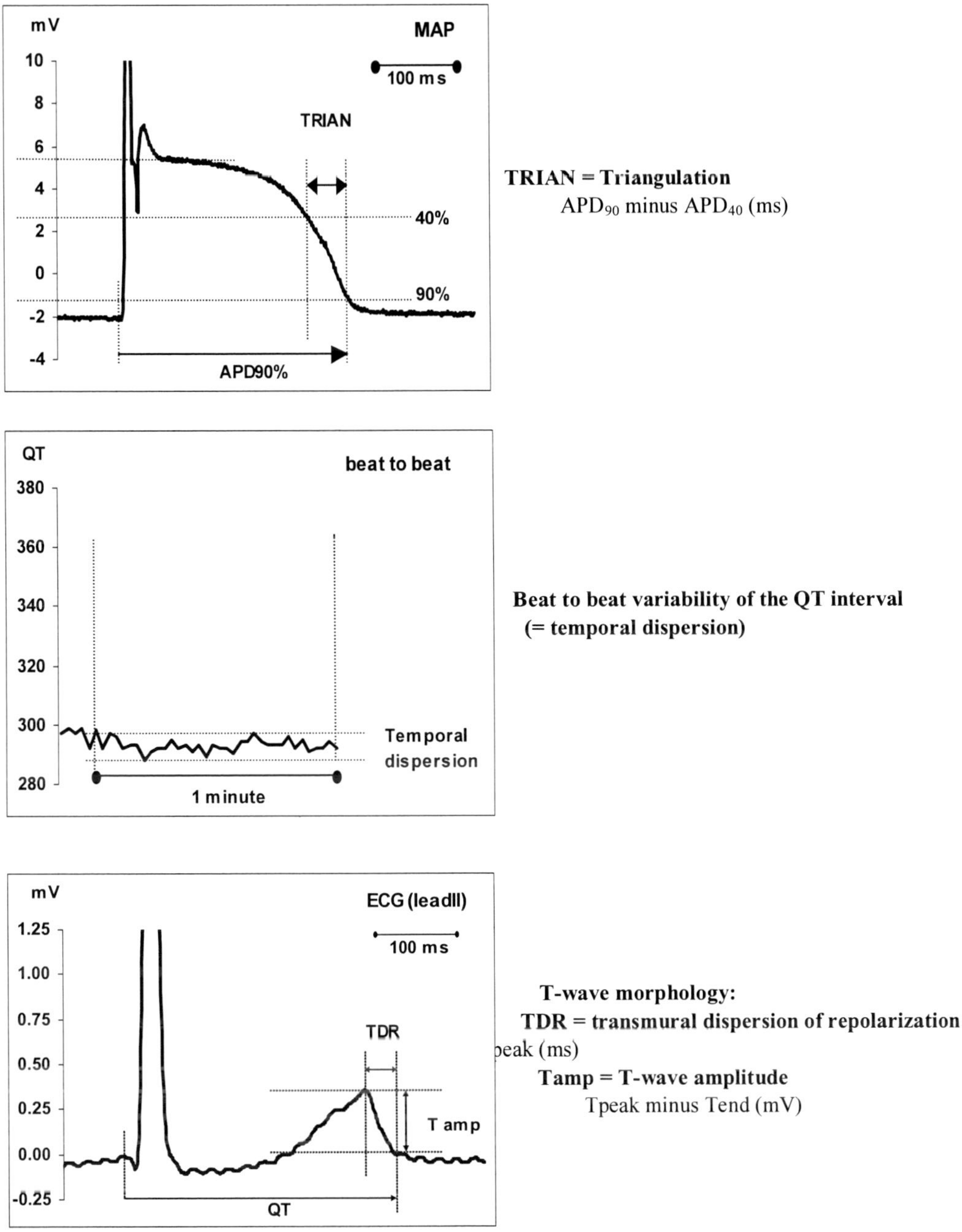

Figure 7. In *vivo indices* derived from *in vitro* proarrhythmia indices and measured in anesthetized dogs from the endocardial right ventricular monophasic action potential (MAP) and the surface ECG: triangulation, beat-to-beat variability and parameters of T-wave morphology (De Clerck and Gallacher 2005, reproduced with permission of the authors).

Studies in normal animals under physiological conditions are stimulated by the new above mentioned *in vitro* findings. Laboratories in academia and the pharmaceutical industry currently intensively investigate the predictive value of beat-to-beat variability of repolarization and other parameters derived from the *in vitro* proarrhythmia indices (Scientific meeting on "Beat-to-beat variability of repolarization to test for the proarrhythmic potential of drugs", Maastricht, The Netherlands, April 14 – 15, 2005). An example of how electrophysiological parameters derived from *in vitro* proarrhythmia indices can be measured in anesthetized dogs is shown in Figure 7. In anesthetized guinea pigs, the study of beat-to-beat alternations of the cardiac monophasic action potential differentiated four torsadogenic drugs from 2 compounds that are safe in man at therapeutic concentration (Fossa et al. 2004). Beat-to-beat variability of repolarization *in vivo* is the macroscopic counterpart of instability as measured under *in vitro* conditions. Although the ionic and cellular mechanisms that underlie the generation of beat-to-beat variability of repolarization and QT interval are not fully understood, the study of this parameter may serve as an additional appropriate approach toward prediction of clinical outcomes. Measurement of beat-to beat-variability of the QT interval can easily be applied to human ECGs. Indeed, it has been shown that beat-to-beat variability measured as T-wave alternans is a powerful predictor of TdP in humans (Brockmeiner et al. 2001).

Anesthetized animals are used when, for example, the compound is poorly tolerated in the chosen species (causing for example tremor or emesis), or when pharmacokinetic/ pharmacodynamic modeling is planned, or when relatively little is known about the compound at the time of evaluation. This raises the complication of the unknown effect of anesthesia on responses to the compound under study, although it is the view of several companies, that at least the anesthetized dog responds to QT effects of drugs in a qualitatively similar extent to the conscious dog.

Interesting observations have recently been reported from a zebrafish model. Milan et al. (2004) observed that 22 of 23 compounds that cause TdP in man produced bradycardia in their zebrafish model. The negative chronotropic effect is obviously due to the role of the hERG channel in the sinus node. The authors suggest that this simple high-troughput assay could become a promising addition to the repertoire of preclinical tests. However, by contrast to the other high throughput assays, the precise concentrations to which the Zebrafishes are exposed are unknown, this constituting an important disadvantage.

Pharmacodynamic Interactions at the Level of the HERG Channel

The voltage-gated potassium channel that generates the I_{Kr} cardiac potassium current is formed by a tetrameric complex of hERG pore-forming α-subunits (Sanguinetti and Mitcheson 2005). The *in vitro* hERG assay is performed with stable mammalian cell lines (HEK, CHO) or *Xenopus* oocytes expressing the α-subunit. What is uncertain is whether human I_{Kr} channels contain ancillary subunits *in vivo*. Two chief contenders for this role are MiNK (encoded by KCNE1) and MiRP1 (KCNE2) (Anantharam and Abbott 2005). There are also reports about a possible *in vivo* interaction between hERG and the α-subunit of I_{Ks} (KvLQT1 encoded by KCNQ1) (Ehrlich et al. 2004). Co-expression of hERG with KvLQT1 significantly altered hERG channel properties. Another recent study has shown that KCR1, a plasma membrane-associated protein that can be immunoprecipitated with hERG, reduces the sensitivity of hERG to blockers (Kupershmidt el al. 2003). This complexity *in vivo* has to be taken into consideration during the evaluation and interpretation in the data with the *in vitro* hERG assay as it is currently performed. Some authors suggest that the molecular composition of I_{Kr} is likely to vary regionally within the heart of one species and also between species (Anantharam and Abbott 2005). Thus, hERG may well exist alone in some cardiomyocytes but with MiNK, MiRP1 and/or other ancillary subunits elsewhere. Add to this the possibility that the I_{Kr} composition varies during the development from the fetus to neonate to adult, and it becomes apparent that attempts to correlate I_{Kr} to a rigid composition may be conceptually flawed.

Pharmacodynamic interactions of compounds at the level of the hERG channel protein on the cell membrane are not well understood. The high activity binding site of hERG blockers is located in the central cavity of the channel (Sanguinetti and Mitcheson 2005). The large pore together with the fourfold symmetry and abundance of aromatic and polar regions that form the binding site allows many different binding modes and interactions. There is no conclusive experimental evidence for other binding sites yet (Sanguinetti 2005) with the exception of peptide toxins which clearly bind to an external site. Allosteric interactions, i.e., influence of gating properties by binding a molecule outside the high affinity binding site, may also influence hERG blocking properties.

Several companies have observed hERG channel activating properties during their screens of NCE for hERG blocking potential. Kang et al. (2005) described the *in vitro* electrophysiological effects of a prototype for this new class of compounds. The compound seems to work by slowing the closure of the hERG channel once it has opened. It slowed current deactivation in stably transfected CHO cells and shortened the QT interval in an isolated heart model. The compound also modified hERG inhibition and action potential prolonging effects of dofetilide. It remains to be clarified which therapeutic potential hERG activators may provide.

Since interactions of chirally active drugs with their pharmacological target are often stereoselective, it appears possible that the hERG blocking activity of a molecule resides predominantly in only one of the enantiomers. Indeed, there is evidence that the hERG block induced by the local anesthetic bupivacaine is stereoselective (Gonzalez et al. 2003). *In vivo*, the QT-prolonging effect of terodiline is mediated by (+)-R-terodiline (Hartigan-Go et al. 1996) and that of prenylamine probably by its (+)-(S)-enantiomer (Bayer et al. 1988).

Interactions with Other Channel Proteins

Compounds showing inhibitory potential in the hERG assay may not be torsadogenic for the human heart. Indeed, verapamil (hERG IC_{50} = 143 nM) and clozapine (hERG IC_{50} = 191 nM) are examples that potently block the hERG channel, but both compounds lack torsadogenic potential (Cavero and Crumb 2001; Warner and Hoffmann 2002). This may be attributed to their additional properties to inhibit, in the same concentration range, the Ca^{2+} and Na^{+} channel, respectively, which theoretically oppose repolarization delay. The explanation of a mitigated hERG channel blocking effect by Ca^{2+} antagonism may not be considered entirely satisfactory when ignoring kinetics of block, since bepridil, another Ca^{2+}

antagonist, also potently blocks the hERG channel (with an IC_{50} of 550 nM) and causes TdP in man (Prystowsky 1992; Redfern et al. 2002). The difference in the torsadogenic potential between these two Ca^{2+} antagonists may also reflect pharmacokinetic differences, however, bepridil has also I_{Ks} blocking properties (Wang et al. 1999). Similarly, the apparently safer clinical cardiac profile of loratadine compared with terfenadine despite their similar potency in blocking the hERG channel (with IC_{50}–values of 173 and 204 nM, respectively) may be related to the molecular mechanism by which they block the hERG channel as well as their relative potency in inhibiting other ion channels like I_{Kr}, I_{Ks} and I_{to} (Cavero and Crumb 2001).

Ranolazine, a new antianginal drug extensively investigated for its lectrophysiological properties, is a particularly good example of mixed cardiac ion channel effects. The ion current inhibitory effects of ranolazine at therapeutic concentrations include IKr (IC50=11.5 AM), late INa, late ICa, peak ICa, and INa–Ca (IC50=5.9, 50, 296, and 91 AM, respectively) and IKs (17% at 30 AM) without associated proarrhythmic properties (Antzelevitch et al., 2004).

Drugs are rarely selective for hERG. Mixed cardiac ion channel inhibition at the low μM range is a frequent effect seen during testing of NCE in early drug development *in vitro*. If the hERG blocking activity of a non-antiarrhythmic drug candidate does not translate into APD and/or QT interval prolongation due to mitigating effects on other cardiac ion channels, one should not feel too comfortable. The likelihood of achieving the right and very delicate balance of ion channel activities during the repolarization phase by good fortune is quite low. We are more likely to end up with a "terfenadine" than a "verapamil" (Redfern et al. 2002).

Channel/Receptor and Intracellular Signaling Cross Talk

Ion channels function within macromolecular complexes mediated by protein-protein interactions. These interactions are manifold and may involve channel accessory subunits, receptors, kinases, phosphatases, scaffolding proteins, and cytoskeleton proteins. The functional effects of these interactions may modify channel expression, trafficking, or channel activity (Kagan and McDonald 2005).

There is growing evidence of a role for hERG in stress related and beat to beat regulation of cardiac excitability. Therefore, hERG interactions with adrenoceptors are of interest. In anesthetized rabbits, TdP arrhythmia only occurs reproducibly when the animals are concomitantly treated with the α_1 adrenergic agonist methoxamine (Carlsson et al. 1993). This indicates an important role of α_1 adrenergic stimulation in the genesis of TdP arrhythmia. Functional coupling of α_{1A} adrenoceptors to hERG was investigated by co-expression of both proteins in CHO cells (Bian et al. 2001). Stimulation of α_1 adrenoceptors with the α_1 agonist phenylephrine caused hERG current reduction. Preliminary data on the mechanism of interaction between hERG and α_{1A} adrenoceptors on the level of intracellular signaling pathways indicate that protein kinase A and C reduce hERG channel activation through intermediate factors (Thomas et al. 2004). In addition, the direct interaction between phosphatidyl-4,5-biphosphate and the channel protein appears to enhance hERG currents (Bian et al. 2001). Increased α_1 adrenergic stimulation may also elevate the cytosolic free

Ca^{2+} concentration and lead to Ca^{2+}-dependent early afterdepolarizations (Carlsson et al. 1996).

Recent studies revealed that I_{Kr} is also regulated by β adrenoceptors. Activation of β adrenoceptors with isoprenaline reduced I_{Kr} amplitude in isolated guinea pig cardiomyocytes (Karle et al. 2002). There is a complex interaction following β adrenoceptor activation between intracellular messengers and the hERG channel protein (Figure 8) (Cui et al. 2000).

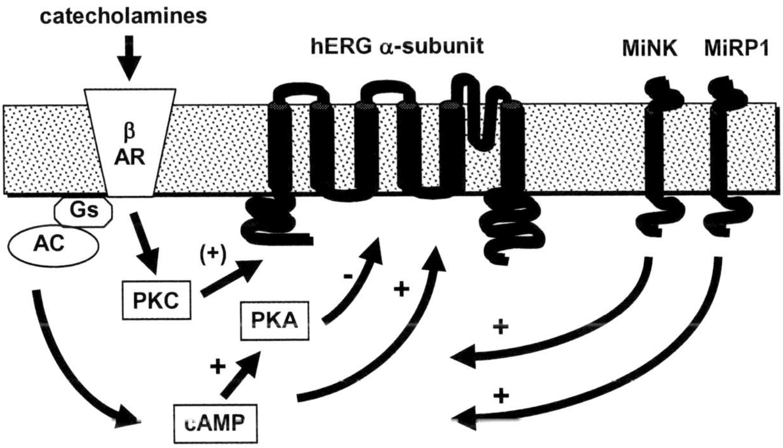

Figure 8. A model illustrating how β adrenergic stimulation modulates hERG channel activity by multiple mechanisms. Catecholamines stimulate β adrenoceptors (β AR) and increase cAMP via G protein (G_s) and adenylate cyclase (AC). The increase in cAMP stimulates hERG via its nucleotide binding domain. This effect can be enhanced by the β-subunits MiNK and MiRP1. cAMP also activates protein kinase (PKA), which reduces hERG currents. Finally, β adrenergic stimulation exerts protein kinase C (PKC) dependent, but PKA independent stimulatory effects on hERG currents; the molecular mechanism of this process has not yet been resolved.

Taken together, available data provide considerable evidence that stimulation of cardiac α or β adrenoceptor reduces I_{Kr}-dependent repolarization. This mechanism provides a basis to understand that hERG blocking activities of molecules may be enhanced by agonistic activities on adrenoceptors. It is important to note that the potential of channel/receptor cross talk of NCE can typically not be detected *in vitro* with the hERG assay in transfected cells, since these cells have a limited expression pattern of receptors.

It is important to note that the potential of channel/receptor cross talk of NCE can typically not be detected in vitro with the hERG assay in transfected cells, since these cells have a limited expression pattern of receptors. Therefore, results of screens for binding against multiple receptors that are usually performed early in the development of NCE are important to fully understand possible interactions with cardiac receptors.

In vivo on the other hand, we face complex interactions between the adrenoceptor interaction of the drug under investigation and endogenous catecholamines possibly released secondarily due to hemodynamic actions and resulting reflex changes of the autonomic tone. How difficult the *in vivo* situation can be is demonstrated by findings with sildenafil and vardenafil. Both compounds are weak hERG blockers relative to the clinical exposure with a safety margin at least 1000-fold above the free concentration after maximum clinical dose, and they do not prolong QT in conscious and anesthetized dogs (www.fda.gov/search.html).

However, these compounds show a slight but significant QT interval prolongation in man (up to 10 ms). They produce mild vasodilation and a reflex increase in heart rate and perhaps contractility, i.e. they cause an increased sympathetic tone which may exaggerate the weak hERG blocking activities of the compounds.

For antipsychotics, effects on hERG appear to be modified by interactions with several other receptors. These interactions may play a role in the manifestation of their torsadogenic potential (Warner and Hoffmann 2002; Taylor 2003) Antipsychotics are often quite potent hERG blockers but they are also multi-receptor drugs and exert their effects by interacting with several receptors like dopamine D_2 and D_4, α_1 and α_2 , 5-HT_{2A} and 5-HT_6 , M_1 and M_4, and H_1 (Richelson 1996).

Little is known about the regulation of hERG channel activity by hormone receptors. In Xenopus oocytes, co-expressing the hERG channel protein and the thyrotropin releasing hormone receptor, Barros et al. (1998) described a modulation of hERG channel gating by activation of the G protein-coupled thyrotropin releasing hormone receptor and protein kinase C activation.

It is clear that there are sex differences in the sensitivity of the heart for TdP arrhythmia. However, conflicting evidence in non-clinical/clinical experiments suggests sex hormones may have a role in increasing the susceptibility of women or reducing the susceptibility of men to TdP (Abi-Gerges et al. 2004).

Taken together, available data provide considerable evidence that stimulation of cardiac G-protein coupled receptors can modulate I_{Kr} dependent repolarization. Potential effects of non-G protein-coupled receptors are largely unknown.

Hypoglycemia and hyperglycemia both can cause prolongation of the QT interval and associated ventricular arrhythmias that are presumably responsible for sudden cardiac death in diabetic patients. Zhang et al. (2003) provided direct evidence that hypoglycemia and hyperglycemia can inhibit the hERG channel under *in vitro* conditions. Their data indicate that inhibition of hERG in hypoglycemia results from underproduction of ATP and in hyperglycemia from overproduction of reactive oxygen species. This example demonstrates that apart from being a well-recognized target for drug inhibition, I_{Kr} can also be influenced by endogenous compounds and this may play a role in the determination of the proarrhythmia risk of hERG blocking drugs under physiological and/or pathophysiological conditions. This raises the question whether one should not only use young healthy animals in preclinical safety testing, but also disease models of the therapeutic indication of the drug under development. This is typically not done, mainly because the predictive value of such disease models for the human pathophysiology is often imperfect, the models are not validated, and thus it is difficult to interpret the obtained results.

From Genes to Channels

Acquired QT prolongation is a common ECG finding in heart diseases, and potassium current down regulation contributes significantly to the enhanced liability of the repolarization process in the failing heart (Näbauer and Kääb 1998).

Prolongation of action potential duration is also a consistent finding in animal models of cardiac hypertrophy and failure (Aronson 1981; Tomaselli et al. 1994). In the canine model of TdP arrhythmia with chronic complete AV block, disturbed ventricular repolarization was found (Volders et al. 1999). In fact, ventricular endocardial monophasic action potential and QT interval were prolonged in these dogs, and a significant downregulation of delayed rectifier K^+ currents (both I_{Kr} and I_{Ks}) was observed. This downregulation could be shown at the level of the current and in its mRNA and protein expression, indicating that acquired QT prolongation and TdP in this model are related to intrinsic repolarization defects, also called electrical remodeling of the ventricles.

From these findings the question arises whether drugs can become torsadogenic via downregulation of delayed rectifier K^+ currents. Multiple processes determine the way in which the nucleotide sequence of the DNA molecule is inserted as channel protein into the membrane of the cardiomyocyte (Roden and Kupershmidt 1998). The first step is gene transcription from DNA to mRNA. The primary transcript is processed extensively in the nucleus before it is translated into a protein in the endoplasmic reticulum. One important process is splicing. hERG undergoes alternative splicing, which results in the formation of two hERG isoforms; only one of them results in functional currents in the heart (Roden and Kupershmidt 1998). The hERG channel protein is synthesized in the lumen of the rough endoplasmic reticulum, where it is inserted into transport vesicles and processed to the cell surface where membrane fusion results in insertion of the protein into the cell membrane. Cytosolic chaperons Hsp70 and Hsp90 are involved in the processing pathway of the hERG protein on the way to the cell surface (Ficker et al. 2005). They are crucial for productive folding of hERG. The assembly of different α-subunits likely occurs prior to transport to the cell surface.

Drugs that inhibit chaperon function produce a another form of acquired long QT syndrome not by direct electrical channel block but by reduced surface expression of the hERG channels (proteins) due to a trafficking defect of hERG. Arsenic trioxide is a prime example of a therapeutic compound that causes QT prolongation, TdP, and sudden death by inhibition of hERG channel maturation (Ficker et al. 2005). Other compounds that reduce hERG currents by trafficking inhibition are geldanamycin and pentamidine (Kuryshev et al. 2005).

Would we identify the cardiac liability of arsenic trioxide, geldanamycin and pentamidine using the current core battery? Most likely not. Even more importantly, how many other drugs are now being developed or are already on the market that impair hERG trafficking? Therefore, the recently introduced HERG-Lite\ screening assay that predicts both channel blockers and trafficking inhibitors is a valuable additional non-clinical tool (Wible et al., 2005)

A group of LQT2 mutations produces trafficking deficient hERG channels that are retained in the endoplasmic reticulum and are thought of as expressing conformational defects recognized by cellular quality control mechanisms. Interestingly, trafficking resumes and functional channels appear on the cell surface after incubation with potent hERG blockers such as astemizole (IC_{50} = 0.9 nM) (Ficker et al. 2005).

One drug that is often discussed in the context of torsadogenicity is amiodarone (Redfern et al. 2002). It is associated with minor electrophysiological effects *in vitro*. However, chronic treatment of dogs induced a moderate prolongation of the QT interval (Merot et al. 1999). Drvota et al. (1998) investigated whether delayed cardiac repolarization by the amiodarone metabolite desethylamiodarone is related to the expression of the channel protein in an isolated guinea pig heart model. Desethylamiodarone prolonged monophasic action potential and QTc in a slowly increasing manner during a 60-min perfusion period. This prolongation of cardiac repolarization was completely abolished by simultaneous treatment with either the protein synthesis inhibitor cycloheximide or the RNA synthesis inhibitor actinomycin D. Since cycloheximide and actinomycin had no effects on cardiac repolarization by themselves, these data indicate that the effect of desethylamiodarone is more dependent on protein synthesis rather than on a direct effect on channel proteins in the membrane (Figure 9). Further mechanistic investigations indicated that the effect of desethylamiodarone on hERG channel expression is mediated via interactions with the nuclear thyroid hormone receptor of (Drvota et al. 1998).

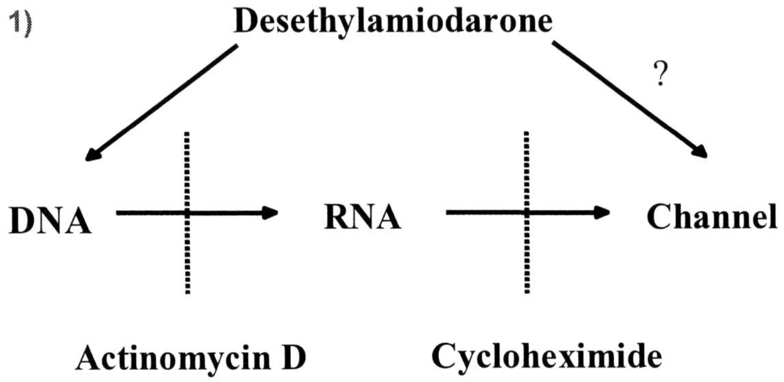

Figure 9. The action of desethylamiodarone on monophasic action potential and QTc is inhibited by either actinomycin D or cycloheximide. If desethylamiodarone would have exerted its action directly on channel proteins, the addition of actinomycin D or cycloheximide would have had no effect (scheme according to data from Drvota et al. 1998).

In another series of experiments Drici et al. (1996) demonstrated that estradiol and dihydrotestosterone treatment of guinea pigs caused a prolongation of the QT interval in *ex vivo* perfused isolated heart preparations. This effect was accompanied by a down-regulation of K^+ channel mRNA (I_{Ks} but not I_{Kr}). These findings indicate that the hormonal milieu of cardiac tissue may be an important regulatory process for the expression of delayed rectifier K^+ channels. Some investigators have found that the difference in QT interval between males and females is due to a shortening of the QT interval that develops in man between puberty and approximately age 55, i.e., the period of high testosterone production (Rautaharju et al. 1992).

The number of hERG channels on the cell surface is determined on the one hand by their production and on the other hand by their degradation. *In vitro* studies suggest that ion channels may undergo rather rapid turnover, with estimated half-lives of hours in cultured cells (Takimoto et al. 1993). Nothing is known whether drugs may augment hERG channel degradation as a theoretically possible mechanism to delay repolarization.

Further studies are necessary to better understand the role of altered gene expression in drug-induced torsadogenesis. This area is an entirely new field of possible drug-induced disturbance of repolarization. It is currently not clear how important these mechanisms are.

Pharmacokinetic Aspects

Drug/drug interactions at the cytochrome P450 level are without question the most important pharmacokinetic aspects for drug-induced torsadogenesis. These interactions are extensively described elsewhere (e.g., Brown et al. 2004) and will not be discussed in this review. Little attention has been paid to the kinetics of drug uptake into the myocardium, despite well known examples of myocardial accumulation of QT prolonging drugs. The myocardial concentration of terfenadine is 260-fold higher than its plasma concentrations and generates tissue concentrations close to the IC_{50} for hERG channel inhibition (Cavero and Crumb 2001). For five antipsychotic drugs, the myocardium to plasma concentrations ranged between 2.2 and 6.4 (Titier et al. 2004). It is also known that most of the macrolide antibiotics accumulate in the heart (Yoshida and Furuta 1999). Minematsu et al. (2001) investigated the relationship between the myocardial concentration of tacrolimus and its QT prolongation in guinea pigs. Distribution of tacrolimus into the ventricles was delayed, eventually reaching a 50-fold higher concentration than in the blood, and it remained high after the end of the infusion. The magnitude of QT prolongation paralleled the concentration of tacrolimus in the ventricular tissue.

There is no clear evidence as to whether an active transport of drugs into the heart exists. Limited information exists on the functional role of efflux transporters in the heart. P-glycoprotein (Pgp) as a drug efflux pump can decrease the cellular concentration of a compound and protect the heart. Indirect evidence for Pgp-mediated transport in the heart has been obtained from enhanced cardiac uptake of anthracyclines after treatment with Pgp inhibitors (Colombo et al. 1996). Weiss and Kang (2002) used a pharmacokinetic/pharmacodynamic model to demonstrate a saturable uptake of idarubicin into the heart and suggested that idarubicin is transported out of the membrane by Pgp before it gets into the cardiomyocyte.

If there are indications of drug/metabolite accumulation in the heart during the development of a new compound, it is necessary to tailor the preclinical *in vivo* testing, since cardiovascular safety is usually tested in a single dose paradigm in telemetered non-rodents. Alternatively, ECG registration during repeat dose toxicity studies can be considered, provided that the animals are conditioned to the manipulation of ECG recording.

The heart is usually considered to be metabolically inert. Indeed, there is very limited information on the metabolic capacity of cardiomyocytes of laboratory animals. Thum and Borlak (2000) recently investigated gene expression and enzyme activity in cultures of adult rat cardiomyocytes. They demonstrated the expression of a number of drug oxidizing enzymes at the gene and protein level, and an increase in the cytochrome P450 level was noted after Aroclor 1254 treatment. The cytochrome P450 expression in cardiomyocyte cultures was, however, clearly lower when compared with hepatocyte cultures, and Aroclor 1254 treatment resulted in lower induction rates in cardiomyocytes than in hepatocytes.

Should the role of drug metabolism and active transport mechanisms in the establishment of QT prolonging effects be investigated in more detail? A hERG assay with an Ames-test like approach, i.e., with the addition of liver microsomes from Arochlor 1254 pretreated rats, is hypothetically plausible. Consideration of intracardiac metabolism and active transport mechanisms may in some cases help to better understand pharmacokinetic drug-drug interactions beyond the hepatic cytochrome P450 level.

The Molecular Basis of HERG Blockade

In this section, the molecular basis of hERG blockade will be discussed, with an emphasis on the underlying factors that promote promiscuous binding. The consequences of blockade on ion channel function and arrhythmogenesis will be addressed from thermodynamic and kinetic perspectives.

Why do so many compounds from distinct structural classes interact with hERG and often display such high selectivity for the hERG channel relative to other human cardiac K^+ channels ? Compounds that exhibit nanomolar activity on hERG often also share similar potency for G protein coupled receptors. It is therefore possible that e.g. serotonin, dopamine and histamine receptors share structural similarities to hERG that are not evident in the amino acid sequences and that these similarities have been inadvertently probed with modern pharmacology in the widespread phenomenon of drug-induced long QT syndrome (Brown and Rampe 2000).

HERG blockade and its pathophysiological consequences are multi-faceted problems. Direct disruption of I_{Kr} is caused by occupation of the internal ion conduction pathway (ICP) of hERG by small organic compounds. Indirect I_{Kr} disruption mechanisms also exist, including genetic mutations in hERG or its accessory proteins. HERG is a homo-tetrameric protein consisting of membrane bound pore and voltage sensing domains (S1-S4) connected to intra-cellular PAS and cyclic nucleotide binding domains. The functional I_{Kr} channel consists of hERG co-complexed with the MiRP1 β subunit. The vast majority of hERG blockers target the α subunit (pore domain), which consists of an approx. 155 residue sequence containing three helices (S5, S6, P), a loop (selectivity filter), and a large insertion between the S5 and P helices (turret) (Sanguinetti & Tristani-Firouzi, 2006). Structures of three bacterial K^+ channel α domains have been solved to date, including voltage sensing KcsA and KvAP, and calcium sensing MthK proteins (Doyle et al., 1998; Jiang et al., 2002b; Jiang et al., 2003). All but the KcsA structure were captured in the open form. Structures of the N-terminal domains (not the pore) of mammalian Kv4.3 and Kv4.2 channels complexed with the T1 subunit of human KChIP1 accessory protein have also been solved (Pioletti et al., 2006; Wang et al., 2007; Scannevin et al., 2004). The crystallographically determined tertiary and quaternary structures of the α subunits are highly conserved among these channels, and are believed conserved throughout the entire K^+ "channelome" (Doyle et al., 1998). A homology model of the open hERG channel was constructed from the 3.2 Å resolution crystal structure of KvAP by Farid et al. (2006). The low resolution of the template crystal, together with uncertainties about detailed structural differences between voltage gated channels, limit the use of this model to exploration of general properties of hERG structure-function and blockade.

The α subunit of KcsA is shown in Figure 10. The S6 helices face toward the interior of the ICP, and S5 helices toward the membrane. The S5-P insertion is located on the extra-cellular surface of the α subunit. The insertion sequence is much longer in hERG than other K^+ channels, and contains an amphipathic helix (Liu et al., 2002). Rotation of Gly648 Φ, Ψ torsion angles in the homology model simulates the transition between activated (open/conducting) and deactivated (closed) forms of the channel (Farid et al, 2006). Superposition of the closed KcsA and open MthK structures is consistent with motion of the C-terminal segment of the S6 helix relative to the stationary N-terminal selectivity filter region (Jiang et al., 2002a). HERG undergoes C-type inactivation upon opening, which is the mechanism of its inward rectification function (resistance to outward current at depolarizing membrane potentials). Specific conformational differences between the activated vs. inactivated (open/non-conducting) forms of hERG are currently unknown, but likely involve changes in the diameter of the selectivity filter ("pore collapse" hypothesis) (Sanguinetti & Tristani-Firouzi, 2006) and interaction between the extra-cellular surface and amphipathic helix of the S5-P insertion (Liu et al., 2002). The Arg rich voltage sensing domain, directly coupled to the S6 helix, cycles back and forth between the two interior faces of the bilayer, as the polarity of the membrane potential reverses between the depolarization and repolarization phases of the action potential (Jiang et al., 2003). Movement of the voltage sensing domain drives the gating mechanism (hinge rotation of the C-terminus of the S6 helix) between open and closed positions. The lipid bilayer is compressed locally upon channel opening, reducing the K^+ diffusion length from approx. 30 to approx. 12 Å, the thickness of the selectivity filter (Jiang et al., 2002a). Ion channels act as "catalysts" to lower the +60 kcal/mol energy barrier (theoretically computed) to ion-lipid diffusion, (Roux & Mackinnon, 1999) allowing the electrochemical gradient to drive the ion flux. A general theoretical mechanism of channel mediated cation transport has been proposed (Roux & Mackinnon, 1999). The theory predicts the existence of a strong electrostatic field within the ICP, which is generated by the dipole moments of the four P helices. Approx. 80% of the ion stabilization energy is derived from these dipole moments. Energies in the absence and presence of the electrostatic field are estimated at approx. 16 and -3.4 kcal/mol for monovalent cations, respectively. Shielding by the membrane further enhances the stabilization energy to -8.5 kcal/mol.

Blocker sensitive sequence positions were mapped experimentally using patch clamp measurements on Ala scanned mutants of the S6 helix for known sets of hERG blockers. Many blockers have been studied to date in the laboratories of Sanguinetti (Chen et al., 2002; Fernandez et al., 2004; Kamiya et al., 2006; Perry et al., 2004; Sanguinetti et al., 2005; Sanguinetti & Mitcheson, 2005), Mitcheson (Mitcheson et al., 2005; Mitcheson et al., 2000a; Mitcheson et al., 2000; Mitcheson et al., 2000b; Mitcheson, 2003), and others (Ficker et al., 2001). A high degree of overlap in mutation sensitive sequence positions was observed for most blockers. In particular, severe loss of potency was observed for Tyr652Ala or Phe656Ala, residues that occur simultaneously at these sequence positions only in members of the EAG K^+ channel family (Chen et al., 2002). Despite this commonality, EAG channels are not susceptible to promiscuous blockade, nor do they possess inactivation function. Chen et al. (2002) and Ficker et al. (2001) set out to determine whether blockade is due to inactivation function per se, or the inactivated hERG conformation. Chen et al. (2002) shifted the sequence positions of Tyr652 and Phe656 in drosophila EAG channels up and down one sequence position relative to wild type. "Tyr down" and "Phe down" EAG mutants gained inactivation function, together with 40- and 10-fold enhancement in cisapride potency, respectively. Ficker et al. (2001) achieved gain of C-type inactivation function in bovine EAG via point mutations, which greatly enhanced sensitivity to blockade by dofetilide. These results suggest that side chain rotamer or local backbone conformational differences of these residues exist between inactivated and activated forms of the channel. The key blocker sensitive positions Val625, Ser624, Tyr652, and Phe656 map to four layers in the ICP of the hERG homology model, as shown in Figure 11. The sensitivity of different blockers to mutation of these key residues is variable. Val625 layer tends to interact with methanesulfonanilide containing blockers (e.g.

MK-499, E-4031, dofetilide) (Kamiya et al., 2006). Bepridil is insensitive to Tyr652Ala (Kamiya et al., 2006). The importance of aromaticity at the Tyr652 layer and hydrophobicity at the Phe656 layer was identified by Fernandez et al. (2004) and Sanguinetti et al. (2005).

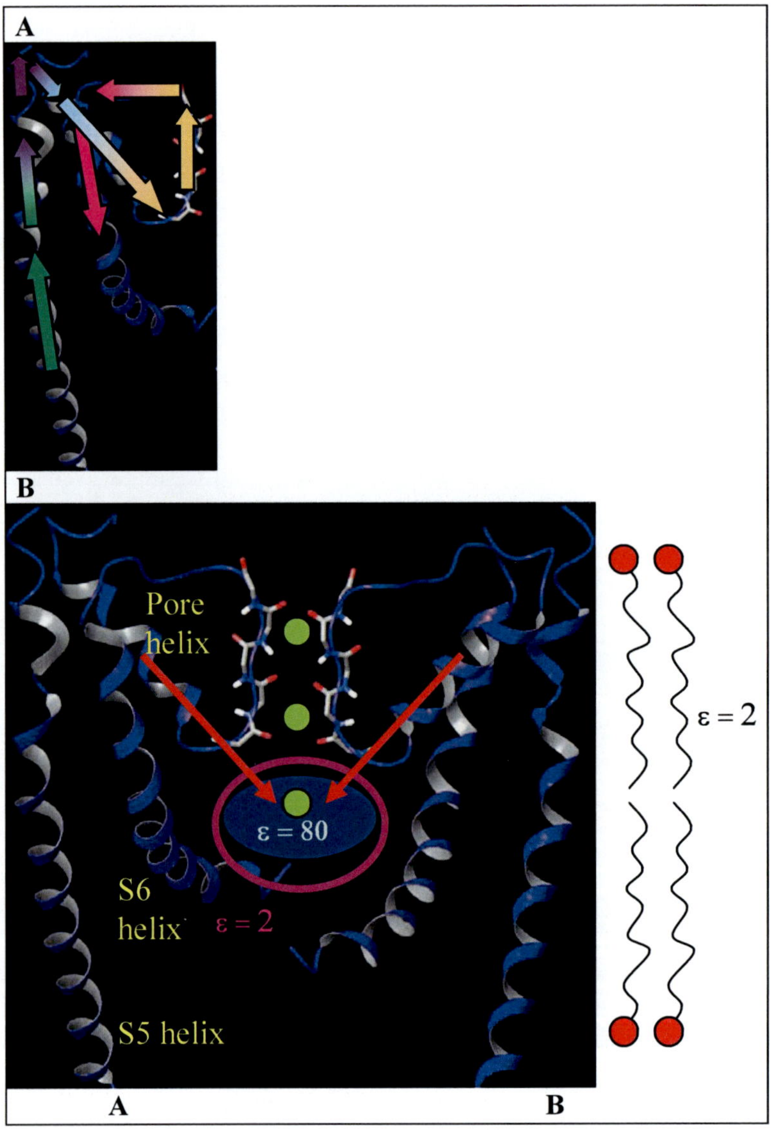

Figure 10. A) Topology of the α subunit monomer viewed perpendicular to the pore axis. The chain traverses along the N-terminal S5 helix (green), S5-P insertion (not shown), P helix (cyan), selectivity loop (orange), and ends at the C-terminal S6 helix (magenta). B) Cutaway of the bacterial K^+ channel KcsA (deactivated form), viewed perpendicular to the pore axis. Arrows depict the dipole moments of the four pore helices. The water filled cavity (blue region) is encased in the double low dielectric environment of the ICP lining (magenta circle) and membrane.

Tyr652 and Phe656 are predicted from the homology model and mutagenesis studies to contribute a large fraction of the hydrophobic lining of the ICP. The blocker accessible cavity runs from the intra-cellular face of the selectivity filter (denoted the "S face") toward the intra-cellular entrance of the ICP (denoted the "E face"). K^+ ions and blockers access the ICP from the E face of the activated channel. Upon closure, the activation gate imposes a hard boundary at the E face, as observed in KcsA crystal structures. The volume of the ICP in the homology model is on the order of 1000 $Å^3$, whereas the volume in non-hERG channels is believed to be smaller due to Pro induced kinking in the S6 helix (Pro106 and Pro108, KcsA numbering) (Keating & Sanguinetti, 2001). Many blockers are trapped upon channel deactivation (e.g. MK-499), suggesting they are capable of fitting within the smaller volume of the ICP in the closed conformation. Bound blockers must either unbind or rearrange upon deactivation, as dictated by the most energetically favored pathway.

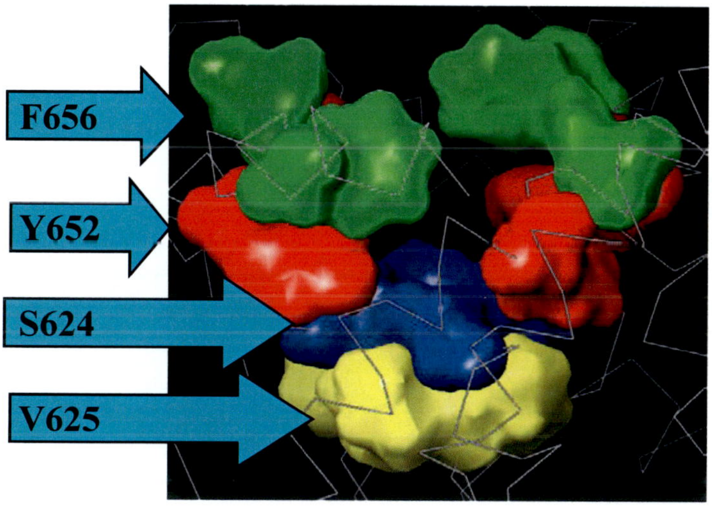

Figure 11. The hERG homology model viewed perpendicular to the central axis of the α subunit. Blockade sensitive residues occur at four levels within the ICP. The binding kinetics may partially reflect the depth at which blockers bind (slower k_{on} and k_{off} at deeper levels).

Patch clamp studies are considered the "gold standard" for hERG blockade assessment. The major advantages of patch clamp include the ability to study blockade for different functional states of the channel, and to observe blockade sensitive changes in kinetic properties. Since compounds enter hERG via its intra-cellular opening, patch clamp measurements implicitly incorporate cell penetration properties that may mask the ion channel interaction component of hERG blockade. Deconvolution of these effects can be difficult. Caco-2, PAMPA, and pharmacokinetic studies may be used to gauge cell penetration contributions (Hidalgo, 2001; Artursson, 1990). However, differences in membrane composition between these systems and cardiac myocytes may limit interpretation of this data in the context of the native biological environment. Radioligand binding (RLB) assays can be used to measure binding affinities of hERG blockers (Chiu et al., 2004). Good correlations between patch clamp and RLB data are often demonstrated, providing further evidence that blockade is a direct consequence of binding in the ICP. RLB data sets are independent of cell penetration, but do not incorporate the effects of channel state on ligand binding. Lack of agreement between RLB and patch clamp data sets may signal large cell penetration effects or state dependent differences between cellular vs. non-cellular hERG preparations. Aside from the data limitations on ligand based modeling approaches, additional reasons for the limited success of these models can be proffered. First, hERG has no known endogenous ligands that bind within the ICP pathway, nor no known function that involves binding of other protein domains as may occur with channels that undergo N-type inactivation. The large, deep, hydrophobic cavity of hERG is likely a major factor in promoting binding of small molecules. However, binding function is discouraged by the low "information content" of the ICP (four-fold symmetry, multiplicity of aromatic side chains, and radially symmetric electrostatic field). Many ligand based 2D and 3D QSAR, and pharmacophore models of hERG blockade have been attempted over the last several years (Bains etal., 2004; Cavalli et al., 2002; Ekins et al., 2002; Pearlstein et al., 2003; Zolotoy et al., 2003). The success of these models has been arguably marginal, in part due to the lack of availability of high quality, self-consistent data sets, and in part due to the unusual properties of the ICP that give rise to promiscuous binding.

So, why does the ICP of hERG bind small molecules in the absence of functional binding properties? Evidence points to the biophysical properties of cation transport as the underlying basis for promiscuous hERG blockade. Two general binding motifs present in the vast majority of all blockers fall prey to the ion transport mechanism of hERG. The first consists of a hydrophobic cation motif that is capable of blocking nearly all K^+ channels. The hydrophobic cation binding mechanism is an unintended byproduct of the strong negative electrostatic potential and hydrophobic lining of the ICP. The second consists of an aryl ring motif that is uniquely involved in blocking hERG. Not surprisingly, the aromatic lining of hERG is the likely basis for binding such blockers. Tyr652 and Phe656 side chains are predicted to compress toward the S face as Gly648 backbone Φ Ψ torsion angles are transitioned to the open conformation of the homology model (Farid et al., 2006). This action increases the effective concentration of aromatic residues in the ICP, and enhances the ability of aryl ring containing blockers to form simultaneous interactions with those residues. Docking calculations performed for several known blockers suggest that the aryl rings of these compounds form multiple simultaneous π-stacking and hydrophobic interactions among these residues (ranging from 4-7 per blocker). V-shaped aromatic ring systems (e.g. diphenylmethane, N-phenylindole) appear especially well suited for packing with Tyr and Phe side chains of the same or different monomers.

The ability of hERG to bind permanently charged hydrophobic cations was demonstrated by Ficker et al. (2002) (e.g. C_{10} tetraethylammonium, hERG IC_{50} = 3.6 μM) (Ficker, Obejero-Paz, Zhao, & Brown, 2002:

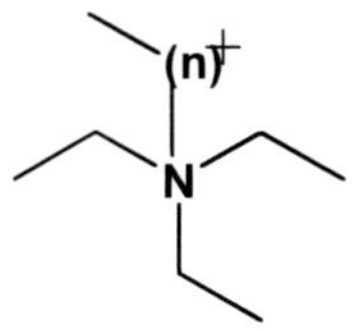

n = 10

Pearlstein et al. (2003) demonstrated that uncharged aryl compounds can also block hERG (e.g. N-fluorophenylisopentylchloroindole, hERG IC_{50} = 1.5 μM):

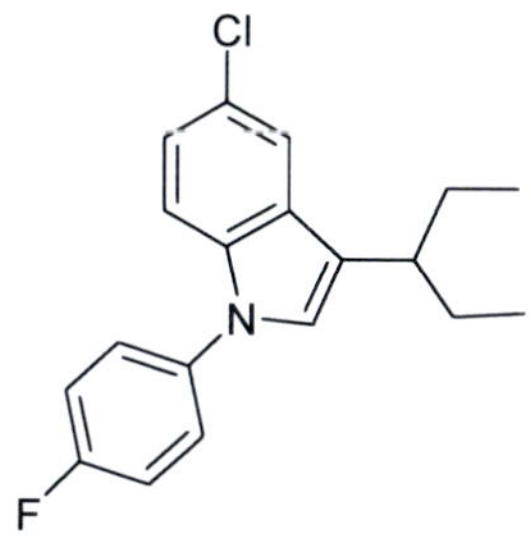

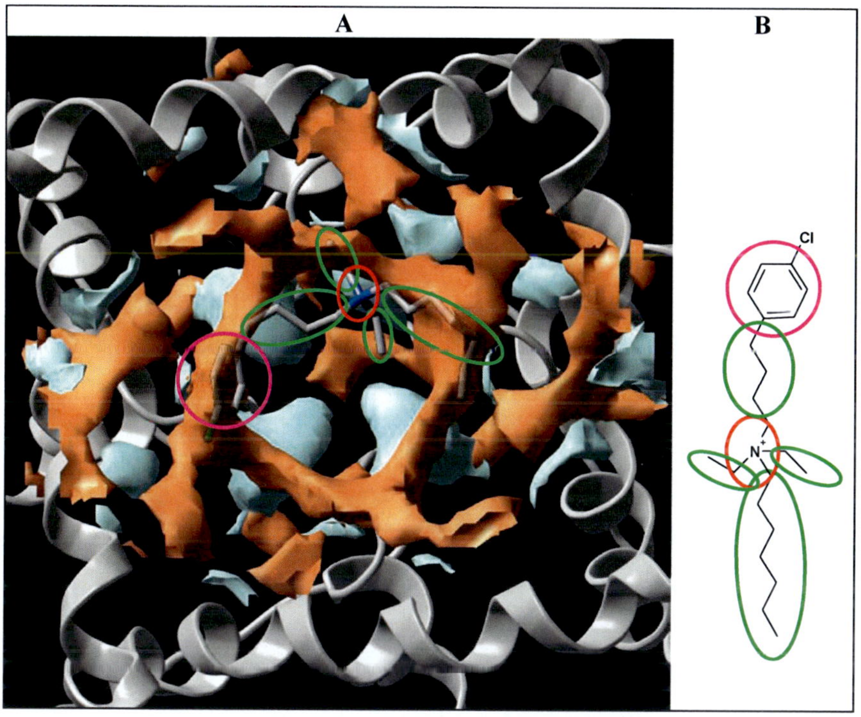

Figure 12. A) The hERG homology model of Farid et al., including a docked pose of clofilium. The structure is oriented parallel to the central axis of the pore, looking from the E face toward the S face direction. The crown shaped hydrophobic (orange) and propeller shaped hydrophilic (cyan) iso-potential energy contour maps are shown within the ICP, as described in the text. The "hub-and-spoke" binding pattern of clofilium is apparent, in which the alkyl chains ("spokes") and basic group ("hub") are buried in the hydrophobic and hydrophilic potentials, respectively. B) 2D structure of clofilium, with hub, spokes, and wheel circled red, green, and magenta, respectively.

Binding of hydrophobic bases and cations is likely similar, although studies of basic compounds in hERG have not been reported. Many drug-like hERG blockers contain combinations of aryl and basic hydrophobic moieties. This is exemplified by N-alkylamine class III anti-arrhythmics, such as ibutilide (hERG IC_{50} = 26 nM) (Perry et al., 2004). Docking studies performed by Farid et al. (2006) suggest that compounds of this nature bind to hERG via a "hub-spoke-wheel" paradigm, in which the basic group serves as the "hub", branched N-alkyl chains as "spokes", and aromatic group(s) as the "wheel". In practice, the hub-spoke-wheel pattern may be abstractly present in many blockers, and difficult to recognize. This binding pattern is mirrored in hydrophobic and hydrophilic iso-potential energy maps computed within the ICP of the hERG homology model. The hydrophobic volume appears "crown shaped", and is largely contributed by the eight aromatic side chains. The hydrophilic volume appears "propeller shaped", and is largely contributed by polar residues at the base of the selectivity filter. The hydrophilic volume is sandwiched between the S face of the cavity and the base of the hydrophobic crown. The basic groups of all docked blockers reside in the hydrophilic propeller adjacent to the S face, proximal to the central axis of the ICP. Aryl and alkyl groups are buried in the hydrophobic crown, and packed with the side chains of Tyr652 and Phe656 (Figures 12 and 13). Iso-potential energy maps computed for tetrabutylammonium (TBA) crystallized in the internal cavity of deactivated KcsA (Lenaeus et al., 2005) are highly consistent with blocker docking poses in the hERG homology model. The cationic group of TBA resides on the central axis of the ICP, with its four butyl groups buried in the hydrophobic crown (collapsed in the closed channel). Radially pseudo-symmetric conformations were predicted for most blockers docked in the homology model, fitting entirely within the volume of the modeled ICP. This is consistent with the ability of many blockers to remain bound ("trapped") upon channel deactivation, although differences in blocker orientation/conformation between the open and closed forms of the channel are likely.

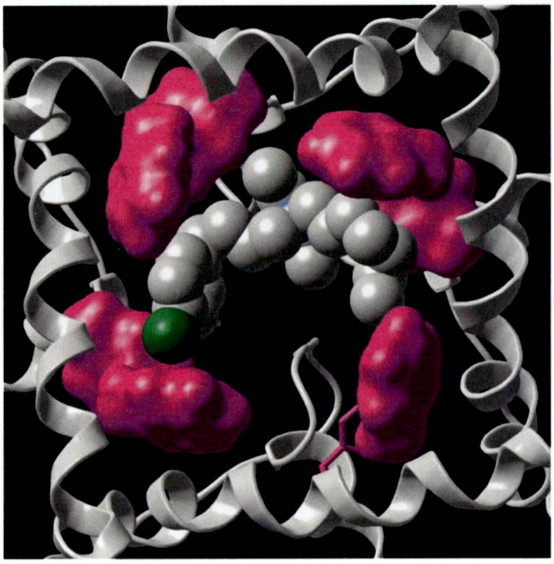

Figure 13. Same as Figure 11, but showing seven multiple simultaneous contacts between clofilium (space filling) and Tyr652/Phe656 (magenta surfaces). Note the three π- stacking interactions predicted between these side chains and the chlorophenyl group of clofilium.

Mitigation of hERG activity in drug candidates is often a challenging problem. Lead series frequently contain an aryl hydrophobic base motif that may adopt a wide variety of chemical forms. Unfortunately, the chemical biology of hERG overlaps with many target classes that have aromatic/hydrophobic and electrostatic binding requirements. A recently published anthology of hERG mitigation case studies underscores the difficulty of achieving net gains in separation between hERG and target activity (Jamieson et al., 2006). The presence of an aryl hydrophobic base motif is indicative of hERG activity, although absolute potency is dependent on the specific chemotype. Quantitative structure-activity relationships within a series are typically flat, but can vary widely between series. For this reason, scaffolds containing an aryl hydrophobic base motif make for poor lead candidates, because small changes are unlikely to yield large impacts on hERG activity. Mitigation of hERG activity via analoging is generally unsuccessful when the following chemical features are present in the scaffold (as dictated by target potency or pharmacokinetic properties):

1) One or more aryl or aliphatic ring systems that are optimal for π-stacking or hydrophobic packing with Tyr652 and/or Phe656.
2) An embedded hub-spoke-wheel motif:
    a) One or more aryl rings occurring with a branched alkyl center.
    b) A basic center substituted with branched or cyclic alkyl groups (esp. when aryl rings also occur in the molecule). Basic centers (e.g. piperidine, piperizine) are often added to enhance solubility and PK properties, but tend to simultaneously enhance hERG activity.
    c) Any of the above features in combination with lipophilic groups that can occupy a large proportion of the hydrophobic crown (e.g. alkyl chains). Heteroatoms and polar groups are often present in these substituents.
    d) Any of the above features in a conformationally flexible scaffold that offers multiple binding configurations. Docking studies suggest that bound conformations allow segregation of polar and hydrophobic groups toward the S and E faces, respectively (Farid et al., 2006). Rigid scaffolds (e.g. MK-499) may have more specific structural requirements.
3) Variation in hERG activity among stereoisomers can occur, but is generally unpredictable.
4) The addition of a carboxylate group tends to reduce hERG activity, but the magnitude of the effect depends on the overall scaffold and substitution position.

The complex relationship between hERG blockade, APD prolongation, and TdP is only beginning to be understood. Inadequate I_{Kr} is the primary cause of TdP, whether drug or mutation induced. Additional factors are for instance reflected in TRIaD, which accounts for the spatial and temporal heterogeneity of APD prolongation and AP propagation in the etiology of TdP. Initiation of TdP is associated with early afterdepolarizations (EADs), characterized by oscillatory fluctuations in membrane potential (possibly multi-focal in origin). EADs reaching suprathreshold depolarization levels can trigger aberrant APs. Proposed mechanisms for EAD generation include decreased extra-cellular $[K^+]$ and intra-cellular Ca^{2+} loading from sacroplasmic reticulum release or abnormal reactivation of $I_{Ca,L}$ channels (Choi et al., 2002). Similar behavior is also observed under ischemic conditions (Lakkireddy et al., 2006). Propagation of EAD induced APs depends on the recruitment of non-refractory Na^+ currents (I_{Na}) along the conduction wave front. The lack of uniform recovery of inactivated SCN5A Na^+ channels, due to variable APD prolongation, may result in heterogeneous zones of refractory and excitable tissue. Advancing AP wave fronts that encounter such tissue may be susceptible to fragmentation, spiraling, and reentry (Starmer et al., 1994; Starmer, Romashko et al., 1995).

The question arises as to how heterogeneous effects on myocardial electrophysiology can be induced by single agent hERG blockade? It is likely that KCNQ1-KCNE1, whose I_{Ks} current accompanies I_{Kr} in phase 2-3 repolarization, plays a key role in this phenomenon

(Tsujimae et al., 2007). KCNQ1 mutations are a major cause of inherited LQT syndrome, suggesting a key role for I_{Ks} in arrhythmia suppression. I_{Ks} is inherently spatially heterogeneous due to variable expression levels of KCNQ1-KCNE1 in endo- midmyo- and epicardium, as well as basal vs. apical myocardium (Pereon et al., 2000). Activation of KCNQ1-KCNE1 is heart rate dependent, with down regulation of I_{Ks} occurring at slower rates (reverse use dependence) (Tsujimae et al., 2007). The overall heterogeneity of I_{Ks} is masked by normal levels of I_{Kr}. However, reduction of I_{Kr} due to blockade or mutations in hERG or MiRP1 can compromise overall outward current reserves, and shift the balance of repolarizing current toward I_{Ks}. The heterogeneous effects of hERG blockade may thus be explained in terms of the fraction of I_{Kr} relative to total repolarization current (Tsujimae et al., 2007):

$$F = I_{Kr}/(I_{Ks} + I_{Kr})$$

Under normal physiological conditions, F is large since $I_{Kr} >> I_{Ks}$. The probability of torsadagenesis is likely enhanced at a threshold value of F corresponding to a critical reduction of I_{Kr}. A safety margin of excess repolarization current capacity ("repolarization reserve") provides natural protection against blockade induced fluctuations in I_{Kr} or I_{Ks}. Partial loss of function mutations in hERG, KCNQ1, MiRP1, or KCNE1 can narrow this repolarization reserve. Arrhythmogenicity was found to be greatly exacerbated by hERG blockade in the presence of MiRP1 mutations (Abbott et al., 1999).

In vitro IC_{50} measurements of binding potency (via RLB) or I_{Kr} reduction (via patch clamp) are typically used to assess hERG blockade. In general, in vivo pharmacological effects are best treated via kinetic, rather than thermodynamic, principles (Copeland et al., 2006). Kinetic behaviors may cooperatively determine the torsadagenic potential of hERG blockade:

1) Pharmacokinetics → rate of buildup and decay in hERG containing tissue compartments.
2) Channel gating kinetics → rate of binding sensitive channel state transitions.
3) Binding kinetics (esp. k_{off}) → rate of buildup and $t_{1/2}$ of bound blocker.

Under this scenario, torsadagenic probability is greatest for compounds that undergo rapid buildup of hERG blockade, and exhibit long recovery times relative to the rate of plasma decay. As for other types of ion channels, hERG blockade is use dependent, building up over several activation/inactivation-deactivation cycles due to lack of continuous accessibility of the binding site. As such, blockade is dependent on both binding kinetics and channel gating kinetics. Mathematical relationships between these processes have been developed for Na^+ channel blockers, including the "modulated" and "guarded" receptor hypotheses (Starmer & Courtney, 1986). The latter is given by:

$$U + D \underset{g\,k_{off}}{\overset{f\,k_{on}}{\rightleftarrows}} B$$

where U and B are unblocked and blocked channel states, respectively, D is the blocker, k_{on} and k_{off} are the binding and unbinding rate constants, respectively, f is the fraction of channels with accessible binding sites, and g is the fraction of bound channels capable of dissociating from the blocker (i.e. untrapped). The parameters f and g account for the dependence of binding on channel gating kinetics. It is apparent that blockers with fast on rates can compensate for smaller fractions of channel states with inaccessible binding sites (e.g. deactivated state). Likewise, those with slow off rates can compensate for large fractions of channel states that promote dissociation (e.g. activated state). Observed rate constants for different blockers studied with patch clamp are indeed quite variable. Tsujimae et al. (2007) described three kinetic classes of compounds in the context of atrial hERG blockade: voltage/time independent (e.g. dofetilide), fast voltage/time dependent (e.g. quinidine), and slow voltage/time dependent (e.g. vesnarinone). Of these blockers, vesnarinone is not torsadagenic. Binding and unbinding rates for bepridil and nikefalant are significantly slower than for E-4031 and dofetilide (Kamiya et al., 2006). Interpretation of binding kinetics via mutagenesis, structure-based modeling, and structure-kinetic relationships may yield new insights about hERG blockade. Slow unbinding equates to persistent hERG blockade, which promotes a convergent set of torsadagenic risk factors: I_{Ks} dominated repolarization current, heterogeneous APD prolongation, aberrant intra-cellular Ca^{2+} loading, EAD generation, degradation of repolarization reserves, and heterogeneous populations of inactivated (refractory) and deactivated (excitable) SCN5A Na^{+} channels. Torsadagenesis may be further enhanced by underlying pathology (e.g. hypertrophy, tissue damage, ischemia) and/or mutations in cardiac channels affecting the repolarization reserve.

For an early assessment of the hERG interaction potential of drug candidates, pharmacophore-based virtual screening procedures may develop as a promising tool. As structural information on the target (hERG and other K^{+} channels) becomes available from X-ray crystallographic studies, it will eventually allow refinement of the pharmacophore and direct performance of "structure-based" virtual screening using pharmacophore constraints (Cavalli et al. 2002). At present, however, *in silico* models cannot replace existing preclinical *in vitro* and *in vivo* testing nor are they considered valuable tools by the health authorities. The closest they may come to is specifying chemical classes that might carry risk (Shah 2005).

Modeling Cardiac Electrogenesis and Torsadogenic Mechanisms under Normal and Pathophysiological Conditions

The ionic currents, pumps and exchangers that contribute to the cardiac action potential can be described using mathematical equations and can be solved on computers. Most of the *in silico* models of cardiomyocytes created over the past 50 years have used Hodgkin-Huxley type kinetic formulations which included mainly sodium and potassium channels. This model has been later adapted to the heart by Denis Noble in 1960. The principle of the model is to define ion concentrations and gradients across the cell membrane by modeling the behavior (gating) of voltage-gated channels and other exchangers, pumps and transporters using mathematical equations. The Luo-Rudy dynamic guinea pig model ventricular cell model was one of the first published ventricular models (Figure 15).

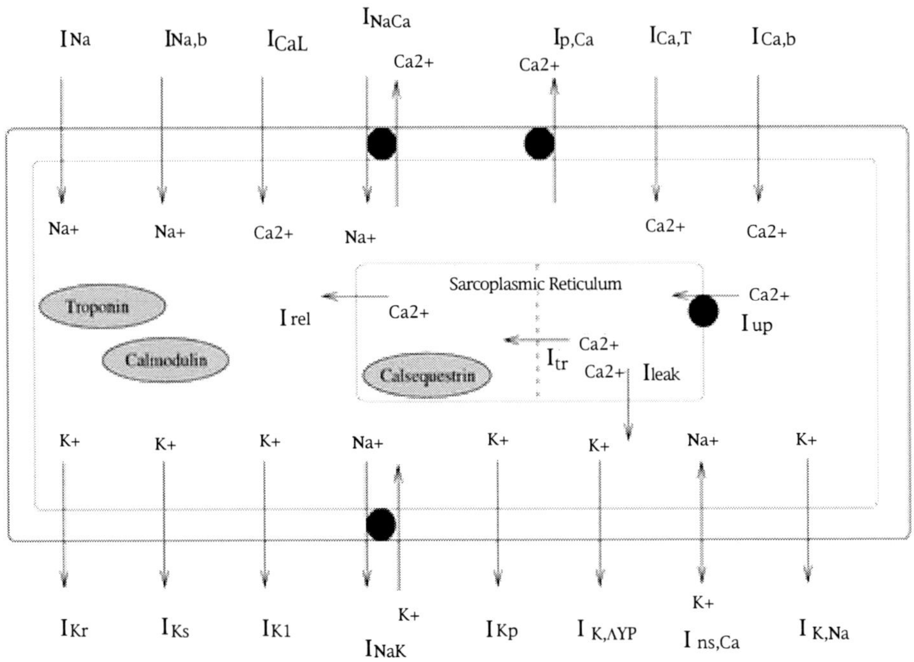

Figure 14. Luo-Rudy guinea pig ventricular myocyte. Schematic diagram for ionic currents, pumps and exchangers included in the second version of the guinea pig ventricular myocyte Luo-Rudy model (LR-II). Sarcoplasmic reticulum (SR) is divided in 2 parts: the network SR (NSR) and the junctional SR (JSR).

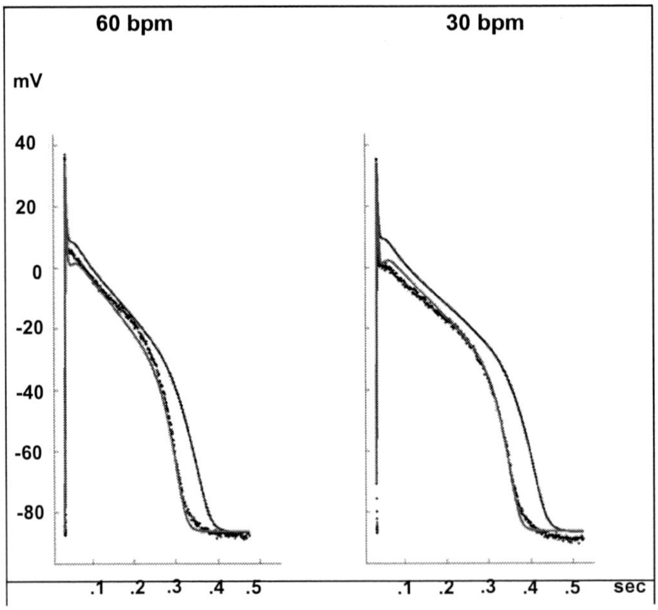

Figure 15. Example of cardiac modeling for action potential recorded from canine dog Purkinje fiber. Typical example of a simulated cardiac action potential from dog Purkinje fiber (original in blue), later on fitted (green) with experimental data (black) at the frequencies of 60 and 30 beats per minute (bpm).

Novel voltage clamp and current clamp experiments have been used for describing the mathematics of individual currents. In this manner, an integrated *in silico* model of the cardiac cell is assembled from individual ion currents and validated by quantitative experimental data (Muzikant and Penland, 2002) using isolated ventricular myocytes or multicellular preparations (Figure 14). Additional parameters must be considered when integrating the cell model into more integrated models (1-D to 3-D), e.g., excitation propagation through coupled cells, local high resistivity between cellular layers, These cellular models are incorporated into 3D cardiac models (Noble 2002) aiming at reproducing cardiac wave propagation and induction of pro-arrhythmic mechanisms of various nature.

Recent modeling efforts related to QT prolongation risk have focused on two different areas. The first effort examined the electrophysiological heterogeneity across the ventricle wall to help test the hypothesis that QT prolongation without accompanying increase in transmural dispersion of repolarization is not arrhythmogenic. The second effort aimed at elucidating how specific mutations in single ion channels affect the electrophysiologic behavior of the integrated cell.

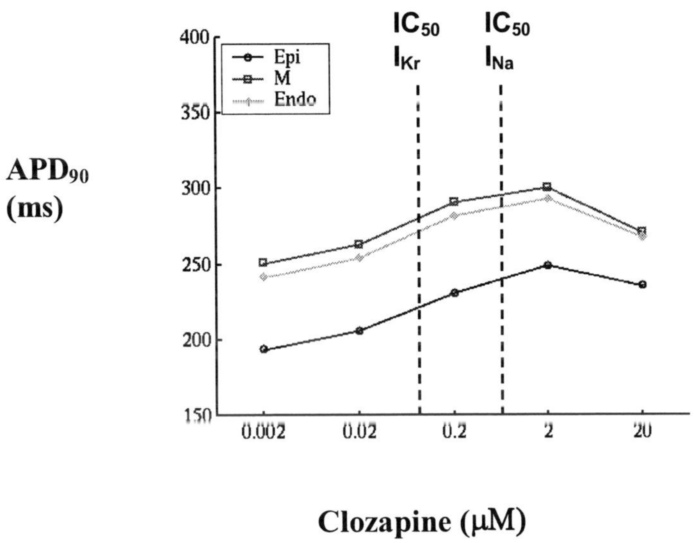

Figure 16. Concentration-dependent effects of clozapine on APD_{90}. Inhibition of I_{Na} limits APD_{90} prolongation induced by I_{Kr}-block. A computer simulation (Cardioprism) of effects on epicardial (Epi), midmyocardial (M) and endocardial (Endo) ventricular cells is shown.

Muzikant and Penland (2002) proposed the in silico model "Cardioprism" using the IC_{50} profile for different ion channels and a library of validated computer models to simulate the effects of compounds on *in vitro* preparations. The library contains *in silico* models of the sinus node, Purkinje fibers, and atrial and ventricular myocytes, including epicardial, midmyocardial and endocardial cells. Furthermore, these models are customized to reflect different species common in preclinical testing, namely rabbits, dogs, and guinea pigs. Using IC_{50}-values for different channels, a picture of how a compound influences the action potential is constructed. Figure 16 illustrates a computer simulation how combined blockade of the I_{Kr} and the I_{Na} can limit the APD prolonging effect of clozapine. Ongoing activities in this field use a reverse engineering approach, i.e., predict the inhibitory potency of NCE on individual cardiac ion channels by using action potentials from multicellular preparations or isolated hearts (Bottino et al., 2006). The Cardioprism model can be considered one of the most advanced techniques of modeling the effects of compounds on cardiac repolarization. However, this *in silico* approach is not supposed to replace existing preclinical screening models but rather to focus on better understanding the mechanisms by which compounds cause TdP and then define more reliable biomarkers for TdP. Interestingly, Cardioprism also allows simulation of the effect of compounds in the clinical situation by taking into consideration risk factors for QT prolongation such as female gender, hypokalemia, the presence of concomitant disease, and drug interaction.

Computer modeling of electrophysiologic information is an important technique for organizing and integrating generated data. The role of *in silico* cardiac modeling in predicting TdP arrhythmia is likely to become increasingly important as a vast amount of data needs to be exploited. An important strength of computer models is to reach down to the genetic level connecting the physiome with the genome (Noble 2002). Available experimental human data (human atrial and/or ventricular cardiac myocytes) is very limited making the validation of human cell model and the project of a complete human-designed modeling platform (tissue and organ level) very challenging.

Limitations of Preclinical Tests for Drug-Induced Torsadogenesis

TdP is a very rare clinical event. It is typically not seen during the development of a new drug until registration, which includes testing in normally less than 5000 patients during clinical phases I -III. Following registration, evidence of the torsadogenic potential of a new drug may be accumulating. Postmarketing, a much higher number of patients is exposed over longer periods of time including patients with risk factors, cardiovascular diseases, co-medication, metabolic impairment and genetically determined enhanced susceptibility. The role of inherited disturbances of the “rhythmome” (genes involved in the regulation of cardiac rhythm) is increasingly better understood. It is estimated that 5 % of patients with drug-induced TdP have subclinical congenital long QT syndrome (Roden 2004). In other words, we know which drugs are associated with TdP and something of how these drugs act to produce TdP, but we do not understand individual patient variability very well. Could safety biomarkers, identified via pharmacogenetic testing of patients with TdP help us characterize these individual liabilities for TdP?

The human heart has a repolarization reserve (Roden 1998). The repolarization reserve is difficult to quantify, but it means a redundancy of physiological systems as a protective mechanism. It is likely that the above mentioned conditions in the target population reduce the repolarization reserve of the heart and this leads in rare and specific cases to TdP. Following this concept, it may be questionable to use healthy young animals with an intact repolarization reserve to predict the torsadogenic potential that occurs in very rare cases under specific conditions in man. On the other hand it appears difficult to mimic the different conditions that may be involved in the initiation of TdP in man.

Summary and Conclusions

None of the currently used preclinical methods have been proven to be fully predictive for the torsadogenic potential of a NCE in man. The role of additional factors in the genesis of TdP arrhythmia beyond hERG inhibition and AP/QT prolongation is increasingly better understood. Based on this emerging knowledge, new methods are evolving that can refine testing for a potential repolarization liability and that may become relevant in the future. Together with regulators, it is necessary to identify the criteria needed to demonstrate the predictive value of new tests in such a way as to mitigate the need for a "thorough QT-study" in phase I.

On the basis of this review, the algorithm for identifying potential torsadogenic compounds can be enhanced (Table 1). The hERG assay will remain the cornerstone in future testing. hERG blockers with a high potency in the low nM range may continue to be problematic to develop. For the potency around 1 μM, evidence has to be provided that the compound is clinically safe for the selected indication at therapeutically relevant exposure. It is necessary to find out whether hERG blockers also affect other cardiac ion channels, since mixed channel inhibition is frequently seen. Several companies observed hERG channel activators as a new class of compounds. It remains to be clarified what therapeutic potential hERG activators may provide. Evolving technologies appear useful to understand torsadogenic mechanisms for ''hERG negative'' compounds.

In *in vitro* models, proarrhythmia indices such as triangulation of the AP, reverse use dependence, instability, and dispersion have proven to be better predictors of torsadogenic potential than simple changes in the duration of the AP and the QT interval.

In vivo models in conscious and anesthetized non-rodents are currently refined by establishing the relevance of parameters such as beat-to-beat-variability and T-wave morphology as derived from the *in vitro* proarrhythmia indices. Animal models of proarrhythmia are to date not recommended for routine evaluation, since the models are insufficiently established to provide any certainty of detecting relevant effects. This holds true for *in vitro* and *in vivo* techniques.

Considerable evidence exists that effects of NCE on cardiac G-protein coupled receptors can modify their hERG blocking activities. In particular, stimulation of α or β adrenoceptors appears to inhibit I_{Kr} dependent repolarization. It is therefore important to find out whether new compounds with hERG blocking activities interact with other cardiac receptors. For this purpose, results of the early screens that test for binding against a wide range of molecular targets can give valuable information.

More experimental data are necessary to further evaluate the role of altered gene expression and trafficking in drug-induced TdP. Recent data indicate that these are relevant mechanisms.

Pharmacokinetic and metabolism data of NCE are crucial for calculating the risk of a torsadogenic potential in man. Consideration of active transport mechanisms in the myocardium and of intracardiac metabolism could help in understanding pharmacokinetic drug-drug interactions beyond the hepatic cytochrome P450 level.

In silico methods possess the potential to improve the prediction of the torsadogenic risk. For the early risk assessment of new drug candidates virtual screening procedures may develop as a promising tool. At present, however, *in silico* methods cannot replace existing preclinical models. The role of *in silico* modeling of TdP arrhythmia is likely to become increasingly important, as the vast amount of data needs to be exploited.

Table 1. Proposed use of evolving technologies to refine the current core battery for testing of the torsadogenic potential of new chemical entities

Test level	Current core battery	Refined/customized algorithm
Channel protein/ isolated cells	Manual hERG assay: investigates important mechanism of drug-induced torsadogenesis, but produces "false positive" and "false negative" data	Automated patch clamp: has the potential to become a valuable HTP screen during lead identification/optimization hERG assay under pathophysiological conditions: currently rarely done, value needs to be further elucidated Pharmacodynamic interactions at the hERG channel (active binding site, allosteric interactions): synergistic or antagonistic effects currently rarely investigated and not well understood Isolated cardiac myocytes: infrequently performed due to technical difficulties Test for stereoselectivity: to be considered if racemate used or other enantiomer formed in vivo Expression of hERG channel on cell surface: to be considered if in vivo findings on repolarization observed (repeat dose test) without in vitro electrophysiological correlate Effects on other cardiac channels than hERG: to be done if hERG block at relevant concentrations does not translate into effects on APD/QT interval or if non-hERG effects on APD and EKG are seen
Repolarization assay in tisues/ isolated organ	Purkinje fiber/papillary muscle: poor correlation with hERG assay and with torsadogenic potential	Isolated heart using indices of proarrhythmia (TRIaD): model can help to differentiate "safe prolongers" from torsadogenic compounds, high predictive value for human torsadogenesis, used by several companies for clinical candidate selection Arterially perfused wedge preparation for measuring effect on M cells and intercellular coupling: best use for mechanistic follow up studies, high predictive value for human torsadogenesis, technically challenging
Whole animal	QT interval in non-rodents: high predictive value for QT prolongation in man, but no specific information on torsadogenic risk	Conscious/anesthetized non-rodents: using parameters derived from in vitro proarrhythmia indices, e.g., beat-to-beat variability, T-wave morphology, have the potential to become highly predictive parameters for human torsadogenesis, can be used for safety margin calculations Proarrhythmia models: predictive value for human torsadogenesis needs to be determined Zebrafish: value as an early HTP screen needs to be further evaluated Effects on autonomic tone: to be investigated on a case by case basis Intracardiac accumulation, transporters, metabolism: to be considered if effects on repolarization are unexpectedly seen at doses that should have high enough safety margin according to hERG assay Torsadogenesis in disease models: use will be the exception, since predictive value for human torsadogenesis is questionable, animal models are often imperfect models for human disease
In silico	Not part of core battery	hERG SAR: currently of limited value, best for investigations within chemical class Modeling of torsadogenesis: important technique for organizing and integrating data

In the end, an integrated assessment of the torsadogenic risk is necessary that includes all relevant preclinical and clinical data. This requires specialist knowledge in this field. The integrated risk assessment must be individualized for each NCE but could be facilitated be the enhanced algorithm (Table 1). We must be open that new torsadogenic mechanisms may be discovered. Some new and unexpected mechanisms such as effects on trafficking and autonomic tone are now well established. Some of the more hypothetical ones are also mentioned in this review.

References

Abbott, G. W., Sesti, F., Splawski, I., Buck, M. E., Lehmann, M. H., Timothy, K. W., Keating, M. T., & Goldstein, S. A. (1999). MiRP1 forms IKr potassium channels with HERG and is associated with cardiac arrhythmia. *Cell*, **97**:175-187

Abi-Gerges N, Philp K, Pollard C, Wakefield I, Hammond TG, Valentin JP (2004) Sex differences in ventricular repolarization: from cardiac electrophysiology to torsades de pointes. *Fundamental Clin Pharmacol* **18**:139-151

Aiba T, Shimizu W, Inagaki M, Noda T, Miyoshi S, Ding WG, Zankow DP, Toyoda F, Matsuura H, Horie M, Sunagawa K (2005) Cellular and ionic mechanism for drug-induced long QT syndrome and effectiveness of verapamil. *J Am Coll Cardiol* **45**: 300-307

Anantharam A, Abbott GW (2005) Does hERG coassamble with a β-subunit? Evidence for roles of MiNK and MiRP. In: Chadwick DJ and Goode J (eds) Novartis Foundation Symposium 266. The hERG Cardiac Potassium Channel: Structure, Function and Long QT Syndrome. John Wiley & Sons Ltd. The Atrium, Southern Gate, Chichester, pp 100-112

Antzelevitch C (2004a) Cellular basis and mechanism underlying normal and abnormal myocardial repolarization and arrhythmogenesis. *Ann Med* **36** (suppl 1):5-14

Antzelevitch C (2004b) Arrhythmogenic mechanisms of QT prolonging drugs: is QT prolongation really a problem? *J Electrocardiol* **37** (suppl):15-24

Antzelevitch, C., Belardinelli, L., Zygmunt, A. C., Burashnikow, A., Diego, J. M., Fish, J. M., et al. (2004). Electrophysiological effects of ranolazine, a novel antianginal agent with antiarrhythmic properties. *Circulation* **100**:904-919

Aronson KS (1981) Afterpotentials and triggered activity in hypertrophied myocardium from rats with renal hypertension. *Circ Res* **48**:720-727

Artursson, P. (1990). Epithelial transport of drugs in cell culture. I: A model for studying the passive diffusion of drugs over intestinal absorptive (Caco-2) cells. *J.Pharm.Sci.* **79**: 476-482

Bains, W., Basman, A., & White, C. (2004). HERG binding specificity and binding site structure: evidence from a fragment-based evolutionary computing SAR study. *Prog Biophys Mol Biol* **86**:205-33

Barros F, Gomez-Varela D, Viloria CG, Palomero T, Giraldez T, Pena P (1998) Modulation of human erg K^+ channel gating by activation of a G protein-coupled receptor and protein kinase C. *J Physiol* **511**:333-346

Bayer R, Schwarzmaler J, Pernice R (1988) Basic mechanism underlying prenylamine-induced torsade de pointes: differences between prenylamine and fendiline due to basic actions of the isomers. *Curr Med Res Opin* **11**:254-272

Belardinelli L, Antzelevitch C, Vos MA (2003) Assessing predictors of drug-induced torsade de pointes. *Trends in Pharmacol Sciences* **24**:61–625

Bian J, Cui J, McDonald TV (2001) HERG K^+ channel activity is regulated by changes in phosphatidyl inositol 4,5-bisphosphonate. *Circ Res* **89**:1168-1176

Bottino D, Penland RC, Stamps A, Traebert M, Dumotier B, Georgiva A, Helmlinger G, Lett GS. (2006) Preclinical cardiac safety assessment of pharmaceutical compounds using an integrated systems-based computer model of the heart. *Prog Biophys Mol Biol* **90**: 414-443

Brockmeier K, Aslan I, Hilbel T, Eberle T, Ulmer HE, Lux RL (2001) T-wave alternans in LQTS: repolarization-rate dynamics from digital 12-lead Holter data. *J Electrocardiol* **34** *(Suppl)*:93-96

Brown A, Rampe D (2000) Drug-induced long QT syndrome: is HERG the root of all evel. *Pharmaceutical news* **7**: 15-20

Brown CS, Farmer RG, Soberman JE, Eichner SF (2004) Pharmacokinetic factors in the adverse cardiovascular effects of antipsychotic drugs. *Clin Pharmacokin* **43**:33-56

Carlsson L, Abrahamson C, Andersson B, Duker G, Schiller Linhardt G (1993) Proarrhythmic effects of the class III agent almokalant: importance of infusion rate, QT dispersion, and early afterdepolarization. *Cardiovasc Res* **27**:2186–2193

Carlsson L, Drews L, Duker G (1996) Rhythm abnormalities related to delayed repolarization in vivo: influence of sarcolemmal Ca^{++} entry and intracellular Ca^{++} overload. *J Pharmacol Exp Ther* **279**:231-239

Cavalli A, Poluzzi E, De Ponti F, Recanatini M (2002) Toward a pharmacophore for drugs inducing the long QT syndrome: insights from a CoMFA study of HERG K^+ channel blockers. *J Med Chem* **45**:3844-3853

Cavero I and Crumb W (2001) Native and cloned ion channels from human heart: laboratory models for evaluating the cardiac safety of new drugs. *Eur Heart J* **3** (supplement K): K53–K63

Cavero I, Mestre M, Guillon JM, Crumb W (2000) Drugs that prolong QT interval as an unwanted effect: assessing their likelihood of inducing hazardous cardiac dysrhythmias. *Exp Opin Pharmacother* **1**:947-973

Charpentier F, Demolombe S, Escande D (2004) Cardiac channelopathies: from men to mice. *Ann Med* **36** (suppl 1):28-34

Chen, J., Seebohm, G., & Sanguinetti, M. C. (2002). Position of aromatic residues in the S6 domain, not inactivation, dictates cisapride sensitivity of HERG and eag potassium channels. *Proc Natl Acad Sci U S A* **99**:12461-12466

Chezalviel Guilbert F, Davy JM, Poirier JM, Weissenburger J (1995) Mexiletine antagonizes effects of sotalol on QT interval duration and its proarrhythmic effects in a canine model of torsade de pointes. *Am J Coll Cardiol* **26**:787-792

Chiu, P. J., Marcoe, K. F., Bounds, S. E., Lin, C. H., Feng, J. J., Lin, A., Cheng, F. C., Crumb, W. J., & Mitchell, R. (2004). Validation of a [3H]astemizole binding assay in HEK293 cells expressing HERG K+ channels. *J.Pharmacol.Sci.* **95**:311-319

Choi, B. R., Burton, F., & Salama, G. (2002). Cytosolic Ca2+ triggers early afterdepolarizations and Torsade de Pointes in rabbit hearts with type 2 long QT syndrome. *J.Physiol* **543**:615-631

Cohen H. Loewenthal U, Kaplan Z (2000) Changes of the autonomic heart rate parameters during treatment with clozapine. *Biol Psychiatry* **47** (Suppl 1):154S

Colombo T, Conzales PO, D'Incalci M (1996) Distribution and activity of doxorubicin combined with SDZ PSC 833 in mice with P388 and P388/DOX leukemia. *Br J Cancer* **73**:866-871

Copeland, R. A., Pompliano, D. L., & Meek, T. D. (2006). Drug-target residence time and its implications for lead optimization. *Nat.Rev.Drug Discov.* **5**:730-739

Cui J, Melman Y, Palma E, Fishman GI, McDonald TV (2000) Cyclic AMP regulates the HERG K^+ channel by dual pathways. *Current Biol* **10**:671-674

DeClerck F, Gallacher D (2005) *Drug-induced effects on dispersion and heterogeneity of ventricular repolarization beyond its duration in anesthetized dogs.* Scientific meeting on "Beat-to-beat variability of repolarization to test for the proarrhythmic potential of drugs", Maastricht, The Netherlands, April 14 – 15, 2005

Doyle, D. A., Morais, C. J., Pfuetzner, R. A., Kuo, A., Gulbis, J. M., Cohen, S. L., Chait, B. T., & Mackinnon, R. (1998). The structure of the potassium channel: molecular basis of K+ conduction and selectivity. *Science* **280**:69-77

Drici MD, Burklow TR, Haridasse V, Glazer RI, Woosley RL (1996) Sex hormones prolong the QT interval and downregulate potassium channel expression in the rabbit heart. *Circulation* **94**:1471-1474

Drici MD, Wang WX, Liu XK (1998) Prolongation of QT interval is isolated feline hearts by antipsychotic drugs. *Psychopharmacology* **18**:607-618

Drvota V, Blange I, Häggblad J, Sylven C (1998) Desethylamiodarone prolongation of cardiac repolarization is dependent on gene expression. A novel antiarrhythmic mechanism. *J Cardiovasc Pharmacol* **32**:645-661

Dumotier B, Georgieva A (2007) Preclinical cardio-safety assessment of torsadogenic risk and alternative methods to animal experimentation. *Cell Biol Toxicol,* in press

Eckardt L, Haverkamp W, Borggrefe M, Breithardt G (1998) Experimental models of torsade de pointes. *Cardiovasc Res* **39**:178-193

Eckardt L, Breithardt G, Haverkamp W (2001) Electrophysiologic characterization of the antipsychotic drug sertindole in a rabbit heart model of torsade de pointes: low torsadogenic potential despite QT prolongation. *J Pharmacol Exper Ther* **300**:64-71

Ehrlich JR, Pourrier M., Weerapura M (2004) KvLQT1 modulates the distribution and biophysical properties of hERG: a novel α-subunit interaction between delayed rectifier currents. *J Biol Chem* **279**:1233-1241

Etkins S, Crumb WJ, Sarazan RD, Wikel JH, Wrighton SA (2002) Three-dimensional quantitative structure-activity relationship for inhibition of human Ether-a-go-go-related gene. *J Pharmacol Exp Ther* **301**:427-434

European Agency for the Evaluation of Medical Products: Committee for Propriety Medicinal Products. *The Assessment of the Potential for QT interval Prolongation by Non-Cardiovascular Medicinal Products.* London 1997.

Farid, R., Day, T., Friesner, R. A., & Pearlstein, R. A. (2006). New insights about HERG blockade obtained from protein modeling, potential energy mapping, and docking studies. *Bioorg.Med.Chem.* **14**:3160-3173

Fermini B, Fossa AA (2003) The impact of drug-induced QT interval prolongation on drug discovery and development. *Nature Reviews Drug Discovery* **2**:439-447

Fernandez, D., Ghanta, A., Kauffman, G. W., & Sanguinetti, M. C. (2004). Physicochemical features of the HERG channel drug binding site. *J Biol Chem* **279**: 10120-27

Ficker E, Dennis A, Kuryshev Y, Wible BA (2005) hERG channel trafficking. In: Chadwick DJ and Goode J (eds) Novartis Foundation Symposium 266. *The hERG Cardiac Potassium Channel: Structure, Function and Long QT Syndrome.* John Wiley & Sons Ltd. The Atrium, Southern Gate, Chichester, pp 75-89

Ficker, E., Jarolimek, W., & Brown, A. M. (2001). Molecular determinants of inactivation and dofetilide block in ether a-go-go (EAG) channels and EAG-related K(+) channels. *Mol.Pharmacol* **60**:1343-1348

Ficker E, Kuryshev Y, Dennis A, Obejero-Paz C, Wang L, Hawryluk P, Wible BA, Brown A (2004) Mechanisms of arsenic-induced prolongation of cardiac repolarization. *Mol Pharmacol* **66**:1-12

Ficker, E., Obejero-Paz, C. A., Zhao, S., & Brown, A. M. (2002). The binding site for channel blockers that rescue misprocessed human long QT syndrome type 2 ether-a-gogo-related gene (HERG) mutations. *J.Biol.Chem.* **277**:4989-4998

Fossa AA, Wisialowski T, Wolfgang E, Wang E, Avery M, Raunig DL, Fermini B (2004) Differential effect of hERG blocking agents on cardiac electrical alternans in the guinea pig. *Eur J Pharmacol* **486**:209-221

Gintant GA, Limberis JT, McDermott JS, Wegner CD, Cox BF (2001) The canine Purkinje fiber: an in vitro model system for acquired long QT syndrome and drug-induced arrhythmogenesis. *J Cardiovasc Pharmacol* **37**:607-618

Gonzalez T, Arias C, Caballero R (2002) Effects of levobupivacaine, ropivacaine and bupivacaine on HERG channels: stereoselective bupivacaine block. *Br J Pharmacol* **137**:1269-1279

Gralinski MR (2000) The assessment of potential for QT interval prolongation with new pharmaceuticals: impact on drug development. *J Pharmacol Toxicol Methods* **43**:91-99

Hammond TG, Carlsson L, Davis AS, Lynch WG, MacKenzie I, Redfern WS, Sullivan AT, Cramm AJ (2001) Methods of collecting and evaluating non-clinical cardiac electrophysiology data in the pharmaceutical industry: results of an international survey. *Cardiovasc Res* **49**:741–750

Haverkamp W, Breithardt G, Camm G (2000) The potential for QT prolongation and proarrhythmia by non-antiarrhythmic drugs: clinical and regulatory implications. *Eur Heart J* **21**:1216-1231

Hartigan-Go K, Bateman DN, Daly AK, Martensson E, Thomas SHL (1996) Stereoselective cardiotoxic effects of terodiline. *Clin Pharmacol Ther* **60**:89-98

Hidalgo, I. J. (2001). Assessing the absorption of new pharmaceuticals. *Curr.Top.Med.Chem.* **1**:385-401

Hondeghem LM, Carlsson L, Duker G (2001) Instability and triangulation of the action potential predict serious proarrhythmia, but action potential duration prolongation is antiarrhythmic. *Circulation* **103**:2004-2013

Hondeghem LM, Hoffmann P (2003) Blinded test in isolated female rabbit heart reliably identifies action potential duration prolongation and proarrhythmic drugs: importance of triangulation, reverse use dependence, and instability. *J Cardiovasc Pharmacol* **41**:14-24.

Hondeghem LM (2005) Estimation of proarrhythmic hazards by QT-prolongation/shortening: QT obsession? DIA Journal, in press

ICH Steering Committee: Safety Pharmacology Studies for Assessing the Potential for Delayed Repolarization (QT Interval Prolongation) by Human Pharmaceuticals. *International Conference on Harmonization of Technical Requirements of Pharmaceuticals for Human Use*. ICH S7B guideline Step 2, June 10, 2004

Jamieson, C., Moir, E. M., Rankovic, Z., & Wishart, G. (2006). Medicinal chemistry of hERG optimizations: Highlights and hang-ups. *J.Med.Chem.* **49**:5029-5046

Jiang, Y., Lee, A., Chen, J., Cadene, M., Chait, B. T., & Mackinnon, R. (2002b). Crystal structure and mechanism of a calcium-gated potassium channel. *Nature* **417**: 515-522

Jiang, Y., Lee, A., Chen, J., Cadene, M., Chait, B. T., & Mackinnon, R. (2002a). The open pore conformation of potassium channels. *Nature* **417** :523-526

Jiang, Y., Lee, A., Chen, J., Ruta, V., Cadene, M., Chait, B. T., & Mackinnon, R. (2003). X-ray structure of a voltage-dependent K+ channel. *Nature* **423**:33-41

Joshi A, Dimino T, Vohra Y, Cui C, Yan GX (2004) Preclinical strategies to assess QT liability and torsadogenic potential of new drugs: the role of experimental models. *J Electrocardiol* **37** (suppl):7-14

Kagan A, McDonald TV (2005) Dynamic control of hERG/I_{Kr} by PKA-mediated interactions with 14-3-3. In: Chadwick DJ and Goode J (eds) Novartis Foundation Symposium 266. *The hERG Cardiac Potassium Channel: Structure, Function and Long QT Syndrome.* John Wiley & Sons Ltd. The Atrium, Southern Gate, Chichester, pp 75 - 89

Kamiya, K., Niwa, R., Mitcheson, J. S., & Sanguinetti, M. C. (2006). Molecular determinants of HERG channel block. *Mol.Pharmacol.* **69**:1709-1716

Kang J, Chen XL, Wang H, Ji J, Cheng H, Incardona J, Reynolds W, Viviani F, Tabart M, Rampe D (2005) Discovery of a small molecule activator of the human Ether-a-go-go-related gene (HERG) cardiac K^+ channel. *Mol Pharmacol* **67**:827-836

Karle CA, Zitron E, Zhang W, Kathoefer S, Schoels W, Kiehn J (2002) Rapid component I_{Kr} of the guinea-pig cardiac deleayed rectifier K^+ current is inhibited by beta1-adrenoceptor activation, via cAMP/protein kinase A-dependent pathways. *Cardiovasc Res* **53**:355-362

Keating, M. T. & Sanguinetti, M. C. (2001). Molecular and cellular mechanisms of cardiac arrhythmias. *Cell* **104**:569-80

Kupershmidt S, Yang IC, Hayashi K (2003) IKr drug response is modulated by KCR1 in transfected cardiac and non-cardiac cell lines. *FASEB J* **17**:2263-2265

Kuryshev YA, Ficker E, Wang L, Hawryluk P, Dennis AT, Wible BA, Brown A, Kang J, Chen XL, Sawamura K, Reynolds W, Rampe D (2005) Pentamidine-induced long QT syndrome and block of hERG trafficking. *J Pharmacol Exp Ther* **312**:316-323

Lakkireddy, V., Bub, G., Baweja, P., Syed, A., Boutjdir, M., & El-Sherif, N. (2006). The kinetics of spontaneous calcium oscillations and arrhythmogenesis in the in vivo heart during ischemia/reperfusion. *Heart Rhythm.* **3**:58-66

Lees-Miller JP, Guo J, Somers JR, Roach DE, Sheldon RS, Rancourt DE (2003) Selective knockout of mouse ERG1 B potassium channel eliminates I(Kr) in adult ventricular myocytes and elicits episodes of abrupt sinus bradycardia. *Mol Cell Biol* **23**:1856-1862

Lenaeus, M. J., Vamvouka, M., Focia, P. J., & Gross, A. (2005). Structural basis of TEA blockade in a model potassium channel. *Nat.Struct.Mol.Biol.* **12**:454-459

Liu, J., Zhang, M., Jiang, M., & Tseng, G. N. (2002). Structural and functional role of the extracellular s5-p linker in the HERG potassium channel. *J.Gen.Physiol* **120**:723-737

London B, Pan X (1998) QT interval prolongation and arrhythmias in heterozygous MERG1-targeted mice. *Circulation* **98**:279(abstract)

Martin RL, McDermott JS, Salmen HJ, Palmatier J, Cox BF, Gintant GA (2004) The utility of hERG and repolarization assays in evaluating deleayed cardiac repolarization: Influence of multi-channel block. *J Cardiovasc Pharmacol* **43**:369-379

Merot J, Charpentier F, Poirier JM, Coutris G, Weissenburger J (1999) Effect of chronic treatment by amiodarone on transmural heterogeneity of canine ventricular repolarization in vivo: interactions with acute sotalol. *Cardiovasc Res* **44**:303-314

Milan DJ, Peterson TA, Ruskin JN, Peterson RT, Calum A, MacRae MB (2004) Drugs that induce repolarization abnormalities cause bradycardia in zebrafish . *Circulation* **107**: 1355 - 1358

Minematsu T, Ohtani H, Yamada Y, Sawada Y, Sato H, Iga T (2001) Quantitative relationship between myocardial concentration of tacrolimus and QT prolongation in guinea pigs: Pharmacokinetic/pharmacodynamic model incorporating a site adverse effect. *J Pharmacokin Pharmacodyn* **28**:533-554

Mitcheson, J., Perry, M., Stansfeld, P., Sanguinetti, M. C., Witchel, H., & Hancox, J. (2005). Structural determinants for high-affinity block of hERG potassium channels. *Novartis.Found.Symp.* **266**:136-150

Mitcheson, J. S. (2003). Drug binding to HERG channels: evidence for a 'non-aromatic' binding site for fluvoxamine. *Br J Pharmacol* **139**:883-884

Mitcheson, J. S., Chen, J., Lin, M., Culberson, C., & Sanguinetti, M. C. (2000a). A structural basis for drug-induced long QT syndrome. *Proc Natl Acad Sci U S A* **97**:12329-33

Mitcheson, J. S., Chen, J., Lin, M., Culberson, C., & Sanguinetti, M. C. (2000b). A structural basis for drug-induced long QT syndrome. *Proc.Natl.Acad.Sci.U.S.A* **97**:12329-12333

Mitcheson, J. S., Chen, J., & Sanguinetti, M. C. (2000). Trapping of a methanesulfonanilide by closure of the HERG potassium channel activation gate. *J Gen Physiol* **115**:229-40

Moss AJ (2003) Long QT syndrome. *JAMA* **289**:2041-2044

Muzikanr AL, Penland RC (2002)Models for profiling the potential QT prolongation risk of drugs. *Current Opin Drug Disc & Devel* **5**:127-135

Näbauer M, Kääb S (1998) Potassium channel down-regulation in heart failure. *Cardiovasc Res* **37**:324-334

Netzer R, Bischoff U, Ebneth A (2003) HTS techniques to investigate the potential effects of compounds on cardiac ion channels at early drug discovery. *Current opinion in Drug Discovery & Development* **6**:462-469

Noble D (2002) Modeling the heart – from genes to cells to the whole organ. *Science* **295**:1678-1682

Pearlstein, R. A., Vaz, R. J., Kang, J., Chen, X. L., Preobrazhenskaya, M., Shchekotikhin, A. E., Korolev, A. M., Lysenkova, L. N., Miroshnikova, O. V., Hendrix, J., & Rampe, D. (2003). Characterization of HERG potassium channel inhibition using CoMSiA 3D QSAR and homology modeling approaches. *Bioorg Med Chem Lett* **13**:1829-35

Pereon, Y., Demolombe, S., Baro, I., Drouin, E., Charpentier, F., & Escande, D. (2000). Differential expression of KvLQT1 isoforms across the human ventricular wall. *Am.J.Physiol Heart Circ.Physiol* **278**:H1908-H1915

Perry, M., De Groot, M. J., Helliwell, R., Leishman, D., Tristani-Firouzi, M., Sanguinetti, M. C., & Mitcheson, J. (2004). Structural determinants of HERG channel block by clofilium and ibutilide. *Mol.Pharmacol.* **66**:240-249

Pioletti, M., Findeisen, F., Hura, G. L., & Minor, D. L., Jr. (2006). Three-dimensional structure of the KChIP1-Kv4.3 T1 complex reveals a cross-shaped octamer. *Nat.Struct.Mol.Biol.* **13**:987-995

Poelzing S, Rosenbaum DS (2005) Celluler mechanisms of torsade de pointes. In: Chadwick DJ and Goode J (eds) Novartis Foundation Symposium 266. *The hERG Cardiac Potassium Channel: Structure, Function and Long QT Syndrome*. John Wiley & Sons Ltd. The Atrium, Southern Gate, Chichester, pp 204-217

Prystowsky EN (1992) Effects of bepridil on cardiac electrophysiologic properties. *Am J Cardiol* **69**:63D–67D

Rautaharju PM, Zhou SH, Wong S, Calhoun HP, Berenson GS, Prineas R, Davignon A (1992) Sex differences in the evolution of the electrocardiographic QT interval with age. *Can J Cardiol* **8**:690-695

Rangno R (1997) Terfenadine therapy: can we justify the risk? *CMAJ* **157**:37-38

Redfern WS, Carlsson L, Davis AS, Lynch WG, MacKenzie I, Palethoroe S, Siegl PKS, Strang I, Sullivan AT, Wallis R, Camm AJ, Hammond TG (2003) Relationship between preclinical cardiac electrophysiology, clinical QT interval prolongation and torsade de pointes for a broad range of drugs: Evidence for a provisional safety margin in drug development. *Cardiovasc Res* **58**:32–45

Richelson E (1996) Preclinical pharmacology of neuroleptics: focus on new generation compounds. *J Clin Psychiatry* **57** (suppl 11):4 - 11

Roden DM (1998) Taking the "idio" out of "idiosynchratic": predicting torsades de pointes. *Pacing Clin Electrophysiol* **21**:1029-1034

Roden DM (2004) Drug-induced prolongation of the QT interval *N Engl J Med* **350**:1013–1022

Roden DM and Kupershmidt S (1999) From genes to channels: normal mechanisms. *Cardiovasc Res* **42**:318-326

Roux, B. & Mackinnon, R. (1999). The cavity and pore helices in the KcsA K+ channel: electrostatic stabilization of monovalent cations. *Science* **285** :100-102

Sanguinetti MC (2005) Closing remarks. In: Chadwick DJ and Goode J (eds) Novartis Foundation Symposium 266. *The hERG Cardiac Potassium Channel: Structure, Function and Long QT Syndrome.* John Wiley & Sons Ltd. The Atrium, Southern Gate, Chichester, pp 286- 287

Sanguinetti, M. C., Chen, J., Fernandez, D., Kamiya, K., Mitcheson, J., & Sanchez-Chapula, J. A. (2005). Physicochemical basis for binding and voltage-dependent block of hERG channels by structurally diverse drugs. In: Chadwick DJ and Goode J (eds) Novartis Foundation Symposium 266. *The hERG Cardiac Potassium Channel: Structure, Function and Long QT Syndrome.* John Wiley & Sons Ltd. The Atrium, Southern Gate, Chichester, pp 159-166

Sanguinetti MS, Mitcheson JS (2005) Predicting drug-hERG channel interactions that cause acquired long QT syndrome. *Trends Pharmacol Sci* **26**:119-124

Sanguinetti, M. C. & Tristani-Firouzi, M. (2006). hERG potassium channels and cardiac arrhythmia. *Nature* **440**:463-469

Scannevin, R. H., Wang, K., Jow, F., Megules, J., Kopsco, D. C., Edris, W., Carroll, K. C., Lu, Q., Xu, W., Xu, Z., Katz, A. H., Olland, S., Lin, L., Taylor, M., Stahl, M., Malakian, K., Somers, W., Mosyak, L., Bowlby, M. R., Chanda, P., & Rhodes, K. J. (2004). Two N-terminal domains of Kv4 K(+) channels regulate binding to and modulation by KChIP1. *Neuron* **41**:587 598

Shah RR (2005) Drug-induced QT interval prolongation: regulatory guidance and perspectives on hERG channel studies. In: Chadwick DJ and Goode J (eds) Novartis Foundation Symposium 266. The hERG Cardiac Potassium Channel: Structure, Function and Long QT Syndrome. John Wiley & Sons Ltd. The Atrium, Southern Gate, Chichester, pp 251- 280

Shah, R. R., & Hondeghem, R. R. (2005). Refining detection of drug-induced proarrhythmia: QT interval and TRIaD. *Heart Rhythm* **2**:758–772.

Starmer, C. F. & Courtney, K. R. (1986). Modeling ion channel blockade at guarded binding sites: application to tertiary drugs. *Am.J.Physiol* **251**:H848-H856

Starmer, C. F., Reddy, M. R., Namasivayam, A., & Singh, M. (1994). Potassium channel blockade amplifies cardiac instability numerical studies of torsades de pointes. *Indian J.Physiol Pharmacol.* **38**:259-266

Starmer, C. F., Romashko, D. N., Reddy, R. S., Zilberter, Y. I., Starobin, J., Grant, A. O., & Krinsky, V. I. (1995). Proarrhythmic response to potassium channel blockade. Numerical studies of polymorphic tachyarrhythmias. *Circulation* **92**:595-605

Takimoto K, Fomina AF, Gealy R, Trimmer JS, Levitan ES, Dexamethasone rapidly induces Kv1.5K^+ channel gene transcription and expression in cloned pituitary cells. *Neuron* **11**:359-369

Taylor D (2003) Ziprasidone in the management of schizophrenia. *CNS drugs* **17**:423-430

Thomas D, Kiehn J, Katus HA, Karle CA (2004) Adrenergic regulation of the rapid component of the cardiac delayed rectifier potassium current, I_{Kr}, and the underlying hERG ion channel. *Basic Res Cardiol* **99**:279-287

Thum T, Borlak J (200) Cytochrome P450 mono-oxygenase gene expression and protein activity in cultures of adult cardiomyocytes of the rat. *Br J Pharmacol* **130**:1745-1752

Titier K, Canal M, Deridet E, Abouelfath A, Gromb S, Molimard M, Moore N (2004) Determination of myocardium to plasma concentration ratios of five antipsychotic drugs: comparison with their ability to induce arrhythmia and sudden death. *Toxicol Appl Pharmacol* **199**:52-60

Tomaselli GF, Beuckelmann DJ, Calkins HG, Berger RD, Kessler PD, Lawrence JH, Kass D, Feldman AM, Marban E (1994) Sudden cardiac death in heart failure. The role of abnormal repolarization. *Circulation* **90**:2534-2539

Tsujimae, K., Suzuki, S., Murakami, S., & Kurachi, Y. (2007). Frequency dependent effects of various IKr blockers on cardiac action potential duration in a human atrial model. *Am.J.Physiol Heart Circ.Physiol, in press*

Valentin JP, Hoffmann P, De Clerck F, Hammong TG, Hondeghem L (2004) Review of the predictive value of the Langendorff heart model (Screenit system) in assessing the proarrhythmic potential of drugs. *J Pharmacol Toxicol Methods* **49**:171-181

VistaGen Therapeutics: http://www.vistagen-inc.com/htm_pages/homepage.htm

Volders PGA, Sipido KR, Vos MA, Spätjens R, Leunissen JDM, Carmeliet E, Wellens HJJ (1999) Downregaulation of delayed rectifier K^+ currents in dogs with chronic complete atrioventricular block and acquired torsades de pointes. *Circulation* **100**:2455-2461

Voss MA, Verduyn SC, Gorgels APM, Lipcsei GC, Wellens HJJ (1995) Reproducible induction of early afterdepolarizations and torsade de pointes arrhythmias by D-sotalol and pacing in dogs with chronic atrioventricular block. *Circulation* **91**:864-872

Wang JC, Kiyosue T, Toyama J (1999) Bepridil differentially inhibits two delayed rectifier K^+ currents, I_{Kr} and I_{Ks}, in guinea-pig ventricular myocytes. *Br J Pharmacol* **128**:1733-1738

Wang, H., Yan, Y., Liu, Q., Huang, Y., Shen, Y., Chen, L., Chen, Y., Yang, Q., Hao, Q., Wang, K., & Chai, J. (2007). Structural basis for modulation of Kv4 K+ channels by auxiliary KChIP subunits. *Nat.Neurosci.* **10**:32-39

Warner B and Hoffmann P (2002) Investigation of the potential of clozapine to cause Torsade de Pointes. *Adv Drug React Toxicol Rev* **21**:189–2003

Weiss M, Kang W (2002) P-glycoprotein inhibitors enhance saturable uptake of idarubicin in the rat heart: Pharmacokinetic/pharmacodynamic modeling. *J Pharmacol Exper Ther* **300**:688-694

Wible, B. A., Hawryluk, P., Ficker, E., Kuryshev, Y. A., Kirsch, G., & Brown, A. M. (2005). HERG-Lite(R): A novel comprehensive highthroughput screen for drug-induced hERG risk. *Journal of Pharmacological and Toxicological Methods,* **52**, 136– 145.

Yan GX, Wu Y, Liu T, Wang J, Marinchak RA, Kowey PR (2001) Phase 2 early afterdepolarization as a trigger of polymorphic ventricular tachycardia in acquired long QT syndrome. *Circulation* **103**:2851-2856

Yoshida H, Furuta T (1999) Tissue penetration properties of macrolide antibiotics – comparative tissue distribution of erythromycin-stearate, clarithromycin, roxithromycin and azithromycin in rats. *Jpn J Antibiot* **52**:497-503

Zangh Y, Han H, Wang J, Wang H, Yang B, Wang Z (2003) Impairment of human Ether-a-go-go-related gene (HERG) K^+ channel function by hypoglycemia and hyperglycemia. *J Biol Chem* **278**:10417-10426

Zolotoy, A. B., Plouvier, B. P., Beatch, G. B., Hayes, E. S., Wall, R. A., & Walker, M. J. (2003). Physicochemical determinants for drug induced blockade of HERG potassium channels: effect of charge and charge shielding. *Curr Med Chem Cardiovasc Hematol Agents* **1**:225-41

In: Progress in Cardiac Arrhythmia Research
Editor: Ira R. Tarkowicz, pp. 67-79

ISBN: 1-60021-796-6

Chapter 2

The Role of Antagonists of the Renin-Angiotensin System in the Prevention of Atrial Fibrillation

Maryse Palardy*[*,ϒ], *Peter G. Guerra and Anique Ducharme
Department of medicine, Montreal Heart Institute Research Center, Montreal (Quebec), Canada

Abstract

Background: Atrial fibrillation (AF) is the most frequently encountered arrhythmia in clinical practice and is associated with increased mortality and morbidity. Its incidence has grown due to the increasing prevalence of risk factors for AF development, which include age, diabetes, hypertension, heart failure (HF), valvular and ischemic heart diseases. Retrospective studies and small prospective trials have suggested a preventive effect of antagonists of the renin-angiotensin system (RAS), including angiotensin-converting enzyme (ACE) inhibitors and angiotensin-II receptor blockers (ARB), on AF occurence.

Method and Results: We performed a systematic literature search on the role of RAS antagonists in the prevention of AF. We looked in particular at the pathophysiology of AF, including the concepts of atrial ionic and anatomical changes induced by AF, called electrical and structural remodelling. We reviewed the published data on the potential beneficial effect of RAS inhibitors on AF occurrence in various experimental and clinical settings.

Conclusions: Inhibition of the renin-angiotensin system seems to prevent AF occurrence in patients with associated disease such as heart failure, hypertension and population with few co-morbidities but persistent AF. The role of these agents in the routine management of AF remains to be determined.

---

* Correspondence concerning this article should be addressed to Dr. Anique Ducharme, Montreal Heart Institute Research Center 5000 Belanger Street East, Montreal (Quebec), Canada, HIT 1C8. Fax: 514-593-2575; Phone: 514-376-3330 ext.3947; E-mail: a_ducharme@icm-mhi.com.
ϒ Dr. Ducharme is supported by the « Fonds de Recherche en Santé du Québec (FRSQ) »

Keywords: atrial fibrillation; angiotensin; angiotensin converting enzyme inhibitors; angiotensin receptor blokers.

Introduction

Atrial fibrillation (AF) is the most common sustained arrhythmia encountered in clinical practice. It has become an important health care burden, its prevalence increasing with the aging of the population, and now affects approximately 10% of octogenarians [1]. Whether AF is an independent predictor of mortality remains controversial [2-5], but it is associated with impaired quality of life, and substantial morbidity from stroke, peripheral embolism and heart failure [6,7]. In patient with LV dysfunction, the presence of AF increases mortality and further progression of left ventricular dysfunction [3]. Even in those with only slightly decreased LVEF [8], the rapid ventricular rates usually secondary to AF can lead to further worsening of LV function, with resulting decline in cardiac index and peak oxygen consumption [9]. Besides heart failure and age, several other conditions, such as diabetes, hypertension, cardio-thoracic surgery, valvular and ischemic heart diseases predispose patients to develop AF.

Despite the increasing prevalence of AF, antiarrhythmic drug therapy has limited efficacy (less than 50%) and important potential adverse effects, as well as risk of inducing proarrhythmias. For these reasons, alternate therapies have been studied, such as antihypertensive drugs, statins [10], fish oils [11], steroids [12], catheter ablation [13], and treatment of sleep apnea [14,15]. In this chapter, we will explore the mechanisms involved in the pathophysiology of atrial fibrillation and focus on experimental and clinical studies demonstrating the effects of RAS inhibitors on AF occurrence.

A Tailored Therapy for Atrial Fibrillation

Even with the development of new antiarrhythmic agents, restoration and maintenance of sinus rhythm still remains a challenge. Whether rhythm control should be the preferred strategy has to be individualized, since recent large scale trials have failed to show a benefit of this strategy over rate control on survival [16-19] or improvement in symptoms [20]. Interestingly, later sub-studies suggested that maintenance of sinus rhythm appears to be an important determinant of survival [21]. However, currently available antiarrhythmic drugs were either ineffective in maintaining sinus rhythm or had adverse effects which offset the mortality benefit of sinus rhythm. Regardless of the chosen strategy (rhythm or rate control), long-term anticoagulation is warranted to reduce embolic risk and stroke-related morbidity [22], in particular in the elderly (75 years or older) who exhibit a stroke rate of 8%/year in AF [23].

In heart failure patients, the best therapeutic option remains to be determined. Sub-analysis of the AFFIRM (Atrial Fibrillation Follow-up Investigation of Rhythm Management) trial found a trend favouring rhythm control in patients with pre-existing heart failure [24]. Likewise, analysis of the subgroup of patients with HF enrolled in RACE [25] (261 patients, mostly NYHA II with preserved systolic function) suggest an advantage of rhythm control if sinus rhythm could be maintained. A multi-center trial (AF-CHF) is currently underway to verify which strategy should be preferred in heart failure patients with depressed systolic function [26]. Nevertheless, the negative inotropic agents used for rate control leaves the patients permanently in AF, which may not be well tolerated by all. Hence, both treatment strategies for AF have limitations, and development of a preventive approach in patients at risk of developing the arrhythmia is attractive.

Cardiac Electrical and Structural Remodeling in AF

AF often begins as paroxysmal, or multiple self-limited episodes, but can evolve into persistent AF. This concept has led to the well-known expression that “AF begets AF”. A pivotal study by Wijffels et al. [27] using a goat model of rapid pacing demonstrated a progressive increase in AF duration with repetitive stimulation. This resulting in a shortening of the atrial refractory period (AERP), enhanced atrial vulnerability and a decreased accommodation capacity of action potential duration to changes in activation rate, suggest the occurrence of an electrical remodelling process independent of the parasympathetic and sympathetic systems. Thus, AF is more likely to happen when atrial effective refractory period (AERP) is short, conduction is slow, or atria enlarge [28].

These AF-induced alterations on action potential are believed to be secondary to an important down-regulation of transient outward K+-current (I_{to}) and inward L-type Ca^{2+} current ($I_{Ca.L}$) density, with up to 70% decline after 6 weeks of tachycardia-induced HF [29,30], while the density of the Na^{+}-Ca^{2+} exchanger (I_{NCX}) and expression of its protein were significantly increased [31]. These changes in ionic currents observed in HF and in atrial tachycardia, are responsible for a marked shortening of the action potential and decreased refractory period [32,33]. In addition, the decline in calcium currents seems to represent an adaptive response in an attempt to counteract atrial tachycardia-induced calcium overload [34]. Thus, these alterations of the atrial electrophysiological properties induced by AF renders the atria vulnerable to further AF, and thereby favours the maintenance of this atrial arrhythmia [35,36], a concept called “electrical remodelling”.

A substantial amount of data suggests that the RAS plays an important role in the atrial remodelling that takes place with development of AF. The role of the RAS on ionic remodelling has been nicely demonstrated in a dog model of rapid atrial pacing, in which angiotensin II infusion was found to markedly delayed the recovery of refractory periods, whereas both captopril and candesartan could prevent early atrial electrical remodelling (occurring within hours), with a reduction of AF duration and attenuation of the effect on the refractory period [37]. Moroever, stimulation of angiotensin II production promotes cardiac fibrosis, contributing to left ventricular (LV) remodeling following myocardial infarction [38,39], and rapid atrial stimulation can increase angiotensin II plasma concentrations in animals [40].

In addition to atrial electrical and LV remodelling, profound structural changes of the atrial tissue may occurred in dogs with HF induced by rapid ventricular pacing, including elevation in atrial angiotensin II concentration, myocytes hypertrophy, apoptosis and extensive interstitial fibrosis [31], thereby interfering with electrical conduction, promoting AF development [41]. The same group [42] also showed that pre-treatment with the ACE inhibitor enalapril leads to an attenuation of conduction heterogeneity, mean duration of AF and atrial fibrosis, with decreased atrial angiotensin-II level and mitogen-activated-protein

(MAP) kinase activation. This effect did not seem to be mediated by improvement in hemodynamic parameters, since the use of combined vasodilatators (hydralazine and isosorbide mononitrates) did not have any effect on structural changes nor on AF development, despite similar decrease in filling pressures. In addition, Sakabe and colleagues have also shown that these HF-induced conduction disturbances and reduction of the effective refractory period were attenuated by pre-treatment with enalapril [43]. Interestingly, Shinagawa et al. [44] demonstrated that these atrial fibrotic modifications induced by five weeks of rapid ventricular pacing persisted, even though the hemodynamics changes, the ventricular function, and atrial dimensions were restored within 5 weeks once rapid ventricular pacing stimulation was stopped [45].

In mildly symptomatic patients (NYHA II) with preserved systolic function undergoing cardiac surgery, the atrial ACE tissue level and angiotensin receptor density were three-fold higher in patients with persistent AF or with a history of AF than in patients with sinus rhythm. Increased tissue levels of activated Erk1/Erk2, a mitogen-activated protein kinase and potent interstitial fibrosis promoter were also noted. In addition, exposure to ACE inhibitors led to a reduction in atrial fibrosis and decreased Erk1/Erk2 levels [46]. Goette and colleagues [47] further demonstrated in atrial biopsies of patients with AF, a down-regulation of AT-1 receptors (promoter of myocardial hypertrophy and extracellular matrix deposition) and up-regulation of the AT2 receptors (inhibitor of proliferation). This phenomenon could be a compensatory mechanism trying to counteract elevated atrial tissue levels of both angiotensin II and ACE [47]. Thus, RAS activation occurs in AF and may induces atrial structural changes, resulting in slow conduction and AF promotion.

In addition to ionic and structural changes, other conditions may predispose to AF, such as atrial stretch, ischemia and genetic predisposition. Acute atrial stretch caused by increased intra-atrial pressure, and sympathetic or parasympathetic stimulation may also trigger AF [48]. Whether atrial enlargement is a consequence of AF or the cause, remains controversial, but AF maintenance requires a critical amount of tissue [49], and atrial dimensions can enlarge during AF and decrease after successful cardioversion [50,51]. Also, atrial stretch markedly increases the irritability of the atrium and predisposes to atrial tachyarrhythmias [52], by modification of the atrial geometrical arrangement, alteration of cell-cell interaction, and activation of stretch-activated channels and I_{Ca} [53]. In rabbits, dilatation of the atria shortens action potentials and increase AF inducibility, whereas releasing the wall stress produces instant cardioversion [54].

Furthermore, in AF occurring in the context of HF, atrial ischemia may decrease excitability thresholds by suppression of I_{Ca}, slower local conduction and promote re-entry, thereby creating a substrate for AF maintenance [55].

Lastly, it has been recently shown that polymorphism of specific allele of the angiotensinogen gene may render the patient prone to AF [56]. Interestingly, these mutations may cause over-expression of atrial angiotensin-II level when the atrial pressure is increased, leading to activation of the MAP-kinases pathway, resulting in atrial fibrosis, reducing atrial effective refractory period, and conduction heterogeneity [56].

Together, these electrical and structural modifications, as well as some possible genetic predisposition, all contribute to the atrial remodelling process, producing an atrial substrate fertile for the development and maintenance of AF.

Clinical Studies Involving RAS Inhibitors and AF Prevention

Retrospective Clinical Trial

In patients with left ventricular dysfunction early after myocardial infarction, data from TRACE (TRAndolapril Cardiac Evaluation) suggested that this ACE inhibitor decreased mortality, morbidity and AF occurence, with significantly more patients developing AF in the placebo than in the trandolapril group, 5.3% and 2.8% respectively, $p<0.05$, (RR=0.45; 95%CI: 0.26-0.76, $p<0.01$ by multivariable analysis) [57]. In a setting of more chronic HF, the impact of enalapril use on the incidence of AF occurrence was evaluated in a single center, retrospective analysis of the SOLVD database [58]. After an average follow up of 2.9 years, an absolute AF risk reduction of 18.6% was shown in the enalapril group, and allocation to enalapril remained the most important predictor of AF prevention by multivariate analysis (HR=0.22, 95%CI: 0.11-0.44, $p<0.0001$). In addition, Maggioni and colleagues recently published a post-hoc analysis of the Val-HeFT trial [59], comparing valsartan and placebo in 5010 patients with symptomatic HF (LVEF <40%, NYHA class II-IV). After 23 months of follow up, patients in sinus rhythm at baseline had an absolute reduction of 2.83% (7.95 versus 5.12%, p=0.0002) in AF incidence with valsartan. While valsartan was an independent predictor of reduction of AF (HR=0.63, 95%CI: 0.49-0.81, p=0.0003), BNP level >97 pg/ml (HR 2.28, 95% CI: 1.75-2.98, $p<0.0001$) and age >70 years (HR=1.51, 95% CI: 1.17-1.95), were increasing the risk. Of note, only a minority of the Val-HeFT population was treated with beta-blockers which is standard of care now.

In a broader population of symptomatic HF patients (NYHA II-IV) with both depressed (LVEF ≤40% either intolerant to- or already on ACE-inhibitors) and preserved systolic function already on a modern pharmacological regimen (including 55% on beta-blockers), the retrospective analysis of CHARM [60] also demonstrated a decreased AF occurrence in the candesartan-treated group compared to placebo (5.55% vs 6.74%, p=0.048, HR=0.81, 95%CI: 0.66-1.0).

In hypertensive patients with electrocardiographic evidence of left ventricular hypertrophy (LVH) enrolled in the LIFE trial [61], AF occurrence was decreased in the losartan compared to the atenolol-treated groups, (respectively 6.8 and 10.1/ 1000 person-years; RR= 0.67, 95%CI: 0.55-0.83, $p < 0.001$), despite similar blood pressure reduction. Patients receiving losartan tended to stay in sinus rhythm longer (1,809 ± 225 vs. 1,709 ± 254 days from baseline, p = 0.057) than those receiving atenolol. Moreover, patients with new-onset AF had two-, three- and fivefold increased rate of cardiovascular events, stroke, and hospitalization for heart failure, respectively. There were fewer composite end points (first occurrence of cardiovascular death, fatal or nonfatal stroke, and fatal or nonfatal myocardial infarction) (n = 31 vs. 51, HR=0.60, 95%CI: 0.38-0.94, p = 0.03) and strokes (n = 19 vs. 38, HR=0.49, 95%CI: 0.29- 0.86, p = 0.01) in patients who developed new-onset AF and treated with losartan instead of atenolol.

Interestingly, like for the HF population, the hemodynamic effect of RAS inhibitors does not seems to be the only mechanism involve for AF prevention in the hypertensive population. A small study of 213 patients with essential hypertension and at least two episodes of symptomatic AF in the last 6 months, but no cardiovascular disease nor diabetes, were randomized to losartan/amiodarone versus amlodipine/amiodarone. Despite similar blood pressure reduction, AF recurrence was reduced only with losartan/amiodarone regimen (11.7% vs 35.0%, P<0.001) [62].

Even in the "real life situation" of a large hypertensive population (10 926 patients), ACE inhibitor utilization had a modest but significant preventive effect of AF incidence when compared to calcium channel blockers [63], mostly in patients with previous history of AF. These patients were healthier, and ischemic heart disease was found in only 15% and HF in less than 4%.

Of note, all these retrospective analyses were carried out in populations with cardiovascular (CV) conditions prone to develop AF (LV dysfunction, symptomatic HF or hypertension with end-organ damage (LVH)). A retrospective study of AFFIRM [64] evaluating the time to first recurrence of AF was not able to show any difference in the AF recurrence attributable to RAS inhibitors use (412 users and 732 non-users) by multivariate analysis (HR=0.91, 95%CI: 0.77-1.09, p=0.31). Patients in the RAS-inhibitor group were more likely to have hypertension, diabetes, coronary artery disease, and congestive heart failure compared to patients not taking RAS inhibitors, all conditions which would make the patient at risk for AF development. Nevertheless, the lower risk of AF recurrence with RAS inhibitors seems to have been limited to patients with congestive heart failure (HR=0.63, 95%CI: 0.43–0.94, p=0.02) or impaired left ventricular function (HR=0.48, 95%CI: 0.24–0.97, p=0.04).

Similar results were observed in the CTAF database (unpublished data), a population similar to AFFIRM. We evaluated the effects of RAS inhibitor utilization in addition to antiarrhythmic agents (amiodarone vs sotalol/propafenone). The CTAF population had mainly paroxysmal AF, normal LVEF, and only 17% had LVH on the baseline ECG, despite a history of hypertension in 46% of the patients. No benefit of RAS inhibitors use on AF recurrence could be demonstrated, even when the analysis was restricted to hypertensive patients.

In the post operative setting, AF (occurring in almost one third of patients after cardiac surgery) may prolong hospitalization length and increases the number of readmissions. In a retrospective analysis of a large longitudinal study [65] of patients undergoing coronary artery bypass graft (CABG) surgery, with or without intervention on the mitral valve, AF was experienced prior to discharge in 32.3%. Peri-operative administration of ACE inhibitors was found to significantly reduce the risk of AF (OR=0.62; 95%CI: 0.48-0.79, p<0.001), and withdrawal of theses agents seems to increase the risk of AF occurrence (OR =1.69; 95% CI 1.38-2.08, p<0.001). AF was surprisingly less frequent in patients with heart failure (OR=0.67, 95%CI: 0.51-0.89, p=0.006), although this is probably attributable to a selection bias, since 45% of these patients were already treated with an ACE inhibitors at baseline.

Finally, ACE inhibitors/ARBs utilization was associated with less development of AF post radiofrequency catheter ablation of the isthmus for recurrent atrial flutter (RR=0.55; 95% CI 0.31-0.97, p=0.04 by multivariable analysis) [66].

The majority of these retrospective studies suggest a beneficial effect on AF occurrence in selected patients with LV dysfunction, hypertension or after cardiac surgery.

Prospective Clinical Trials

The use of RAS antagonists has been studied prospectively in combination with amiodarone for "facilitated" cardioversion in persistent AF. These small studies enrolled a broader and somewhat healthier population, similar to AFFIRM and CTAF populations, and demonstrated a preventive effect of RAS blockade on AF recurrence. Ueng et al. [67] compared the effect of enalapril and amiodarone to amiodarone alone in 145 patients with persistent AF (>3months duration), undergoing electrical cardioversion. After 270 days of follow up, AF occurred in 25.7% and 42.7% of the patients, respectively (p=0.021). Using a similar design, Madrid et al. [68] randomized 154 patients with persistent AF to either amiodarone/irbesartan, or amiodarone alone, and demonstrated a 20% absolute reduction of AF recurrence at 2 month with the combination, which was maintained at 12 months. Lastly, a recently published study suggested that the use of an ACE inhibitor can prevent the progression of paroxysmal AF into chronic AF [69].

The underlying mechanisms explaining the success of this "facilitated cardioversion" are not fully understood. The concept of atrial stunning suggests that myocytes calcium abnormalities correlate with decrease fiber shortening, and are likely to explain the transient contractile dysfunction frequently observed after cardioversion. This stunning can last for few weeks after cardioversion despite electrical restoration of sinus rhythm, and is associated with an increased incidence of thrombus formation [70,71]. In a small study [72], pre-treatement with irbesartan ≥2 weeks before electrical cardioversion significantly decreased atrial stunning, as evidenced by improved LA appendage emptying velocity and decreased amount of LA spontaneous echo contrast observed by transoesophageal echocardiography. Other factors such as AF duration (>1-2 weeks), ischemic heart disease, LA diameter (>51 mm), also increase duration and severity of LA stunning [73]. Thus trying to decrease the stunning duration could reduce the risk of early embolic events and recurrence of AF.

Since the studies evaluating the impact of RAS inhibition on AF prevention or facilitated electrical cardioversion were either retrospective or small, they may not have been adequately powered to provide a definitive answer to this question. There is a need for randomized large trial to address this question and asses which subgroup of the population would benefit the most from RAS inhibition. In the mean time, three meta-analysis of importance have confirmed the protective effect of the ACE inhibitors and ARBs on incidence of AF [74-76], with a more pronounced preventive impact in patients with heart failure or complicated hypertension. Two ongoing randomized trials of ARBs have AF prevention as a secondary endpoint, these include ACTIVE (Atrial Fibrillation Clopidogrel Trial with Irbesartan for Prevention of Vascular Events), and ONTARGET/ TRANSCEND (Ongoing Telmisartan Alone and in Combination with Ramipril Global Endpoint Trial/Telmisartan Randomized Assessment in ACE Intolerant Subjects with Cardiovascular Disease) [77]. The only randomized, prospective placebo-controlled trial aiming to test as a primary endpoint, whether valsartan can reduce AF, is GISSI-Atrial Fibrillation [78] and will randomize 1402 patients. A substudy of GISSI-AF is also planned to help clarify the effect of AT1-receptor blockers valsartan on neurohormones and LA dimensions. We hope these trials will shed light on the question.

Conclusion

AF occurring in the context of HF may result in an increase in both morbidity and mortality. As we have shown in this review, this new avenue of AF prevention with ARBs or ACE inhibitors may be a useful adjunct to treatments strategies using antiarrhythmic agents. It seems, however, that the preventive effect of RAS inhibitors on AF recurrence may be limited to population with LV dysfunction, ischemic cardiomyopathy, or left ventricular hypertrophy (LVH). The role of these agents for "facilitated cardioversion" is intriguing, but extrapolation of these results to the larger population of patients with AF with few or no comorbidities should be done with caution.

References

[1] Benjamin EJ, Levy D, Vaziri SM, D'Agostino RB, Belanger AJ, Wolf PA. Independent risk factors for atrial fibrillation in a population-based cohort. The Framingham Heart Study. *JAMA* 1994; 271(11):840-844.

[2] Mathew J, Hunsberger S, Fleg J, Mc SF, Williford W, Yusuf S. Incidence, predictive factors, and prognostic significance of supraventricular tachyarrhythmias in congestive heart failure. *Chest* 2000; 118(4):914-922.

[3] Dries DL, Exner DV, Gersh BJ, Domanski MJ, Waclawiw MA, Stevenson LW. Atrial fibrillation is associated with an increased risk for mortality and heart failure progression in patients with asymptomatic and symptomatic left ventricular systolic dysfunction: a retrospective analysis of the SOLVD trials. Studies of Left Ventricular Dysfunction. *J Am Coll Cardiol* 1998; 32(3):695-703.

[4] Crijns HJ, Tjeerdsma G, de Kam PJ et al. Prognostic value of the presence and development of atrial fibrillation in patients with advanced chronic heart failure. *Eur Heart J* 2000; 21(15):1238-1245.

[5] Olsson LG, Swedberg K, Ducharme A et al. Atrial fibrillation and risk of clinical events in chronic heart failure with and without left ventricular systolic dysfunction: results from the Candesartan in Heart failure-Assessment of Reduction in Mortality and morbidity (CHARM) program. *J Am Coll Cardiol* 2006; 47(10):1997-2004.

[6] Lip GY, Boos CJ. Antithrombotic treatment in atrial fibrillation. *Heart* 2006; 92(2): 155-161.

[7] Benjamin EJ, Wolf PA, D'Agostino RB, Silbershatz H, Kannel WB, Levy D. Impact of atrial fibrillation on the risk of death: the Framingham Heart Study. *Circulation* 1998; 98(10):946-952.

[8] Dorian P. The future of atrial fibrillation therapy. *J Cardiovasc Electrophysiol* 2006; 17 Suppl 2:S11-S16.

[9] Daoud EG, Weiss R, Bahu M et al. Effect of an irregular ventricular rhythm on cardiac output. *Am J Cardiol* 1996; 78(12):1433-1436.

[10]Young-Xu Y, Jabbour S, Goldberg R et al. Usefulness of statin drugs in protecting against atrial fibrillation in patients with coronary artery disease. *Am J Cardiol* 2003; 92(12):1379-1383.

[11]Mozaffarian D, Psaty BM, Rimm EB et al. Fish intake and risk of incident atrial fibrillation. *Circulation* 2004; 110(4):368-373.

[12]Dernellis J, Panaretou M. Relationship between C-reactive protein concentrations during glucocorticoid therapy and recurrent atrial fibrillation. *Eur Heart J* 2004; 25(13):1100-1107.

[13]Haissaguerre M, Jais P, Shah DC et al. Spontaneous initiation of atrial fibrillation by ectopic beats originating in the pulmonary veins. *N Engl J Med* 1998; 339(10):659-666.

[14]Gami AS, Pressman G, Caples SM et al. Association of atrial fibrillation and obstructive sleep apnea. *Circulation* 2004; 110(4):364-367.

[15]Kanagala R, Murali NS, Friedman PA et al. Obstructive sleep apnea and the recurrence of atrial fibrillation. *Circulation* 2003; 107(20):2589-2594.

[16]Wyse DG, Waldo AL, DiMarco JP et al. A comparison of rate control and rhythm control in patients with atrial fibrillation. *N Engl J Med* 2002; 347(23):1825-1833.

[17]Van G, I, Hagens VE, Bosker HA et al. A comparison of rate control and rhythm control in patients with recurrent persistent atrial fibrillation. *N Engl J Med* 2002; 347(23):1834-1840.

[18]Carlsson J, Miketic S, Windeler J et al. Randomized trial of rate-control versus rhythm-control in persistent atrial fibrillation: the Strategies of Treatment of Atrial Fibrillation (STAF) study. *J Am Coll Cardiol* 2003; 41(10):1690-1696.

[19]Opolski G, Torbicki A, Kosior DA et al. Rate control vs rhythm control in patients with nonvalvular persistent atrial fibrillation: the results of the Polish How to Treat Chronic Atrial Fibrillation (HOT CAFE) Study. *Chest* 2004; 126(2):476-486.

[20]Hohnloser SH, Kuck KH, Lilienthal J. Rhythm or rate control in atrial fibrillation--Pharmacological Intervention in Atrial Fibrillation (PIAF): a randomised trial. *Lancet* 2000; 356(9244):1789-1794.

[21]Corley SD, Epstein AE, DiMarco JP et al. Relationships between sinus rhythm, treatment, and survival in the Atrial Fibrillation Follow-Up Investigation of Rhythm Management (AFFIRM) Study. *Circulation* 2004; 109(12):1509-1513.

[22]Fuster V, Ryden LE, Cannom DS et al. ACC/AHA/ESC 2006 Guidelines for the Management of Patients with Atrial Fibrillation: a report of the American College of Cardiology/American Heart Association Task Force on Practice Guidelines and the European Society of Cardiology Committee for Practice Guidelines (Writing Committee to Revise the 2001 Guidelines for the Management of Patients With Atrial Fibrillation): developed in collaboration with the European Heart Rhythm Association and the Heart Rhythm Society. *Circulation* 2006; 114(7):e257-e354.

[23]Risk factors for stroke and efficacy of antithrombotic therapy in atrial fibrillation. Analysis of pooled data from five randomized controlled trials. *Arch Intern Med* 1994; 154(13):1449-1457.

[24]Blackshear JL, Safford RE. AFFIRM and RACE Trials: Implications for the Management of Atrial Fibrillation. *Card Electrophysiol Rev* 2003; 7(4):366-369.

[25]Hagens VE, Crijns HJ, van Veldhuisen DJ et al. Rate control versus rhythm control for patients with persistent atrial fibrillation with mild to moderate heart failure: results from the RAte Control versus Electrical cardioversion (RACE) study. *Am Heart J* 2005; 149(6):1106-1111.

[26]Roy D. Rationale for the Atrial Fibrillation and Congestive Heart Failure (AF-CHF) trial. *Card Electrophysiol Rev* 2003; 7(3):208-210.

[27]Wijffels MC, Kirchhof CJ, Dorland R, Allessie MA. Atrial fibrillation begets atrial fibrillation. A study in awake chronically instrumented goats. *Circulation* 1995; 92(7):1954-1968.

[28]Rensma PL, Allessie MA, Lammers WJ, Bonke FI, Schalij MJ. Length of excitation wave and susceptibility to reentrant atrial arrhythmias in normal conscious dogs. *Circ Res* 1988; 62(2):395-410.

[29]Nattel S, Li D. Ionic remodeling in the heart: pathophysiological significance and new therapeutic opportunities for atrial fibrillation. *Circ Res* 2000; 87(6):440-447.

[30]Van Wagoner DR, Pond AL, Lamorgese M, Rossie SS, McCarthy PM, Nerbonne JM. Atrial L-type Ca2+ currents and human atrial fibrillation. *Circ Res* 1999; 85(5):428-436.

[31]Li D, Melnyk P, Feng J et al. Effects of experimental heart failure on atrial cellular and ionic electrophysiology. *Circulation* 2000; 101(22):2631-2638.

[32]Le Grand BL, Hatem S, Deroubaix E, Couetil JP, Coraboeuf E. Depressed transient outward and calcium currents in dilated human atria. *Cardiovasc Res* 1994; 28(4):548-556.

[33]Nattel S, Khairy P, Schram G. Arrhythmogenic ionic remodeling: adaptive responses with maladaptive consequences. *Trends Cardiovasc Med* 2001; 11(7):295-301.

[34]Yue L, Feng J, Gaspo R, Li GR, Wang Z, Nattel S. Ionic remodeling underlying action potential changes in a canine model of atrial fibrillation. *Circ Res* 1997; 81(4):512-525.

[35]Nattel S. New ideas about atrial fibrillation 50 years on. *Nature* 2002; 415(6868): 219-226.

[36]Daoud EG, Bogun F, Goyal R et al. Effect of atrial fibrillation on atrial refractoriness in humans. *Circulation* 1996; 94(7):1600-1606.

[37]Nakashima H, Kumagai K, Urata H, Gondo N, Ideishi M, Arakawa K. Angiotensin II antagonist prevents electrical remodeling in atrial fibrillation. *Circulation* 2000; 101(22):2612-2617.

[38]Schnee JM, Hsueh WA. Angiotensin II, adhesion, and cardiac fibrosis. *Cardiovasc Res* 2000; 46(2):264-268.

[39]Ruiz-Ortega M, Lorenzo O, Ruperez M et al. Role of the renin-angiotensin system in vascular diseases: expanding the field. *Hypertension* 2001; 38(6):1382-1387.

[40]Willems R, Sipido KR, Holemans P, Ector H, Van de WF, Heidbuchel H. Different patterns of angiotensin II and atrial natriuretic peptide secretion in a sheep model of atrial fibrillation. *J Cardiovasc Electrophysiol* 2001; 12(12):1387-1392.

[41]Li D, Fareh S, Leung TK, Nattel S. Promotion of atrial fibrillation by heart failure in dogs: atrial remodeling of a different sort. *Circulation* 1999; 100(1):87-95.

[42]Li D, Shinagawa K, Pang L et al. Effects of angiotensin-converting enzyme inhibition on the development of the atrial fibrillation substrate in dogs with ventricular tachypacing-induced congestive heart failure. *Circulation* 2001; 104(21):2608-2614.

[43]Sakabe M, Fujiki A, Nishida K et al. Enalapril prevents perpetuation of atrial fibrillation by suppressing atrial fibrosis and over-expression of connexin43 in a canine model of atrial pacing-induced left ventricular dysfunction. *J Cardiovasc Pharmacol* 2004; 43(6):851-859.

[44]Shinagawa K, Shiroshita-Takeshita A, Schram G, Nattel S. Effects of antiarrhythmic drugs on fibrillation in the remodeled atrium: insights into the mechanism of the superior efficacy of amiodarone. *Circulation* 2003; 107(10):1440-1446.

[45]Shinagawa K, Shi YF, Tardif JC, Leung TK, Nattel S. Dynamic nature of atrial fibrillation substrate during development and reversal of heart failure in dogs. *Circulation* 2002; 105(22):2672-2678.
[46]Goette A, Staack T, Rocken C et al. Increased expression of extracellular signal-regulated kinase and angiotensin-converting enzyme in human atria during atrial fibrillation. *J Am Coll Cardiol* 2000; 35(6):1669-1677.
[47]Goette A, Arndt M, Rocken C et al. Regulation of angiotensin II receptor subtypes during atrial fibrillation in humans. *Circulation* 2000; 101(23):2678-2681.
[48]Leonardi M, Bissett J. Prevention of atrial fibrillation. *Curr Opin Cardiol* 2005; 20(5):417-423.
[49]West TC, LANDA JF. Minimal mass required for induction of a sustained arrhythmia in isolated atrial segments. *Am J Physiol* 1962; 202:232-236.
[50]Sanfilippo AJ, Abascal VM, Sheehan M et al. Atrial enlargement as a consequence of atrial fibrillation. A prospective echocardiographic study. *Circulation* 1990; 82(3): 792-797.
[51]Van Gelder IC, Crijns HJ, van Gilst WH, Hamer HP, Lie KI. Decrease of right and left atrial sizes after direct-current electrical cardioversion in chronic atrial fibrillation. *Am J Cardiol* 1991; 67(1):93-95.
[52]Solti F, Vecsey T, Kekesi V, Juhasz-Nagy A. The effect of atrial dilatation on the genesis of atrial arrhythmias. *Cardiovasc Res* 1989; 23(10):882-886.
[53]Allessie MA, Boyden PA, Camm AJ et al. Pathophysiology and prevention of atrial fibrillation. *Circulation* 2001; 103(5):769-777.
[54]Ravelli F, Allessie M. Effects of atrial dilatation on refractory period and vulnerability to atrial fibrillation in the isolated Langendorff-perfused rabbit heart. *Circulation* 1997; 96(5):1686-1695.
[55]Sinno H, Derakhchan K, Libersan D, Merhi Y, Leung TK, Nattel S. Atrial ischemia promotes atrial fibrillation in dogs. *Circulation* 2003; 107(14):1930-1936.
[56]Tsai CT, Lai LP, Lin JL et al. Renin-angiotensin system gene polymorphisms and atrial fibrillation. *Circulation* 2004; 109(13):1640-1646.
[57]Pedersen OD, Bagger H, Kober L, Torp-Pedersen C. Trandolapril reduces the incidence of atrial fibrillation after acute myocardial infarction in patients with left ventricular dysfunction. *Circulation* 1999; 100(4):376-380.
[58]Vermes E, Tardif JC, Bourassa MG et al. Enalapril decreases the incidence of atrial fibrillation in patients with left ventricular dysfunction: insight from the Studies Of Left Ventricular Dysfunction (SOLVD) trials. *Circulation* 2003; 107(23):2926-2931.
[59]Maggioni AP, Latini R, Carson PE et al. Valsartan reduces the incidence of atrial fibrillation in patients with heart failure: results from the Valsartan Heart Failure Trial (Val-HeFT). *Am Heart J* 2005; 149(3):548-557.
[60]Ducharme A, Swedberg K, Pfeffer MA et al. Prevention of atrial fibrillation in patients with symptomatic chronic heart failure by candesartan in the Candesartan in Heart failure: Assessment of Reduction in Mortality and morbidity (CHARM) program. *Am Heart J* 2006; 152(1):86-92.
[61]Wachtell K, Lehto M, Gerdts E et al. Angiotensin II receptor blockade reduces new-onset atrial fibrillation and subsequent stroke compared to atenolol: the Losartan Intervention For End Point Reduction in Hypertension (LIFE) study. *J Am Coll Cardiol* 2005; 45(5):712-719.

[62]Fogari R, Mugellini A, Destro M et al. Losartan and prevention of atrial fibrillation recurrence in hypertensive patients. *J Cardiovasc Pharmacol* 2006; 47(1):46-50.

[63]L'Allier PL, Ducharme A, Keller PF, Yu H, Guertin MC, Tardif JC. Angiotensin-converting enzyme inhibition in hypertensive patients is associated with a reduction in the occurrence of atrial fibrillation. *J Am Coll Cardiol* 2004; 44(1):159-164.

[64]Murray KT, Rottman JN, Arbogast PG et al. Inhibition of angiotensin II signaling and recurrence of atrial fibrillation in AFFIRM. *Heart Rhythm* 2004; 1(6):669-675.

[65]Mathew JP, Fontes ML, Tudor IC et al. A multicenter risk index for atrial fibrillation after cardiac surgery. *JAMA* 2004; 291(14):1720-1729.

[66]Anne W, Willems R, Van der MN, Van de WF, Ector H, Heidbuchel H. Atrial fibrillation after radiofrequency ablation of atrial flutter: preventive effect of angiotensin converting enzyme inhibitors, angiotensin II receptor blockers, and diuretics. *Heart* 2004; 90(9):1025-1030.

[67]Ueng KC, Tsai TP, Yu WC et al. Use of enalapril to facilitate sinus rhythm maintenance after external cardioversion of long-standing persistent atrial fibrillation. Results of a prospective and controlled study. *Eur Heart J* 2003; 24(23):2090-2098.

[68]Madrid AH, Bueno MG, Rebollo JM et al. Use of irbesartan to maintain sinus rhythm in patients with long-lasting persistent atrial fibrillation: a prospective and randomized study. *Circulation* 2002; 106(3):331-336.

[69]Hirayama Y, Atarashi H, Kobayashi Y et al. Angiotensin-converting enzyme inhibitor therapy inhibits the progression from paroxysmal atrial fibrillation to chronic atrial fibrillation. *Circ J* 2005; 69(6):671-676.

[70]Omran H, Jung W, Rabahieh R et al. Left atrial chamber and appendage function after internal atrial defibrillation: a prospective and serial transesophageal echocardiographic study. *J Am Coll Cardiol* 1997; 29(1):131-138.

[71]Fatkin D, Kuchar DL, Thorburn CW, Feneley MP. Transesophageal echocardiography before and during direct current cardioversion of atrial fibrillation: evidence for "atrial stunning" as a mechanism of thromboembolic complications. *J Am Coll Cardiol* 1994; 23(2):307-316.

[72]Dagres N, Karatasakis G, Panou F et al. Pre-treatment with Irbesartan attenuates left atrial stunning after electrical cardioversion of atrial fibrillation. *Eur Heart J* 2006; 27(17):2062-2068.

[73]Khan IA. Atrial stunning: determinants and cellular mechanisms. *Am Heart J* 2003; 145(5):787-794.

[74]Madrid AH, Peng J, Zamora J et al. The role of angiotensin receptor blockers and/or angiotensin converting enzyme inhibitors in the prevention of atrial fibrillation in patients with cardiovascular diseases: meta-analysis of randomized controlled clinical trials. *Pacing Clin Electrophysiol* 2004; 27(10):1405-1410.

[75]Healey JS, Baranchuk A, Crystal E et al. Prevention of atrial fibrillation with angiotensin-converting enzyme inhibitors and angiotensin receptor blockers: a meta-analysis. *J Am Coll Cardiol* 2005; 45(11):1832-1839.

[76]Kalus JS, Coleman CI, White CM. The impact of suppressing the renin-angiotensin system on atrial fibrillation. *J Clin Pharmacol* 2006; 46(1):21-28.

[77]Teo K, Yusuf S, Sleight P et al. Rationale, design, and baseline characteristics of 2 large, simple, randomized trials evaluating telmisartan, ramipril, and their combination in high-risk patients: the Ongoing Telmisartan Alone and in Combination with Ramipril Global

Endpoint Trial/Telmisartan Randomized Assessment Study in ACE Intolerant Subjects with Cardiovascular Disease (ONTARGET/TRANSCEND) trials. *Am Heart J* 2004; 148(1):52-61.

[78]Disertori M, Latini R, Maggioni AP et al. Rationale and design of the GISSI-Atrial Fibrillation Trial: a randomized, prospective, multicentre study on the use of valsartan, an angiotensin II AT1-receptor blocker, in the prevention of atrial fibrillation recurrence. *J Cardiovasc Med (Hagerstown)* 2006; 7(1):29-38.

In: Progress in Cardiac Arrhythmia Research
Editor: Ira R. Tarkowicz, pp. 81-108

ISBN: 1-60021-796-6

Chapter 3

Arrhythmogenicity of Anti-Ro/SSA-Antibodies: From the Newborn to the Adult?

Pietro Enea Lazzerini, Pier Leopoldo Capecchi and Franco Laghi Pasini

Department of Clinical Medicine and Immunological Sciences, Divisions of Clinical Immunology, University of Siena, Italy

Abstract

The Ro-ribonucleoproteins (52- and 60-kDa) are the main intracellular targets of the anti-Ro/SSA-antibodies, frequently detected in autoimmune rheumatic diseases, particularly Sjögren's syndrome, and systemic lupus erythematosus, but occasionally also in asymptomatic individuals. Passive trans-placental passage of anti-Ro/SSA-antibodies from mother to foetus is associated with a peculiar syndrome named *neonatal lupus*, where the congenital heart block (CHB) represents the most severe clinical feature. In fact, CHB is responsible of significant mortality (about 20%) and morbidity, with over 60% of surviving affected children requiring pace-maker. In anti-Ro/SSA-positive mothers, the risk of giving birth to a newborn with CHB is around 1-2 %, with a recurrence risk in a subsequent child of 10-16%.

On this basis, great scientific interest arose about the pathogenetic mechanisms underlying CHB development, aimed at identifying possible therapeutic targets. In the inflammatory theory, the occurrence of apoptosis during the development of foetal heart represents the pivotal factor in the beginning of the pathogenetic cascade, thus resulting in translocation of Ro/SSA-antigens to cell surface where they are bound by maternal autoantibodies. The subsequent phagocytosis of opsonized cells by tissue macrophages induces the secretion of pro-inflammatory and pro-fibrotic cytokines producing cardiac damage and irreversible scarring. Other authors proposed an electrophysiological theory, in which anti-Ro/SSA-antibodies block specific ion channels critically involved in the function of the atrio-ventricular (AV) node. In fact, it has been demonstrated that purified anti-Ro/SSA antibodies induce AV-block in isolated human foetal heart and inhibit inward calcium fluxes through L-type calcium-channels in human heart ventriculocytes.

More recently, other cardiac rhythm disturbances different from CHB have been reported in children born from anti-Ro/SSA-positive mothers, among which sinus bradycardia and corrected QT (QTc)-interval prolongation. The pathogenetic mechanisms of such abnormalities are also largely unknown, even if experimental data suggest an electrophysiological interference on both T- and L-type calcium-channels in the genesis of sinus bradycardia.
Although anti-Ro/SSA-antibodies have been traditionally considered dangerous only for the foetal heart, recent studies demonstrated the presence of QTc prolongation at the electrocardiogram also in anti-Ro/SSA-positive adults affected with connective tissue diseases (CTD), as a possible sign of cardiac damage. This feature may be of particular clinical relevance, being the QTc prolongation an established risk factor for life-threatening arrhythmias and sudden death in the general population. On this basis, studies aimed at defining the incidence of complex ventricular arrhythmias and their relationship with the QTc prolongation in anti-Ro/SSA-positive CTD patients are presently in progress.

1. Introduction

Connective tissue diseases (CTD) are a group of chronic inflammatory diseases of immuno-pathological origin characterized by autoantibody synthesis and systemic involvement. Among the different body districts involved, heart and vascular system are common targets of the disease, with relevant prognostic implications in terms of morbidity and mortality. Cardiac rhythm disturbances, i.e. conduction defects and tachyarrhythmias, represent a common manifestation of such cardiovascular damage in the clinical setting [1].

The underlying arrhythmogenic mechanisms are probably multiple and intriguing, even though the myocardial fibrosis frequently observed at the pathological examination seems to play a pivotal role. In fact, myocardial fibrosis, that is produced directly by inflammatory processes, or indirectly as a consequence of coronary artery occlusive disease, may affect the conduction system also representing the pathological substrate for reentry circles [1].

Among the CTD-associated rhythm disorders, congenital heart block (CHB), which is the main feature of neonatal lupus, a rare syndrome related to the transplacental passage of autoantibodies from anti-Ro/SSA-positive mothers to their newborns, seems to acknowledge a peculiar mechanism of disease possibly dependent on a direct arrhythmogenicity of maternal autoantibodies [1].

In the present chapter, we systematically reviewed: (i) the clinical aspects and the pathogenetic mechanisms regarding the anti-Ro/SSA associated cardiac rhythm disorders, including the more recently described foetus-neonatal EKG abnormalities different from CHB; (ii) the arising data from the literature concerning the possible arrhythmogenicity of anti-Ro/SSA antibodies also in adult patients.

2. Anti-Ro/SSA Antibodies: General Considerations

2.1. Molecular Targets

The first description of anti-Ro/SSA antibodies was made over 45 years-ago, when they have been identified as precipitating autoantibodies reacting with undefined antigens contained in salivary and lacrimal gland's extracts of patients affected with Sjogren's syndrome (SS) [2,3]. At the present, it is well known that the main intra-cellular target recognized by such antibodies is represented by the Ro ribonucleoproteins (Ro RNP), constituted by two different Ro proteins of 52 and 60 kDa, and small cytoplasmic RNAs termed human Y-RNAs (hYRNAs) [4].

In humans, Ro 60 kDa protein is encoded by a 1.8 kb gene, located on chromosome 19, and possesses a RNA binding domain [5,6]; conversely, Ro 52 kDa protein, which is encoded by a gene located on chromosome 11 [7], shows zinc finger and leucine zipper domains without a specific RNA binding site [8]. Another differential element between such two molecules is represented by the conformation dependence. In fact, the auto-epitopes recognized by anti-60 kDa Ro/SSA antibodies are highly conformational and the antibody binding is largely lost with the denaturation of the protein. On the contrary, anti-52 kDa Ro/SSA antibodies recognize only linear epitopes, usually placed in the leucine zipper site, which are not expressed on the surface of the naïve protein [9-12]. At the moment, the function of Ro 60 and 52 kDa proteins has not been fully elucidated, even if a role in the hYRNA transport and/or in the regulation of RNA polymerase III is hypothesized [13].

The hYRNAs include four low-molecular weight molecules (28-38 kDa) synthesized by the RNA polymerase III and named hY1, hY3, hY4 and hY5, respectively [14,15]. Such molecules, mostly located in the cytoplasmic compartment (70%) and few in the nuclear compartment, present at the 5' extremity the noncovalent fixation site for the Ro 60 kDa protein [16].

Finally, hYRNAs also bind at the 3'extremity the La/SSB antigen, a 48 kDa phosphorylated protein located in nucleus and cytoplasm, playing a pivotal role in RNA polymerase III transcription process as a termination factor [16]. All these molecules, considered as a whole, result in the formation of a heterogeneous antigenic structure named Ro/La RNP complex.

2.2. Clinical Associations

Anti-Ro/SSA antibodies represent a common finding in patients affected with several autoimmune disorders, particularly SS and systemic lupus erythematosus (SLE).

The prevalence of anti-Ro/SSA antibodies in patients with primary SS (pSS) is generally high, even if the different studies report a large variability of results (ranging from 30 to 95%) [17-23]. Discordance is present also in the studies investigating the relationship between such antibodies and the clinical manifestations of the disease. In fact, even though some authors reported a higher prevalence of adenopathies, Raynaud's phenomenon, cutaneous vasculitis, cytopenia [17,23], salivary involvement [23,24] and precocious atherosclerosis [21] in anti-Ro/SSA positive pSS patients, other authors did not find any correlation with particular organ manifestations [19,20].

In SLE patients, a positivity for anti-Ro/SSA antibodies was found in about 30-50% of the subjects [18,25,26], with a significant association with peculiar features of the disease such as non-erosive deforming Jaccoud's arthropathy [27], interstitial pneumonitis [28], cardiac valvular [29] and hepatic involvement [30]. Also the skin may be a target of such antibodies, as suggested by the high prevalence of positive patients in subacute cutaneous lupus erythematosus (SCLE) [31]. Finally, anti-Ro/SSA antibodies showed a strong relationship with late onset SLE, a peculiar form of the disease affecting people over 50 years, characterized by a lower frequency of renal damage and a benign clinical behaviour [32].

Although SS and SLE represent the paradigmatic anti-Ro/SSA-associated diseases, a positivity for such antibodies can be occasionally detected in the course of other disorders also not necessarily of rheumatologic interest. Anti-Ro/SSA antibodies are demonstrable in 3-15% of the patients affected with rheumatoid arthritis (RA) who commonly present a peculiar clinical feature characterized by extra-articular manifestations including not only xerophthalmia and xerostomia, but also episcleritis and amyloidosis [33-35]. Similarly, anti-Ro/SSA antibodies are present in a number of subjects with systemic sclerosis (SSc) (3-11%) [36,37], polymyositis-dermatomyositis (PM/DM) (5-15%) [38,39], and undifferentiated connective tissue disease (UCTD) (8-30%) [40], frequently suffering of sicca symptoms and with a high risk to develop a severe pulmonary disease [41,42].

Not only rheumatic autoimmune diseases are associated with circulating anti-Ro/SSA antibodies, since autoantibodies are detectable in 5-35% of the patients with primary biliary cirrhosis [43-45]. In these cases, a higher prevalence of sicca syndrome and extra-hepatic features is encountered [43,46].

Finally, anti-Ro/SSA antibodies can be rarely demonstrated also in healthy individuals. In two large studies, the first conducted on 5,000 sera from female blood donors between the ages of 20 and 50 years, and the second on 800 asymptomatic pregnant women, anti-Ro/SSA positivity revealed a similar frequency of about 0.5% [47,48].

3. Neonatal Lupus

Differently from the adults, in which the specific pathogenetic role of anti-Ro/SSA antibodies has not been fully elucidated as yet, in the newborn the direct injuring activity of such antibodies has been clearly demonstrated. In fact, the trans-placental passage of anti-Ro/SSA (and anti-La/SSB) antibodies from positive mothers to their babies is responsible of a peculiar syndrome named neonatal lupus (NLE), characterized by an immune-mediated damage of several specific body districts, i.e. skin, liver, blood and heart [49].

3.1. Extra-Cardiac Manifestations

The cutaneous disease has been the firstly discovered manifestation of NLE, and it gave the syndrome the name [50]. In fact, although the other signs of NLE are not habitually observed in adult patients with SLE, the clinical and histological features of the skin involvement remind the cutaneous lupus. The typical lesion of NLE is an annular or polycyclic erythematous plaque of about 1 cm in diameter, erupting few days or weeks after birth in the skin of the head, frequently initiated or exacerbated by sun exposure, and then spontaneously resolving [51]. The pathological examination of the lesion shows the same findings classically detected in adults with SCLE, a cutaneous subset of lupus strongly associated with anti-Ro/SSA antibodies [52].

Hepatobiliary and hematologic manifestation of NLE occur less frequently (both in about 10% of the cases) and, differently from cutaneous involvement which exists as the sole disease feature in most children, they are habitually present together with other NLE symptoms [49]. Fulminant hepatic failure, transient cholestasis with direct hyperbilirubinemia and mild to moderate transaminase elevations constitute the possible forms of liver involvement [53], whereas thrombocytopenia represents the main, nevertheless usually clinically silent, hematologic feature of NLE [54].

3.2. Cardiac Manifestations

Despite the clinical relevance of some of the above mentioned manifestations, heart involvement is the main factor leading to a severe prognosis in children affected with NLE [49]. In fact, some babies develop abnormalities of the cardiac conduction system and/or a dilated cardiomyopathy (DCM) which are frequently life-threatening, so that the mortality rate of cardiac NLE is about 20% [55].

Conduction disturbances consist on different degrees of atrio-ventricular (AV) block collectively named congenital heart block (CHB), representing the more widely recognized feature of the heart disease in the course of NLE [49]. Cardiomyopathy, when present, classically arises in the clinical setting early after the birth in association with CHB; however, less frequently a late-onset dilated cardiomyopathy is described developing despite the early implantation of cardiac pacemaker [56]. The pathogenesis of DCM is not well understood, but recent data strengthen the hypothesis that it may be the consequence of an antibody-mediated inflammatory process responsible of a diffuse injury of the myocardium [57]. In the absence of conduction defects, also the occurrence of endocardial fibroelastosis is rarely reported, a poorly understood disease of the endomyocardium that often progresses to end-stage heart failure and death. The diffuse deposition of IgG and the presence of a T-cell infiltrate throughout the myocardium suggest that, also in this case, the trans-placental passage of maternal autoantibodies may induce an immune reaction responsible of the damage [58].

4. Anti-Ro/SSA-Associated Cardiac Rhythm Disorders in the Foetus and Newborn

4.1. Congenital Heart Block

With the term of congenital heart block (CHB), as recently proposed, an atrioventricular block is defined diagnosed in the uterus, at birth or within the neonatal period, i.e. 0-27 days after birth [59]. CHB can occur in association with structural heart disease or in the setting of structurally normal heart. In the latter eventuality, CHB develops in the great majority of the cases (over 85%) in foetuses or newborns from mothers positive for anti-Ro/SSA (and/or anti-Ro/SSB) antibodies, independently from the fact that they suffer of a rheumatic disease or, conversely, they are perfectly asymptomatic [60]. Although anti-Ro/SSA-associated CHB is generally complete, less frequently first or second degree AV blocks can be also observed [61].

4.1.1. Epidemiology, Clinical Spectrum and Prognostic Implications

Complete CHB has an incidence in the general population of about 1/15-20,000 in live-born infants [60], but if we consider the presence of such a rhythm disorder among the newborns from mothers positive for circulating anti-Ro/SSA antibodies, the incidence increases to 1-2% [62,63]. The risk of recurrence of CHB in a subsequent pregnancy is also predictable, and ranges between 10 and 16% [55,64,65]. CHB develops in the uterus, between 16 and 24 weeks of gestation and then emerges at the birth mainly as complete, i.e. third-degree AV block [55]. However, as previously stated, also less severe degrees of AV block are detectable in newborns with CHB [61,64]. In fact, Askanase and coll. [61], evaluating nearly 200 children with CHB, reported a first-degree or a second-degree AV block in about 5% and 2% of the cases, respectively. Interestingly, the prospective evaluation of such children demonstrated a progression to a complete CHB in the half of the subjects, underlying the importance of an electrocardiographic monitoring in newborns from anti-Ro/SSA positive mothers also in the presence of a normal heart rate.

The recent development of a new Doppler-echocardiographic method estimating the PR interval duration on the basis of the delay between the onset of the hemodynamic events caused by atrial (mitral A wave) and ventricular depolarization (aortic pulsed Doppler tracing), allowed the evaluation of the AV conduction already during pregnancy [66]. On this basis, Sonesson and coll. [67] demonstrated a high prevalence (33%) of signs of first-degree AV block in foetuses from 24 mothers with anti-Ro/SSA 52 kD antibodies, prospectively followed between 18 and 24 weeks of gestation. Two out of these eight foetuses showed a progression of the block degree, with evolution in complete CHB or second-degree AV block, respectively, whereas the remaining six foetuses had a spontaneous normalization of the PR interval before or shortly after the birth. Notably, the foetus developing the second-degree block demonstrated an improvement of the AV conduction (return to a first-degree block) after treatment with betamethasone. The presence of anti-Ro/SSA-related AV disturbances during the prenatal period were reported by other authors [68], even if the prevalence of the first-degree AV block resulted significantly lower (2/66, 3%), as a possible consequence of technical difference in the measurement of PR interval [69]. Finally, the spectrum of the possible AV conduction delays detected in anti-Ro/SSA foetuses also includes, as recently reported, the Luciani-Wenckenbach phenomenon [70].

As regards the prognostic implications of CHB, once it becomes complete it is permanent and, although some babies are able to compensate for the slow heart rate, they require the implantation of a life-long pacemaker in over the 60% of the cases [55]. The mortality rate is about 15-20%; it is related to the development of complete CHB and is predominant *in utero* and in the first months of life [55,64,65] . An element of crucial relevance in its determinism is represented by the heart rate, since that Groves and coll. demonstrated as a ventricular rate lower than 55 beats/minute was associated with greater likelihood of poor outcome for the development of cardiac failure [71].

4.1.2. Pathogenesis

Despite the large amount of studies investigating the mechanisms of damage implied in the onset of CHB in foetuses passively acquiring anti-Ro/SSA antibodies during pregnancy, at the moment the pathogenesis of such disturb has not been fully elucidated. However, two main theories currently arise from the research, one based on an inflammatory-driven injury of the conduction tissue, the second related to the peculiar properties of the electrophysiologic interference demonstrated for anti-Ro/SSA antibodies. Indeed, such theories not necessarily are to consider as mutually exclusive, but the different mechanisms could cooperate in the determinism of the several aspects constituting the clinical spectrum of CHB.

4.1.2.1. Inflammatory Theory

This theory hypothesizes that anti-Ro/SSA antibodies may trigger an inflammatory process involving the conduction system responsible of tissue damage and, finally, resulting in the fibrosis of the AV node.

A lot of experimental evidence confirms the relevance of both these components, imflammation and fibrosis, in the heart affected with CHB. Autopsy investigations performed in foetuses and babies with complete CHB revealed the presence of a large spectrum of lesions of the conduction system, including myocarditis, haemorrhage, necrosis, fibrosis and calcification [72,73]. More frequently, such lesions produce a discontinuity between the atrium and the AV node, even if the interruption may occasionally be situated between the AV node and the main His bundle, or within the bundle, itself. [74,75]. In this context, deposition of IgG and complement, infiltration of macrophages, multinucleated giant cells and lymphocytes as signs of the inflammatory involvement, have been clearly demonstrated [73,76-79].

Recently, a great interest is arising about the specific mechanisms linking the presence of anti-Ro/SSA antibodies in the foetal heart and the development of inflammation and fibrosis. In this view, many studies strongly suggested the pivotal role played by the cardiocyte apoptosis in the beginning and maintenance of the pathogenetic cascade leading to CHB. In fact, Ro/SSA antigen is normally inaccessible for antibody binding, as it is sequestered within the cell. However, during the normal development of foetal heart, the occurrence of physiologic apoptosis is associated to the translocation of Ro/SSA (and La/SSB) to the surface of cardiac myocytes, thus facilitating the recognition of the antigen by circulating maternal anti-Ro/SSA antibodies [80,81]. Moreover, recent studies demonstrated that in CHB hearts apoptosis is not only detectable but exaggerated with respect to normality (more than 30-fold in septal tissue) as a result of an impaired clearance of apoptotic cardiocytes related to their opsonization by maternal autontibodies [73,82].

It is thought that the binding of Ro/SSA antigen on the cell surface by cognate antibodies ("opsonization") represents the trigger event of the inflammatory response supporting the cardiac injury. In fact, many experimental data support the view that opsonized apoptotic cardiomyocytes undergo phagocytosis by tissue macrophages and, as a consequence, such cells produce inflammatory and profibrosing cytokines, including TNFα and TGFβ [83,84]. In particular, TGFβ seems the crucial molecule in the determinism of the signature lesion of CHB, i.e. the fibrosis of the AV node. In fact, it has been demonstrated that such cytokine exerts a modulating activity on cardiac fibroblast, inducing an increased expression of smooth muscle actin (SMAc) indicating a scarring myofibroblast phenotype [84,85]. In accordance, the immunohistology of human CHB heart revealed intense TGFβ staining and predominant SMAc-positive infiltrate in the areas of fibrosis and microcalcification of the conduction system [73]. Moreover, human foetal cardiac fibroblasts exposed to supernatants obtained from macrophages incubated with opsonized apoptotic cardiocytes markedly enhanced the SMAc expression, and this effect was blocked by anti-TGFβ antibodies [85].

It must be outlined that the presence of maternal autoantibodies although necessary is not sufficient to produce the above depicted pathologic cascade, and its clinical consequences. In fact, as previously stated, even though nearly every mother with an affected child has circulating anti-Ro/SSA (and/or anti-La/SSB) antibodies [60], only about 1-2% of mothers with antibodies will have a child with complete CHB [62,63]. Nevertheless, such mothers show a prevalence of about 300 times higher than the general population (1/20,000), with a further relative increase of about 10 times when the risk of recurrence in a subsequent pregnancy is considered (10-20%) [55,64,65]. Such data strongly suggest a great relevance of genetic factors in the susceptibility of the foetus to the damaging effect of the maternal antibodies, and recent data seem to support this view. In particular, the human gene encoding for TGFβ (chromosome 19) is highly polymorphic, and the Leu^{10} allele (leucine → proline at codon 10) is associated with high amounts of TGFβ [86]. On this basis, Clancy and coll. [87] evaluated the frequency of the polymorphism Leu^{10} in 88 children, 40 of them affected with CHB, demonstrating that such an allele was significantly higher in the CHB group. Thus, the authors hypothesized that an exaggerated TGFβ secretion putatively resulting from a peculiar genetic profile may represent a crucial factor in the clinical determinism of CHB. However, a very recent study on twins and triplets discordant for the disease suggests that additional pathogenetic mechanism(s) are also likely to play a role. In fact, Cimaz and coll. [88] investigated the TGFβ polymorphisms in 2 families in which one of the mothers gave birth to triplets (1 affected with complete CHB, 1 with incomplete CHB and 1 unaffected), and the other gave birth to twins (1 affected with complete CHB, 1 unaffected). The profibrotic genotype was detected in the twin with complete CHB but not in the healthy twin, while all of the triplets displayed the same TGFβ genotype at codon 10. Moreover, peripheral blood mononuclear cells from the two children with complete CHB exhibited higher spontaneous and mitogen-stimulated TGFβ secretion than was observed in their siblings.

4.1.2.2. Electrophysiological Theory

The possibility that anti-Ro/SSA antibodies could exert a direct interference on the electrophysiology of the foetal conduction system arose about 15 years ago starting from the seminal findings of Alexander and coll. [89] and Garcia and coll. [90]. The former authors reported that superfusion of newborn rabbit ventricular papillary muscles with IgG-enriched fractions from sera containing anti-SSA/Ro-SSB/La antibodies specifically reduced the plateau phase of the action potential; then, the second group of researchers, using isolated adult rabbit hearts, showed that IgG fractions with anti-SSA/Ro-SSB/La antibodies induced conduction abnormalities and reduced Ca^{++} currents.

On this basis, a great scientific interest recently involved this topic resulting in a large amount of experimental data supporting the relevance of a perturbation in the cardiac electric activity in the pathogenesis of the autoantibody-associated CHB.

The aptitude of anti-Ro/SSA antibodies to induce AV conduction disturbances throughout a direct arrhythmogenic effect has been clearly demonstrated in several models, either in vitro and in vivo. The report of Boutjdir and coll. [91] is particularly impressive, in that the authors provided evidence that the perfusion of isolated beating human foetal heart with anti-52-kD Ro/SSA antibodies affinity-purified from sera of mothers whose children have CHB induced complete AV block in about 30 minutes. Reperfusion of the heart with antibody-free solution resulted in slow recovery of the heart block, that was induced again after the heart superfusion with IgG-enriched fractions from mothers with affected children. In the same study, the authors also demonstrated that anti-52-kD Ro/SSA antibodies inhibited L-type calcium currents ($I_{Ca}L$) at the whole-cell and single channel level. Finally, they showed that immunization of female mice with recombinant 52-kD Ro/SSA protein generated high-titre antibodies that crossed the placenta during a subsequent pregnancy, producing varying degrees of AV conduction abnormalities, including complete AV block, in the pups.

Consistent results were subsequently obtained in a rat heart model (Langendorff beating heart), with the adjunctive demonstration that the blocking activity of such antibodies on cardiac myocytes was selectively exerted on $I_{Ca}L$, without any significant effect on other specific potassium (I_{k1}, I_{to}) and sodium (I_{Na})currents [92]. Moreover, immunoblot data clearly showed cross-reactivity of purified IgG with the α_{1C} subunit of the L-type calcium channel, representing the pore forming subunit, in engineered Xenopus oocytes [93].

Such data, considered as a whole, strongly suggest that anti-Ro/SSA antibodies may produce AV conduction abnormalities in foetuses, including complete CHB, as a consequence of a direct and selective interaction with the α_{1C} subunit of myocardial L-type calcium channels resulting in an inhibition of the related inward current, crucially involved in the electrophysiological activity of the AV node cells. This view may also explain the particular vulnerability of the foetal heart, being both cardiac $I_{Ca}L$ density and α_{1C} subunit mRNA levels significantly higher (two- to four-fold and four- to nine-fold, respectively) in the adult than human foetal heart [94-96]. Moreover, sarcoplasmic reticulum is less abundant in foetal than in adult cardiac cells, thus making excitation-contraction coupling critically dependent on transsarcolemmal calcium entry [97].

Although such a theory apparently does not seem able to account for the pathological findings, including inflammation, apoptosis and fibrosis, characterizing the development of complete CHB, recent data proposed an alternative pathogenetic cascade possibly linking the channel binding and the cardiac tissue damage. In fact, cardiocytes from pups born to anti-Ro/SSA immunized rodents exhibited reduced L-type calcium current density accompanied by a similar decrease in calcium channel protein, thus suggesting a channel down-regulation as a consequence of the chronic exposure to maternal antibodies during pregnancy [98,99]. Moreover, it has been demonstrated that anti-Ro/SSA antibodies binding cultured cardiomyocytes produced a progressive decrease in frequency of calcium oscillation, resulting in accumulating levels and overload of intracellular calcium, with subsequent loss of contractility and ultimately apoptosis and cell death [100]. Interestingly, such effects were selectively induced by using anti-Ro/SSA antibodies direct to a specific epitope within the leucine zipper amino acid sequence 200-239 (p200) of the Ro52 protein [100]. These data appear in accordance with clinical studies suggesting that the risk of CHB in offspring is higher in women in whom the anti-Ro/SSA activity is targeted to the 52 kDa rather than the 60 kDa component of the antigen [101,102,103], especially in those women in which the antibody response is directed to p200 sequence [102]. As a further confirmation of this view, Salomonsson and coll. found a significant correlation between the prolongation of the foetal AV time and the level of antibodies to p200 in 25 pregnant anti-Ro52-positive women. More in detail, mothers of foetuses developing second- and third-degree AV block were found among those with the highest levels of p200 antibodies, whereas in mothers of less affected foetuses, the Ro52 antibody response was mainly directed to another peptide (p176) of the Ro52 protein [100].

On this basis, the intriguing hypothesis that the p200 Ro52 sequence is structurally and antigenically homologue to the α_{1C} subunit of myocardial L-type calcium channels may be proposed, as suggested by data from a computer-based analysis of the amino acid sequence from the SWISS-PROT database between 52 kDa Ro/SSA, 60 kDa Ro/SSA and 48 kDa La/SSB proteins and the α_{1C} subunit. In fact, the study revealed that most the homology is with 52 kDa component, and, in particular, when a 3-dimensional representation of the α_{1C} subunit structure was used, numerous homologous epitopes are found in the extracellular loops [98].

However, at the moment, no definite target for CHB-inducing antibodies has been clearly identified and, as a further confirmation of the complexity of the pathogenetic phenomena involved, some studies recently proposed that maternal antibodies may affect the calcium channel function in an indirect manner, through the block of specific modulating receptors. In particular, such studies focused the attention on the putative role of serotoninergic 5-hydroxytriptamine (5-HT) receptors in the development of CHB.

The 5-HT_4 receptor is expressed and functional in both human and murine foetal heart cells, where serotonin induces stimulation of the L-type calcium current [104,105]. These data are in accordance with the fact that serotonin exerts positive chronotropic and inotropic effects in the adult human atrium and 5-HT_4 receptor engagement leads to the stimulation of adenyl cyclase activity, activation of cAMP-dependent protein kinase A, and phosphorylation of several key proteins involved in excitation-contraction coupling, among which those of cardiac L-type calcium channels [106,107]. Eftekhari and coll. reported that antibodies reactive with the 5-HT_{4A} receptor, cloned from human adult atrium, also bound 52 kDa Ro/SSA protein. More in detail, the authors identified a peptide in the C-terminus of the 52 kDa molecule (amino acids 365-382) that shared some similarity with the 5-HT_4 receptor, and was recognized by sera from mothers of children of CHB. Such amino acid sequence was reported to be crossreactive with antibodies to a synthetic peptide corresponding to the second extracellular loop of the human 5-HT_4 receptor (amino-acid residues 165-185). Moreover, affinity-purified 5-HT_4 antibodies antagonized the serotonin-induced L-type calcium channel activation in human atrial cells [108]. In a subsequent study, the same researchers substantiated in vivo their findings with the induction of first- and second-degree AV blocks in pups of mice immunized with the above depicted 5-HT_4 receptor-derived synthetic peptide [105]. On this bases, in a recent collaborative study, the prevalence of anti-5-HT_4 receptor autoantibodies in mothers of children with CHB was assessed. Although the presence of anti-5-HT_4 receptor was more prevalent in mothers with affected children than in controls, only 12 out of such 75 mothers (16%) presented these autoantibodies in their sera. Interestingly, in a mother with an isolated child with CHB but who had no detectable anti-Ro/SSA 52 kDa antibodies, reactivity with the 5-HT_4 receptor was noted [109].

In conclusion, considering the results of these studies as a whole, while 5-HT_4 receptor autoantibodies do not have the predictive value of anti-Ro/SSA antibodies, their presence may contribute to the pathogenesis of disease in a minor subset of mothers whose children have CHB.

The accurate dissection of the above depicted theories permits the individuation of elements possibly linking such two apparently alternative points of view of the pathogenesis of CHB. In particular, it is evident as the occurrence of an exaggerated cardiomyocyte apoptosis in foetal heart exposed to anti-Ro/SSA antibodies is a key step in both the pathogenetic cascades. Nevertheless, while such a phenomenon constitutes the initiating event in the inflammatory theory, it represents the final result of the persistent disturb of calcium homeostasis secondary to the electrophysiological interference of anti-Ro/SSA antibodies. As a consequence, a putative unifying theory may be proposed in which the autoantibody-mediated functional block of $I_{Ca}L$ produces the early and reversible (spontaneously or after transplacental steroid therapy) abnormalities of the AV conduction, such as first- and second-degree AV block. Therefore, if a sufficiently prolonged channel block takes place, the secondary ionic dysregulation leads to cell apoptosis that, in its turn, may result in the translocation of Ro/SSA-antigens to cell surface where they are bound by maternal autoantibodies triggering the inflammatory cascade. At this time, probably, the conduction disturbances are still theoretically reversible with an appropriate treatment. Differently, a progression to fibrosis and calcification leading to a permanent conduction injury with the clinical outcome of a complete heart block (third-degree AV block) occurs, particularly in foetuses carrying specific susceptibility genes (Figure 1).

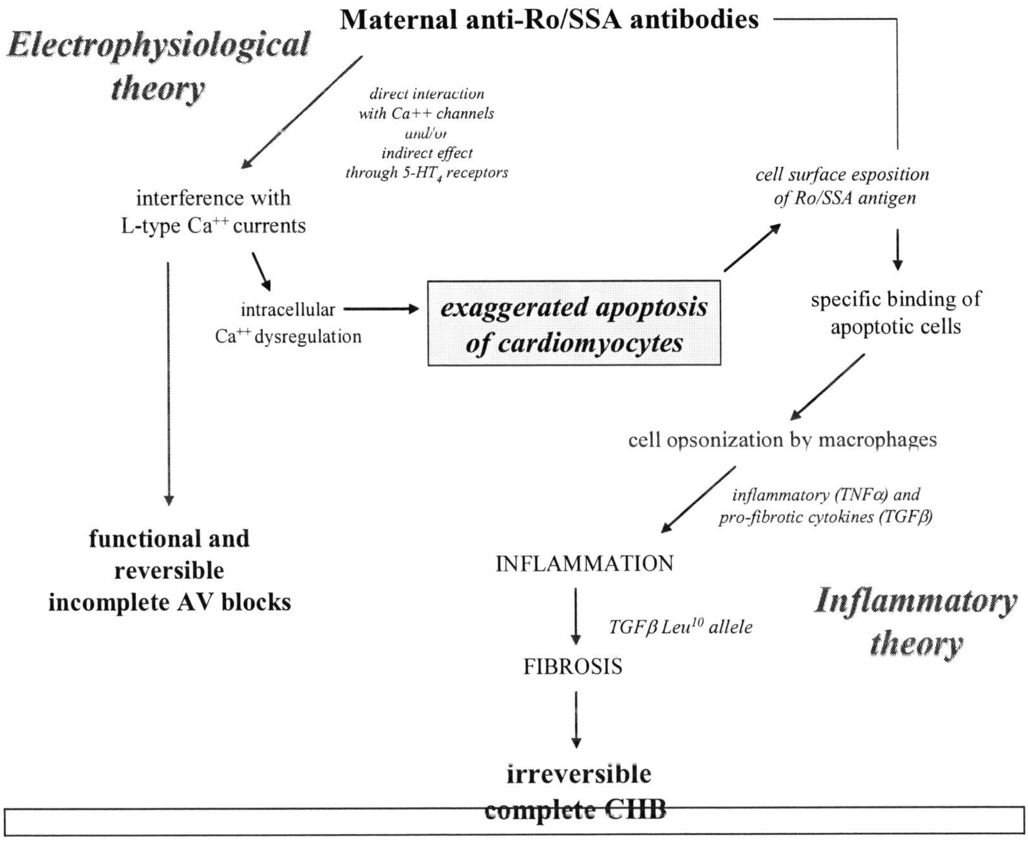

Figure 1. Pathogenesis of CHB: proposal for an unifying theory.

4.2. Sinus Bradycardia

Although CHB represents the main cardiac rhythm disorder associated with anti-Ro/SSA antibodies in foetus and newborn, recent in vitro and in vivo studies suggested that also the sino-atrial (SA) node might be involved in the spectrum of the conduction abnormalities observed. In fact, the Boutjdir's research group demonstrated that perfusion of Langendorff perfused rabbit hearts with IgG from mothers with CHB children caused sinus bradycardia preceding AV block using surface EKG and optical action potentials [110]. Successively, the same researchers observed a significant sinus bradycardia in the animal models of CHB developed by either passive transfer of positive IgG into pregnant mice [111] or by active immunization of female mice [91] or rabbits [93] with Ro/SSA antigen.

4.2.1. Clinical Findings

After some anecdotal case reports describing sinus bradycardia in a foetus [112], and in infants [113,114] with anti-Ro/SSA antibodies, Brucato and coll. [115] prospectively followed 21 pregnancies in autoantibody-positive mothers, performing EKGs in the newborns in the first days after birth. In 3 cases (about 15%), a significant sinus bradycardia was observed (heart rate less than third centile for age). Remarkably, in all cases bradycardia disappeared within 10 days after birth, without any sequelae. Such results were subsequently confirmed by the same authors in an extension of the study finally involving a group of 24 children [62]. However, conflicting data have been reported by a recent study of Costedoat-Chalumeau and coll. [63] that compared EKGs in 58 consecutive children aged 0 to 2 months born to anti-Ro/SSA positive mothers with an age-matched control group of 85 infants born to anti-Ro/SSA positive mothers with connective tissue diseases (CTD). The authors did not find any significant difference in mean heart rate, and this remained true at 2 to 4 months of life.

On the basis of the above mentioned data, the clinical relevance of sinus bradycardia appears not to be fully elucidated at this moment, and larger controlled studies are needed to address adequately this topic.

4.2.2. Pathogenesis

The possible pathogenetic mechanisms supporting the development of anti-Ro/SSA-associated sinus bradycardia have been recently investigated, and the available studies strongly suggest also in this case the relevance of an electrophysiological interference on specific cardiac ion channels.

Pacemaker activity in SA node cells is dependent on several ionic currents, among which the role of T-type ($I_{Ca}T$) calcium current operative in the late phase of the diastolic depolarization seems particularly relevant. On the basis of these premises, Xiao and coll. [93] demonstrated the inhibitory effect of IgG from mothers with CHB children on $I_{Ca}T$ expressed in Xenopus oocytes. To further strengthen these findings, the same research group tested the effect of such antibodies also on spontaneously beating SA node myocytes reporting the rapid onset of sinus bradycardia (from 155 to 66 bpm after 2 minutes of perfusion), only partially recovered after the subsequent superfusion of the cells with antibody-free solution. These results were associated with the concomitant reduction of the phase 4 diastolic depolarization of the action potential and the inhibition of $I_{Ca}T$ [116].

Recent data suggest that also the L-type calcium current ($I_{Ca}L$) is significantly involved in the genesis of sinus bradycardia. More in detail, it has been demonstrated that spontaneous diastolic depolarization of SA node cells is selectively regulated by a specific variant of the

L-type calcium channel carrying the subunit α_{1D} in the place of α_{1C} [117]. Qu and coll. [118] reported that α_{1D}-calcium channels are expressed in the human foetal heart and α_{1D}-$I_{Ca}L$ is inhibited by IgG from mothers with CHB children. Interestingly, western blot data showed the direct binding between maternal antibodies and α_{1D}-calcium channel protein [118].

Although such data are consistent with the hypothesi that anti-Ro/SSA antibodies exert a negative chronotropic effect on foetal heart as a consequence of a direct blockage of the calcium channels, another study proposes the hypothesis of an indirect antibody modulation of such currents throughout an interference with the 5-HT_4 receptor activity. In fact, the immunization of female mice with synthetic peptides deriving from amino acid sequences of the serotoninergic 5-HT_4 receptor induces classical signs of neonatal lupus in their pups, such as skin rush and AV conduction disturbances, but also sinus bradycardia in almost 30% of the cases [105].

Finally, human foetal autopsies from CHB subjects revealed calcification of the SA node [74,77]; thus the possibility cannot ruled out that, similarly to what happens in the AV node, not only functional electrophysiological phenomena, but also an inflammatory injury may in some cases occur also in such a district, resulting in scarring and calcium deposition.

4.3. QT Interval Prolongation

The prolongation of the heart rate-corrected QT interval (QTc) completes the spectrum of the possible electrocardiographic abnormalities associated with the positivity of anti-Ro/SSA antibodies in the foetus and newborn. The detection of such an asymptomatic electrocardiographic abnormality may have a relevant clinical impact, since the prolongation of QTc in the neonatal period and infancy represents a risk factor for arrhythmic sudden infant death [119]

4.3.1. Clinical Findings

The possible association between complete CHB and QTc prolongation is known since more than 25 years ago, when Esscher and Michaelsson [120] reported an elevated prevalence of such disturbance in 273 affected children (21.6%). In the same period, some isolated case reports have been also described in which infants with complete CHB and QTc prolongation presented life-threatening arrhythmias (ventricular tachycardia and/or ventricular fibrillation) requiring permanent pacing [121,122]. However, in those years the precise pathogenetic relationship between CHB and anti-Ro/SSA antibodies was still unknown and, as a consequence, no information is available about the autoantibody pattern of the investigated children (and mothers). Indeed, a recent paper depicted the case of a foetus with autoimmune-mediated CHB (anti-Ro/SSA positivity documented in the mother) developing ventricular tachycardia. Interestingly, the early postnatal EKG evaluation of the newborn revealed the prolongation of the QT interval [123].

The first description of a specific association between anti-Ro/SSA antibodies and QTc prolongation, independently from the presence of complete CHB, has been made more recently by Cimaz and coll. [124]. They reported a significant elongation of QTc in 21 asymptomatic children born to anti-Ro/SSA positive mother, but without CHB, in comparison to 7 infants born to anti-Ro/SSA negative mothers with CTD (442 vs 403 msec). More in detail, 9 out 21 (43%) babies of the first group had QTc values above the upper normal limit of 440 msec (97.5th percentile), whereas all the infants without antibodies had QTc within normal limits. Moreover, also the mean QTc values in anti-Ro/SSA patients were higher than 440 msec (442 vs 403 msec in controls). Interestingly, QTc prolongation resolved spontaneously during the first year of life in concomitance with the disappearance of acquired maternal antibodies [125]. Consistent results were afterwards obtained by other authors, who adjunctively demonstrated a further increase of QTc in those children having siblings with CHB [126]. However, a more recent paper disagrees with the previous studies. In fact, Costedoat-Chalumeau and coll. [63] investigating 58 consecutive children aged to 0 to 2 months born to anti-Ro/SSA-positive mothers in comparison with 85 age-matched babies from anti-Ro/SSA-negative CTD mothers, did not report any significant difference in QTc between the 2 groups.

4.3.2. Pathogenesis

Differently from the other anti-Ro/SSA associated rhythm disturbances, the understanding of the pathophysiological mechanisms supporting the development of QTc prolongation is at the moment very scant. In fact, although the concomitant disappearance of the QTc prolongation and the acquired maternal autoantibodies during the first year of life described by Cimaz and coll. [125] strongly suggests a functional and reversible mechanism, probably of electrophysiological origin, nevertheless specific data linking this EKG abnormality and the impairment of definite ionic currents in the heart are not currently available.

However, it is now well known that in the course of the so-called familial *long QT syndrome (LQTS)*, a congenital disorder predisposing individuals to potentially fatal ventricular arrhythmias, the mutations involve genes encoding specific potassium and sodium channels [127]. Moreover, several drugs are able to induce an acquired LQTS by the block of the rapid component of the delayed rectifier potassium current (I_{Kr}) [127]. On this basis, a plausible hypothesis may be that anti-Ro/SSA antibodies interfere not only with calcium but also with specific potassium channels, then resulting in the observed QTc prolongation. In fact, even if in vitro experiments demonstrated that such antibodies do not affect potassium currents such as the inward rectifier potassium current (I_{K1}), the transient outward current (I_{to}), and the slow component of the delayed rectifier potassium current (I_{Ks}) [92,93], no data are presently available about the specific effect of anti-Ro/SSA antibodies on I_{Kr}. Thus, the possibility of a selective blocking activity of the maternal antibodies on this latter current cannot be ruled out.

Finally, an interference of anti-Ro/SSA antibodies on the activity of 5-HT_4 receptors may be also suggested. In fact, mice immunized with peptides corresponding to the second extracellular loop of the human 5-HT_4 receptor, gave birth to pups presenting the clinical feature of neonatal lupus including, in the 27% of the cases, an increased QT interval at the 2-day-EKG analysis [105].

5. Anti-Ro/SSA-Associated Cardiac Rhythm Disorders in the Adult

Traditionally, adult heart has been considered resistant to the pathogenetic effect of anti-Ro/SSA antibodies even though, despite the hypotheses tentatively proposed, the putative mechanisms of such presumptive resistance are substantially unknown at the moment. However, recent data from our Institution and other research groups have newly fired the debate about this topic.

5.1. Conduction Disturbances

It is commonly believed that the anti-Ro/SSA positivity does not influence the prevalence of conduction disturbances in adult patients. However, interesting findings emerge from the systematic review of the literature concerning the possible relationship between abnormalities of the AV node function and circulating anti-Ro/SSA antibodies in adult CTD patients.

In fact, although rarely, the occurrence of a complete (third-degree) AV block in anti-Ro/SSA positive adults has been described. Lee and coll. [128] reported the case of a 39-year-old woman with Sjogren's syndrome, positive for both anti-60-kD and 52-kD Ro/SSA antibodies, in which complete heart block appeared in the absence of other specific risk factors. More recently, in a prospective study aimed to assess the prevalence of CHB in infants from 100 mothers with anti-Ro/SSA antibodies, Brucato and coll. [62] recorded one mother (anti-60-kD positive) who abruptly developed a complete "idiopathic" block, requiring implantation of pacemaker. Interestingly, she previously delivered two healthy babies, without any EKG abnormality. Beside such two evocative examples, other authors depicted case reports hypothesizing a causal association between complete AV block and anti-Ro/SSA antibodies, particularly in the course of systemic lupus erythematosus (SLE). In fact, even though the onset of third-degree AV block in SLE patients represent an exceptional event, in more of these few cases it occurs in anti-Ro/SSA positive subjects. More in detail, considered as a whole, less than 15 SLE patients with such rhythm disorder have been currently described in literature but, among these, a positivity was detectable in 5 out of 7 subjects (71%) specifically tested for the presence of anti-Ro/SSA antibodies [129-139]. Finally, Behan and coll. reported circulating anti-Ro/SSA antibodies in a fatal case of dermatomyositis with complete heart block [140].

The overall prevalence of conduction disturbances in adult patients with anti-Ro/SSA antibodies, including less severe degrees of AV block, bundle branch and fascicular blocks, has been also investigated, but the results are conflicting. Logar and coll. [141], evaluating 67 SLE patients (36 anti-Ro/SSA positive), found a significantly higher prevalence of conduction defects in anti-Ro/SSA positive than in anti-Ro/SSA negative patients, and healthy controls. EKG abnormalities were detected in 6/36 (17%) of positive patients (vs. 1/31 of negative patients and 1/50 (2%) of healthy controls), represented by first-degree AV block (4 cases), left anterior hemiblock (3 cases), and right bundle branch block (2 cases). Consistent data have been obtained in patients with polymyositis. In fact, conduction disorders have been detected in 13 out 55 patients under study, of which 9 (69%) resulted positive for anti-Ro/SSA antibodies. Interestingly, 4 out of 5 patients presenting a complete heart block were anti-Ro/SSA seropositive [142].

In contrast with these results, two subsequent studies reported no differences in the prevalence of conduction defects on the basis of the anti-Ro/SSA positivity of the patients [143,144]. In particular, Gordon and coll. [144] analyzed the EKG in 111 consecutive patients with CTD, 49 of which anti-Ro/SSA positive, and 19 mothers who had children with complete CHB. Conduction abnormalities were demonstrated in only three patients, all affected with SLE: two cases of first-degree AV block (one anti-Ro/SSA positive) and one case with complete heart block (anti-Ro/SSA negative, with evidence of myocarditis). Moreover, no significant difference was present in the mean PR interval and QRS duration between anti-Ro/SSA positive and anti-Ro/SSA negative patients. Finally, Lodde and coll. [145] reported a first-degree AV block in about 10% of patients affected with primary Sjogren's syndrome (SS) (5/51), significantly associated with anti-La/SSB antibodies but unrelated to the presence of anti-Ro/SSA antibodies.

In conclusion, although the association between anti-Ro/SSA antibodies and conduction disturbances is undoubtedly less evident in adults than in infants, the possibility that also the adult cardiac conduction tissue may be affected by such antibodies cannot be presently ruled out. A different degree of vulnerability of the adult heart, rather than an absolute resistance, may be a conceivable hypothesis. Further investigation are needed to clarify this topic, possibly defining factors and mechanisms involved in the peculiar susceptibility to anti-Ro/SSA antibodies that seems to exist in a few number of adult subjects.

5.2. QT Interval Prolongation

Starting from the above mentioned consideration that anti-Ro/SSA antibodies have been associated with QTc prolongation in infants, our group recently investigated whether these antibodies may also affect cardiac repolarization in the adult. To this aim, comparing 57 patients with CTD (31 anti-Ro/SSA positive and 26 anti-Ro/SSA negative as controls) in an EKG-resting study, we found a significant prolongation of the corrected-QT-interval (QTc) (445 vs 419 msec) and a high incidence (58%) of QTc values above the upper limit of normal (440 msec) in anti-Ro/SSA positive subjects with respect to controls [146]. Since the incidence of cardiac arrhythmias and sudden death in patients with CTD is higher than that in general population [1], we evaluated also the possible influence of anti-Ro/SSA antibodies on other established risk factors possibly involved in the occurrence of life-threatening arrhythmias in these subjects, i.e. heart rate variability (HRV) impairment and presence of ventricular late potentials (VLP) [147]. Interestingly, although a preponderant proportion of subjects under study showed a reduction in HRV, with a concomitant alteration in the sympathovagal balance as sympathetic prevalence, and presence of VLP, these abnormalities were equally distributed in the two groups. Such further results seem to suggest a selective arrhythmogenic effect of anti-Ro/SSA antibodies on the QTc-related electrophysiological phenomena, but also that anti-Ro/SSA-positive patients may represent, within the context of the CTD patients, a subgroup of subjects with a particularly high risk of developing malignant arrhythmias [146].

Conversely, a later study of Castedoat-Chalumeau and coll. [148] evaluating 32 anti-Ro/SSA positive in comparison with 57 anti-Ro/SSA negative CTD patients described no differences in QTc interval duration. Indeed, the authors studied a very selected cohort of patients consisting almost exclusively of patients with SLE (close to 90% in each groups) and, as a consequence, the absence of difference between the two groups may be related to a peculiar "resistance" of SLE patient to the hypothesized electrophysiologic effects of these antibodies. In fact, in another similar study performed by Gordon and coll. [144], in which the SLE patients preponderance was still significant (about 70% overall) but less extreme, the QTc in the anti-Ro/SSA positive group was reported to be longer than in the anti-Ro/SSA negative group, and this difference, although not significant, indeed approached significance ($p=0.063$).

The question has been recently addressed by a study of Pineau and coll. [149] performed on 150 SLE patients (38.3% anti-Ro/SSA-positive) aimed at examining whether the presence of anti-Ro/SSA antibodies was associated with an increased risk of QTc prolongation. The authors, in agreement with our results, reported that the anti-Ro/SSA positivity was highly associated with prolongation of QTc interval. More in detail, in a multivariate analysis considering all statistically significant confounders (age, disease duration, disease activity score and disease damage index) they demonstrated that the presence of anti-Ro/SSA antibodies implied odds 12.6 times higher of having such EKG abnormality.

Since the prolongation of the QTc has been identified as an important risk factor for arrhythmic sudden death in the general population [147,150], the association between anti-Ro/SSA antibodies and QTc prolongation in adult CTD patients suggests the hypotheses that these subjects may be particularly predisposed to the development of life-threatening arrhythmias. Moreover, on the basis of the consideration that specific drugs commonly employed in the treatment of CTD may also increase the QTc interval (i.e. hydroxychloroquine and iloprost) [151,152], the definition of the arrhythmic risk in such patients appears of still more particular interest. Although no prospective trials concerning this issue are currently available, a study investigating the prevalence of ventricular arrhythmias in anti-Ro/SSA-positive CTD and their relationship with the QTc duration is now in progress in our Institution.

6. Conclusion

The arrhythmogenicity of anti-Ro/SSA antibodies for the foetal heart and their crucial role in the development of CHB is now well established, representing a paradigmatic model of passively acquired autoimmunity. Conversely, more investigation is required to definitely assess the specific pathogenetic mechanisms involved in the onset and progression of the antibody-dependent cardiac damage responsible for the conduction system impairment. Nevertheless, both inflammatory injury and electrophysiological interference seem to play a crucial role in the determinism of CHB (Figures 1 and 2).

Moreover, in recent years a great interest arose about new cardiac rhythm disturbances, such as sinus bradycardia and QTc interval prolongation, described as associated with anti-Ro/SSA positivity in the foetus and newborn and likely dependent on electrophysiological mechanisms (Figure 2). However, in this case, the opinions are more conflicting.

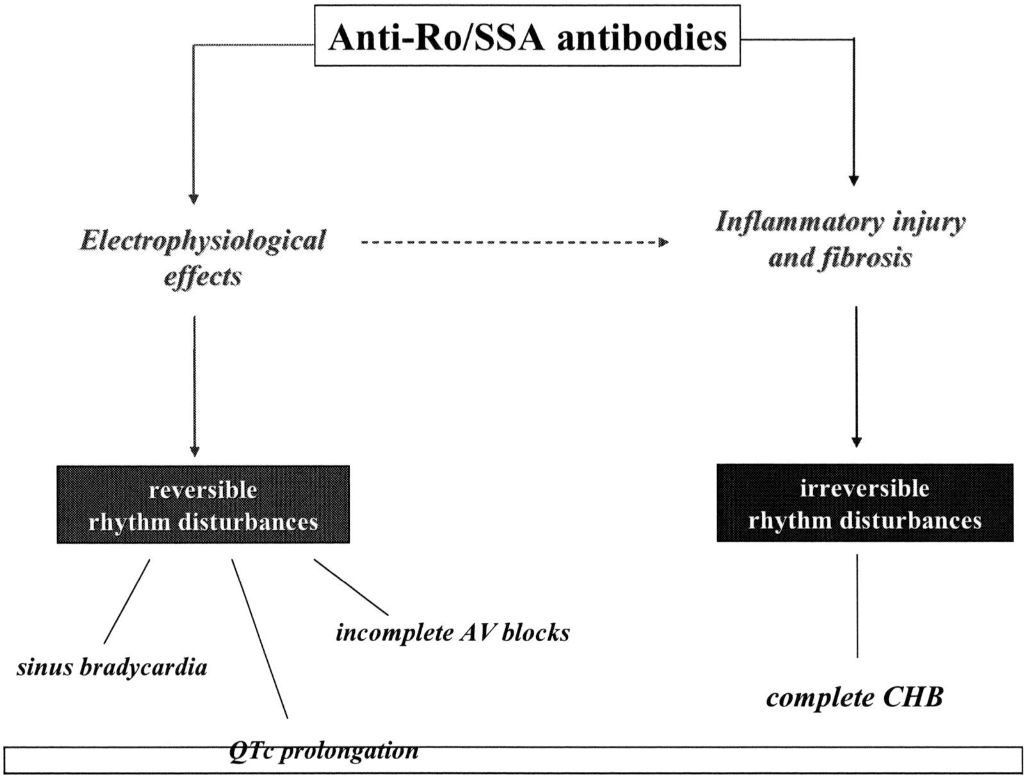

Figure 2. A bird's eye on the putative mechanisms involved in the pathogenesis of the anti-Ro/SSA-associated rhythm disorders in infants and adults.

Finally, intriguing data suggest that also the adult heart, traditionally considered protected from the arrhythmogenic injury of the anti-Ro/SSA antibodies, may represent a possible target in this autoimmune pattern. The prolongation of the QTc interval seems the most frequent abnormality observed in adult with anti-Ro/SSA-positive CTD, even though it is still a matter of debate. The putative implication that this finding may be assumed as a risk factor for arrhythmic sudden death is not currently known, but preliminary data from our research group suggest a relationship between anti-Ro/SSA antibodies, QTc prolongation and prevalence of complex ventricular arrhythmias in adult CTD patients.

References

[1] Lazzerini PE, Capecchi PL, Guideri F, Acampa M, Galeazzi M, Laghi Pasini F. Connective tissue diseases and cardiac rhythm disorders: an overview. *Autoimmun Rev* 2006, 5, 306-313.

[2] Jones B. Lacrimal and salivary precipitating antibodies in Sjogren's syndrome. *Lancet* 1958, 195, 773-776.

[3] Anderson JR, Gray KG, Beck JS. Precipitating autoantibodies in Sjogren's disease. *Lancet* 1961, 2, 456-460.

[4] Franceschini F, Cavazzana I. Anti-Ro/SSA and anti-La/SSB antibodies. *Autoimmunity* 2005, 38, 55-63.

[5] Ben-Chetrit E, Gandy BJ, Tan EM, Sullivan KF. Isolation and characterization of a cDNA clone encoding the 60-kD component of the human SS-A/Ro ribonucleoprotein autoantigen. *J Clin Invest* 1989, 83, 1284-1292.

[6] McCauliffe DP, Zappi E, Lieu TS, Michalak M, Sontheimer RD, Capra DJ. A human Ro/SS-A autoantigen is the homolougue of calreticulin and is highly homologous with onchocercal RAL-1 antigen and an aplysia "memory molecule". *J Clin Invest* 1990, 86, 332-335.

[7] Frank MB, Itoh K, Fujisaku A, Pontarotti P, Mattei MG, Neas BR. The mapping of the human 52-kD Ro/SSA autoantigen gene to human chromosome 11, and its polymorphisms. *Am J Hum Genet* 1993, 52, 183-191.

[8] Chan EKL, Hamel JC, Buyon JP, Tan EM. Molecular definition and sequence motifs of the 52-kD component of human SS-A/Ro autoantigen. *J Clin Invest* 1991, 87, 68-76.

[9] Itoh Y, Reichlin M. Autoantibodies to the Ro/SSA antigen are conformation dependent. I: anti-60 kD antibodies are mainly directed to the native protein; anti-52 kD antibodies are mainly directed to the denatured protein. *Autoimmunity* 1992, 14, 57-65.

[10] Boire G, Craft J. Biochemical and immunological heterogeneity of the Ro ribonucleoprotein particles. Analysis with sera specific for the RohY5 particle. *J Clin Invest* 1989, 84, 270-279.

[11] Boire G, Lopez-Longo FJ, Lapointe S, Menard HA. Sera from patients with autoimmune disease recognize conformational determinants on the 60-kD Ro/SS-A protein. *Arthritis Rheum* 1991, 84, 722-730.

[12] Itoh Y, Itoh K, Frank MB, Reichlin M. Autoantibodies to the Ro/SSA antigen are conformation dependent. II: Antibodies to the denatured form of 52 kD Ro/SSA are a cross reacting subset of antibodies to the native 60 kD Ro/SSA molecule. *Autoimmunity* 1992, 14, 89-95.

[13] Meyer O. Anti-SSA/Ro and anti-SSB/La antibodies. What's new? *Ann Med Interne* 2002, 153, 520-529.

[14] Hendrick JP, Wolin SL, Rinke J, Lerner MR, Steiz JA. Ro small cytoplasmic ribonucleoproteins are a subclass of La ribonucleoproteins: further characterization of the Ro and La small ribonucleoproteins from uninfected mammalian cells. *Mol Cell Biol* 1981, 1, 1138-1149.

[15] Wolin SL, Steitz JA. The Ro small cytoplasmic ribonucleoproteins: identification of the antigenic protein and its binding on the Ro RNAs. *Proc Natl Acad Sci USA* 1984, 81, 1996-2000.

[16] Van Venrooij WJ, Slobbe RL, Pruijn GJM. Structure and function of La and Ro RNPs. *Mol Biol Rep* 1993, 18, 113-121.

[17] Harley JB, Alexander EL, Bias WB, Fox OF, Provost TT, Reichlin M, Yamagata H, Arnett FC. Anti-Ro (SS-A) and anti-La (SS-B) in patients with Sjogren's syndrome. *Arthritis Rheum* 1986, 29, 196-206.

[18] Tsay GJ, Wang CL, Chen TY, Huang CN, Hsu TC. SS-A/Ro antibodies in Chinese patients with systemic lupus erythematosus and Sjogren's syndrome. *J Formos Med Assoc* 1996, 95, 905-910.

[19] Tzioufas AG, Wassmuth R, Dafni UG, Guialis A, Haga HJ, Isenberg DA, Jonsson R, Kalden JR, Kiener H, Sakarellos C, Smolen JS, Sutcliffe N, Vitali C, Yiannaki E,

Moutsopoulos HM. Clinical, immunological, and immunogenetic aspects of autoantibodies production against Ro/SSA, La/SSB and their linear epitopes in primary Sjogren's syndrome (pSS): a European multicentre study. *Ann Rheum Dis* 2002, 61, 398-404.

[20] Locht H, Pelck R, Manthorpe R. Clinical manifestations correlated to the prevalence of autoantibodies in a large (n=321) cohort of patients with primary Sjogren's syndrome: a comparison of patients initially diagnosed according to the Copenhagen classification criteria with the American-European consensus criteria. *Autoimmun Rev* 2005, 4, 276-281.

[21] Vaudo G, Bartoloni Bocci E, Shoenfeld Y, Schillaci G, Wu R, Del Papa N, Vitali C, Delle Monache F, Marchesi S, Mannarino E, Gerli R. Precocious intimamedia thickening in patients wiyhprimay Sjogren's syndrome. *Arthritis Rheum* 2005, 52, 3890-3897.

[22] Ruiz-Tiscar JL, Lopez-Longo FJ, Sanchez-Ramon S, Santamaria B, Urrea R, Carreno L, Estecha A, Vigil D, Fernandez-Cruz E, Rodriguez-Mahou M. Prevalence of IgG anti-{alpha}-fodrin antibodies in Sjogren's syndrome. *Ann N Y Acad Sci* 2005, 1050, 210-216.

[23] Nardi N, Brito-Zeron P, Ramos-Casals M, Aguilò S, Cervera R, Ingelmo M, Font J. Circulating auto-antibodies against nuclear and non-nuclear antigens in primary Sjogren's syndrome. Prevalence and clinical significance in 335 patients. *Clin Rheumatol* 2006, 25, 341-346.

[24] Haga HJ. Clinical and immunological factors associated with low lacrimal and salivary flow rate in patients with primary Sjogren's syndrome. *J Rheumatol* 2002; 29, 305-308.

[25] Yee C, Hussein H, Skan J, Bowman S, Situnayake D, Gordon C. Association of damage with autoantibody profile, age, race, sex and disease duration in systemic lupus erythematosus. *Rheumatology* 2003, 42, 276-279.

[26] Faria AC, Barcellos KS, Andrade LE. Longiyudinal fluctuation of antibodies to extractable nuclear antigens in systemic lupus erythematosus. *J Rheumatol* 2005, 32, 1267-1272.

[27] Franceschini F, Cretti L, Quinzanini M, Rizzini FL, Cattaneo R. Deforming arthropathy of the hands in systemic lupus erythematosus is associated with antibodies to SSA/Ro and to SSB/La. *Lupus* 1994, 3, 419-422.

[28] Hedgepeth MT, Boulware DW. Interstitial pneumonitis in antinuclear antibody-negative systemic lupus erythematosus: a new clinical manifestation and possible association with anti-Ro (SSA) antibodies. *Arthritis Rheum* 1988,51, 545.

[29] Shahin AA, Shahin HA, Hamid MA, Amin MA. Cardiac involvement in patients with systemic lupus erythematosus and correlation of valvular lesion with anti-Ro/SS-A and anti-La/SS-B antibody levels. *Mod Rheumatol* 2004, 14, 117-122.

[30] Lu MC, Li KJ, Hsieh SC, Wu CH, Yu CL. Lupus-related advanced liver involvement as the initial presentation of systemic lupus erythematosus. *J Microbiol Immunol Infect* 2006, 39, 471-475.

[31] McCauliffe DP. Cutaneous disease in adults associated with anti-Ro/SS-A autoantibody production. *Lupus* 1997, 6, 158-166.

[32] Catoggio LR, Skinner RP, Smith G, Maddison PJ. Systemic lupus erythematosus in the elderly. Clinical and serological characteristics. *J Rheumatol* 1984, 11, 175-181.

[33] Skopuli FN, Andonopoulos AP, Moutsopoulos HM. Clinical implications of the presence of anti-Ro(SSA) antibodies in patients with rheumatoid arthritis. *J Autoimmun* 1988, 3, 381-388.
[34] Franceschini F, Cavazzana I, Malacarne F, Airò P, Cattaneo R, Del Papa N, Radice A, Sinico A. Anti-Ro/SSA antibodies in rheumatoid arthritis (RA). *Arthritis Res Ther* 2003, 5 (suppl 1), 8.
[35] Cavazzana I, Franceschini F, Qiunzanini M, Manera C, Del Papa N, Maglione W, Comina D, Radice A, Sinico RA, Cattaneo R. Anti-Ro/SSA antibodies in rheumatoid arthritis: clinical and immunological associations. *Clin Exp Rheumatol* 2006, 24, 59-64.
[36] Drosos AA, Andonopoulos AP, Costopoulos JS, Stravopoulos ED, Papadimitriou CS, Moutsopoulos HM. Sjogren's syndrome in progressive systemic sclerosis. *J Rheumatol* 1988, 15, 965-968.
[37] Fujimoto M, Shimozuma M, Yazawa N, Kubo M, Ihn H, Sato S, Tamaki T, Kikuchi K, Tamaki K. Prevalence and clinical relevance of 52 kDa and 60 kda Ro/SSA autoantibodies in Japanese patients with systemic sclerosis. *Ann Rheum Dis* 1997, 56, 667-670.
[38] Rutjes SA, Vree Egberts WTM, Jongen P. Anti-Ro 52 antibodies frequently co-occur with anti-Jo1 antibodies in sera from patients with idiopathic inflammatory myopathy. *Clin Exp Immunol* 1997, 109, 32-40.
[39] Kubo M, Ihn H, Asano Y, Yamane K, Yazawa N, Tamaki K. Prevalence of 52 kD and 60 kD autoantibodies in Japanese patients with polymyositis/dermatomyosistis. *J Am Acad Dermatol* 2002, 47, 148-151.
[40] Mosca M, Tani C, Neri C, Baldini C, Bombardieri S. Undifferentiated connective tissue disease (UCTD). *Autoimmun Rev* 2006, 6, 1-4.
[41] Breit SN, Cairns D, Szentirmay A, Callaghan T, Murray D, Wacher T, Gibson PJ, Marks G, Bryant DH, Teates M, Fernandez V, Penny R. The presence of Sjogren's syndrome is a major determinant of pattern of interstitial lung disease in scleroderma and other connective tissue disease. *J Rheumatol* 1989, 16, 8.
[42] La Corte R, Lo Monaco A, Locaputo A, Dolzani F, Trotta F. In patients with antisynthetase syndrome the occurrence of anti-Ro/SSA antibodies causes a more severe interstitial lung disease. *Autoimmunity* 2006, 39, 249-253.
[43] Penner E. Demonstration of immune complexes containing the ribonucleoprotein antigen Ro in primary biliary cirrhosis. *Gastroenterology* 1986, 90, 724-727.
[44] Chou MJ, Lee SL, Chen TY, Tsay GJ. Specificity of antinuclear antibodies in primary biliary cirrhosis. *Ann Rheum Dis* 1995, 54, 148-151.
[45] Muratori P, Muratori L, Ferrari R, Cassani F, Bianchi G, Lenzi M, Rodrigo L, Linares A, Fuentes D, Bianchi FB. Characterization and clinical impact of antinuclear antibodies in primary biliary cirrhosis. *Am J Gastroenterol* 2003, 98, 431-437.
[46] Dorner T, Held C, Trebeljahr G, Lukowsky A, Yamamoto K, Hiepe F. Serologic characteristics in primary biliary cirrhosis associated with sicca syndrome. *Scand J Gastroenterol* 1994, 29, 655-660.
[47] Fritzler MJ, Pauls JD, Kinsella TD, Bowen TJ. Antinuclear, anticytoplasmic, and anti-Sjogren's syndrome antigen A (SS-A/Ro) antibodies in female blood donors. *Clin Immunol Immunopathol* 1985, 36, 120-128.

[48] Harmon CE, Lee LA, Huff JC, Norris DA, Weston WL. The frequency of autoantibodies to the SS-A/Ro antigen in pregnancy sera. *Arthritis Rheum* 1984, 27, S20.

[49] Lee LA. Transient autoimmunity related to maternal autoantibodies: neonatal lupus. *Autoimmun Rev* 2005, 4, 207-213.

[50] McCuistion CH, Schoch Jr EP. Possible discoid lupus erythematosus in newborn infant: report of a case with subsequent development of acute systemic lupus erythematosus in mother. *Arch Dermatol* 1954, 70, 782-785.

[51] Weston WL, Morelli JG, Lee LA. The clinical spectrum of anti-Ro-positive cutaneous neonatal lupus erythematosus. *J Am Acad Dermatol* 1999, 40, 675-681.

[52] David-Bajar KM, Bennion SD, DeSpain JD, Golitz LE, Lee LA. Clinical, histologic, and immunofluorescent distinctions between subacute cutaneous lupus erythematosus and discoid lupus erythematosus. *J Invest Dermatol* 1992, 99, 251-257.

[53] Lee La, Sokol RJ, Buyon JP. Hepatobiliary disease in neonatal lupus: prevalence and clinical characteristics in cases enrolled in a national registry. *Pediatrics* 2002, 109, E11.

[54] Watson R, Kang JE, May M, Hudak M, Kickler T, Provost TT. Thrombocytopenia in the neonatal lupus syndrome. *Arch Dermatol* 1088, 124, 560-563.

[55] Buyon JP, Hiebert R, Copel J, Craft J, Friedman D, Katholi M, Lee LA, Provost TT, Reichlin M, Rider L, Rupel A, Saleeb S, Weston WL, Skovron ML. Autoimmune-associated congenital heart block: demographics, mortality, morbidity and recurrence rates obtained from a national neonatal lupus registry. *J Am Coll Cardiol* 1998, 31, 1658-1666.

[56] Moak JP, Barron KS, Hougen YJ, Wiles HB, Balaji S, Sreeram N, CohenMH, Nordenberg A, Van Hare GF, Friedman RA, PREZ M, Cecchin F, Schneider DS, Nehgme RA, Buyon JP. Congenital heart block: development of late-onset cardiomyopathy, a previously underappreciated sequela. *J Am Coll Cardiol* 2001, 37, 238-242.

[57] Villain E, Coastedoat-Chalumeau N, Marijon E, Boudjemline Y, Piette JC, Bonnet D. Presentation and prognosis of complete atrioventricular block in childhood, according to maternal antibody status. *J Am Coll Cardiol* 2006, 48, 1682-1687.

[58] Neld LE, Silverman ED, Smallhorn JF, Taylor GP, Mullen JBM, Benson LN, Hornberger LK. Endocardial fibroelastosis associated with maternal anti-Ro and anti-La antibodies in the absence of atrioventricular block. *J Am Coll Cardiol* 2002, 40, 796-802.

[59] Brucato A, Jonzon A, Friedman D, Allan LD, Vignati G, Gasparini M, Stein JI, Montella S, Michaelsson M, Buyon J. Proposal for a new definition of congenital complete atrioventricular block. *Lupus* 2003, 12, 427-435.

[60] Buyon JP. Neonatal lupus syndromes. In: Lahita R, editor. *Systemic lupus eruthematosus*, 4th ed. San Diego, CA: Elsevier Academic Press. 2004, 449-484.

[61] Askanase AD, friedman DM, Copel J, Dische MR, Dubin A, starc TJ, Katholi MC, Buyon JP. Spectrum and progression of conduction abnormalities in infant born to mothers with anti-SSa/Ro-SSB/La antibodies. *Lupus* 2002, 11, 145-151.

[62] Brucato A, Frassi M, Franceschini F, Cimaz R, Faden D, Pisoni MP, Muscara M, Vignati G, Stramba-Badiale M, Catelli L, Lojacono A, Cavazzana I, Ghirardello A, Vescovi F, Gambari PF, Doria A, Meroni PL, Tincani A. Risk of congenital complete

heart block in newborns of mothers with anti-Ro/SSA antibodies detected with counterimmunoelectrophoresis: a prospective study of 100 women. *Arthritis Rheum* 2001, 44, 1832-1835.

[63] Costedoat-Chalumeau N, Amoura Z, Lupoglazoff JM, Thi Huong du L, Denjoy I, Vauthier D, Sebbouth D, Fain O, Georgi-Lavialle S, Ghillani P, Musset L, Wechsler B, Duhaut P, Piette JC. Outcome of prgnancies in patients with anti-Ro/SSA antibodies: a study of 165 pregnancies, with special focus on electrocardiographic variations in the children and comparison with a control group. *Arthritis Rheum* 2004, 50, 3187-3194.

[64] Brucato A, Gasparini M, Vignati G, Riccobono S, De Juli E, Quinzanini M, Bortolon C, Coluccio E, Massari D. Isolated congeniital complete heart block: longterm outcome of children and immunogenetic study. *J Rheumatol* 1995, 22, 541-543.

[65] Eronen M, Siren MK, Ekblad H, Tikanoja T, Julkunen H, Paavilainen T. Short- and long-term outcome of children with congenital complete heart block diagnosed in utero or as a newborn. *Pediatrics* 2000, 106, 86-91.

[66] Glickstein JS, Buyon J, Friedman D. Pulsed Doppler echocardiographic assessment of the fetal PR interval. *Am J Cardiol* 2000, 86, 236-239.

[67] Sonesson SE, Salomonsson S, Jacobsson LA, Bremme K, Wahren-Herlenius M. Signs of first-degree heart block occur in one-third of fetuses of pregnant women with anti-SSA/Ro 52-Kd antibodies. *Arthrits Rheum* 2004, 50, 1253-1261.

[68] Friedman D, Buyon J, Copel J, Kim M. PR interval and dexamethasone evaluation: an ongoing prospective fetal echocardiographic study in neonatal lupus. I – observational study. [Abstract] *Lupus* 2004, 13, 760.

[69] Costedoat-Chalumeau N, Amoura Z, Villain E, Cohen L, Piette JC. Anti-SSA/Ro antibodies and the heart: more than complete heart block? A review of electrocardiographic and myocardial abnormalities and treatment optios. *Arthritis Res Ther* 2005, 7, 69-73.

[70] Raboisson MJ, Fouron JC, Sonesson SE, Nyman M, Proulx F, Gamache S. Fetal Doppler echocardiographic diagnosis and successful steroid therapy of Luciani-Wenckebach phenomenon and endocardial fibroelastosis related to maternal anti-Ro and anti-La antibodies. *J Am Soc Echocardiogr* 2005, 18, 375-380.

[71] Groves AMM, Allan LD, Rosenthal E. Outcome of isolated congenital heart block diagnosed in utero. *Heart* 1996, 75, 190-194.

[72] Michaelsson M. Congenital complete atrioventricular block. *Prog Pediatr Cardiol* 1995, 4, 1-7.

[73] Clancy RM, Kapur RP, Molad Y,Askanase AD, Buyon JP. Immunohistological evidence supports apoptosis, IgG deposition, and novel machrophage/fibroblast crosstalk in the pathologic cascade leading to congenital heart block. *Arthritis Rheum* 2004, 50, 173-182.

[74] Ho SY, Esseher E, Anderson RH, Michaelsson M. Anatomy of congenital heart block and relation to maternal anti-Ro antibodies. *Am J Cardiol* 1986, 58, 291 294.

[75] Anderson RH, Wenick ACG, Losekoot TG, Becker AE. Congenitally complete heart block. *Circulation* 1977, 56, 90-98.

[76] Herreman G, Galezewski N. Maternal connective tissue disease and congenital heart block. *N Engl J Med* 1985, 312, 1329

[77] Litsey SE, Noonan JA, O'Connor WN, Cottrill CM, Mitchell B. Maternal connective tissue disease and congenital heart block. Demonstration of immunoglobulin in cardiac tissue. *N Eng J Med* 1985, 312, 98-100.

[78] Lee LA, Coulter S, Erner S, Chu H. Cardiac immunoglobulin deposition in congenital heart block associated with maternal anti-Ro antibody. *Am J Med* 1987, 83, 793-796.

[79] Fesslova V, Mannarino S, Salice P, Boschetto C, Trespidi L, Acaia B, Mosca F, Cimaz R, Meroni PL. Neonatal lupus: fetal myocarditis progressing to atrioventricular block in triplets. *Lupus* 2003, 12, 775-778.

[80] Miranda-Carus ME, Tseng CE, Rashbaum W, Ochs RL, Casiano CA, Di Donato F, Chan EKL, Buyo JP. Accessibility of SSA/Ro and SSB/La antigens to maternal antibodies in apoptotic human fetal cardiac myocytes. *J Immunol* 1998, 161, 5061-5069.

[81] Tran HB, Ohlsson M, Beroukas D, Hiscock J, Bradley J, Buyon JP, Gordon TP. Subcellular redistribution of La(SS-B) autoantigen during physiologic apoptosis in the fetal mouse heart and conduction system: a clue to the pathogenesis of congenital heart block. *Arthritis Rheum* 2002, 46, 202-208.

[82] Clancy RM, Neufing PJ, Zheng P, O'Mahony M, Nimmerjahn F, Gordon TP, Buyon JP. Impaired clearance of apoptotic cardocytes is linked to anti-SSA/Ro and –SSB/La antibodies in the pathoenesis of congenital heart block. *J Clin Invest* 2006, 116, 2413-2422.

[83] Miranda-Carus ME, Askanase AD, Clancy RM, Di Donato F, Chou TM, Libera MR, Chan EKL, Buyon JP. Anti-SSA/Ro and anti-SSB/La autoantibodies bind the surface of apoptotic fetal cardiocytes and promote secretion of tumor necrosis factor α by macrophages. *J Immunol* 2000, 165, 5345-5351.

[84] Clancy RM, Buyon JP. Clearance of apoptotic cells: TGF-beta in the balance between inflammation and fibrosis. *J Leukoc Biol* 2003, 74, 959-960.

[85] Clancy RM, Askanase AD, Kapur RP, Chiopelas E, Azar N, Miranda-Carus ME, Buyon JP. Trandifferentiation of cardiac fibroblasts: a fetal factor in anti-SSA/Ro-SSB/La antibody-mediated congenital heart block. *J Immunol* 2002, 169, 2156-2163.

[86] Awad MR, El-Gamel , Hasleton P, Turner DM, Sinnott PJ, Hutchinson IV. Genotypic variation in the transforming growth factor-beta1 gene: association with transforming growth factor-beta1 production, fibrotic lung disease, and graft fibrosis after lung transplantation. *Transplantation* 1998, 66, 1014-1020.

[87] Clancy RM, Backer CB, Yin X, Kapur RP, Molad Y, Buyon JP. Cytokine polymorphisms and histologic expression in autopsy studies: contribution of TNFα and TGFβ1 to the pathogenesis of autoimmune-associated congenital heart block. *J Immunol* 2003, 171, 3253-3261.

[88] Cimaz R, Borghi MO, Gerosa M, Biggioggero M, Raschi E, Meroni PL. Transforming growth factor beta1 in the pathogenesis of autoimmune congenital complete heart block: lesson from twins and triplets discordant for the disease. *Arthritis Rheum* 2006, 54, 356-359.

[89] Alexander EL, Buyon JP, Provost TT, Guarnieri T. Anti-Ro/SSA antibodies in the pathophysiology of congenital heart block in neonatal lupus syndrome, an experimental model. In vitro electrophysiologic and immunocytochemical studies. *Arthritis Rheum* 1992, 35, 176-189.

[90] Garcia S, Nascimento JHM, Bonfa E, Levey R, Oliveirn SF, Tavares AV, Campos deCarvalho AC. Cellular mechanism of the conduction abnormalities induced by serum from anti-Ro/SSA positive patients in rabbit hearts. *J Clin Invest* 1994, 93, 718-724.
[91] Boutjdir M, Chen L, Zhang ZH, Tseng CE, DiDonato F, Rashbaum W, Morris A, El-Sherif N, Buyon JP. Arrhythogenicity of IgG and anti-52-kD SSA/Ro affinity-purified antibodies from mothers of children with congenital heart block. *Circulation Res* 1997, 80, 354-362.
[92] Boutjdir M, Chen L, Zhang ZH, Tseng CE, El-Sherif N, Buyon JP. Serum and immunoglobulin G from the mother of a child with a congenital heart block induce conduction abnormalities and inhibit L-type calcium channels in a rat heart model. *Pediatr Res* 1998, 44, 11-19.
[93] Xiao GQ, Hu K, Boutjdir M. Direct inhibition of expressed cardiac L- and T-type calcium channels by IgG from mothers whose children have congenital heart block. *Circulation* 2001, 103, 1599-1604.
[94] Cohen NM, Lederer WJ. Calcium current in single human cardiac myocytes. *J Cardiovasc Electrophysiol* 1993, 4, 422-437.
[95] Bkaily G, Sculptureanu A, Jacques D, Economos D, Menard D. Apamin, a highly potent fetal L-type Ca current blocker in single heart cell. *Am J Physiol* 1992, 262, H463-H471.
[96] Qu Y, Boutjdir M. Gene expression of SERCA2a and L-and T-type Ca channels during human heart development. *Pediatr Res* 2001, 50, 569-574.
[97] Maylie JG. Excitation-contraction coupling in neonatal and adult myocardium of cat. *Am J Physiol* 1982, 242, H834-H843.
[98] Qu Y, Xiao GQ, Chen L, Boutjdir M. Autoantibodies from mothers of children with congenital heart block downregulate cardiac L-type Ca channels. *J Mol Cell Cardiol* 2001, 33, 1153-1163.
[99] Xiao GQ, Qu Y, Hu K, Boutjdir M. Down-regulation of L-type calcium channel in pups born to 52 kDa SSA/Ro immunized rabbits. *FASEB J* 2001, 15, 1539-1545.
[100] Salomonsson S, Sonesson SE, Ottoson L, Muhallab S, Olsson T, Sunnerhagen M, Kuchroo VK, Thoren P, Herlenius E, Waheren-Herlenius M. Ro/SSA autoantibodies directly bind cardiomyocytes, disturb calcium homeostasis, and mediate congenital heart block. *J Exp Med* 2005, 201, 11-17.
[101] Julkunen H, Miettinen A, Walle TK, Chan EK, Eronen M. Autoimmune response in mothers with congenital and postnatally diagnosed isolated heart block: a population based study. *J Rheumatol* 2004, 31, 183-189.
[102] Salomonsson S, Dorner T, Theander E, Bremme K, Larsson P, Wharen-Herlenius M. A serologic marker for fetal risk of congenital heart block. *Arthritis Rheum* 2002, 46, 1233-1241.
[103] Fritsch C, Hoebeke J, Dali H, Ricchiuti V, Isenberg DA, Meyer O, Muller S. 52-kDa Ro/SSA epitopes preferentially recognized by antibodies from mothers of children with neonatal lupus and congenital heart block. *Arthritis Res Ther* 2005, 8, R4.
[104] Buyon JP, Clancy R, Di Donato F, Miranda-Carus ME, Askanase AD, Garcia J, Qu Y, Hu K, Yue Y, Chan EKL, Boutjdir M. Cardiac 5-HT_4 serotoninergic receptors, 52 kD SSA/Ro and autoimmune associated congenital heart block. *J Autoimmun* 2002, 19, 79-86.

[105] Eftekhari P, Roegel JC, Lezoualc'h F, Fischmeister R, Imbs JL, Hoebeke J. Induction of neonatal lupus in pups of mice immunized with synthetic peptides derived from amino acid sequences of the serotoninergic 5-HT_4 receptor. *Eur J Immunol* 2001, 31, 573-579.

[106] Blondel O, Vandecasteele G, Gastineau M, Leclerc S, Dahmoune Y, Lonaglois M, Fischmeister R. Molecular and functional characterization of a 5-HT_4 receptor cloned from human atrium. *FEBS Lett* 1997, 412, 465-474.

[107] Ouadid H, Seguin J, Dumuis A, Bockaert J, Nargeot J. Serotonin increases calcium current in human atrial myocytes via the newly described 5-hydroxytryptamine4 receptors. *Mol Pharmacol* 1992, 41, 346-351.

[108] Eftekhari P, Salle L, Lezoualc'h F, Mialet J, Gastineau M, Briand JP, Isenberg DA, Fournie GJ, Argibay J, Fischmeister R, Muller S, Hoebeke J. Anti-SSA/Ro52 autoantibodies blocking the cardiac 5-HT_4 serotoninergic receptor could explain neonatal lupus congenital heart block. *Eur J Immunol* 2000, 30, 2782-2790.

[109] Kamel R, Eftekhari P, Clancy R, Buyon JP, Hoebeke J. Autoantibodies against the serotoninergic 5-HT_4 receptor and congenital heart block: a reassessment. *J Autoimmun* 2005, 25, 72-76.

[110] Restivo M, Kozhevnikov DO, Boutjdir M. Optical mapping of activation patterns in an animal model of congenital heart block. *Am J Physiol Heart Circ Physiol* 2000, 99, 1914-1918.

[111] Mazel JA, El-Sherif N, Buyon JP, Boutjdir M. Electrocardiographic abnormalities in a murine model injected with IgG from mothers of children with congenital heart block. *Circulation* 1999, 99, 1914-1918.

[112] Fox R, Lumb MR, Hawkins DF. Persistent foetal sinus bradycardia associated with maternal anti-Ro/SSA antibodies. Case report. *Br J Obstet Gynaecol* 1990, 97, 1151-1153.

[113] Cimaz R, Airoldi ML, Careddu P, Careddu P, Centinaio G, Catelli L, Franceschini F, Meroni PL. Transient neonatal bradicardia without heart block associated with anti-Ro antibodies. *Lupus* 1997, 6, 487-488.

[114] Menon A, Silverman ED, Gow RM, Hamilton RM. Chronotropic competence of the sinus node in congenital complete heart block. *Am J Cardiol* 1998, 82, 1119-1121.

[115] Brucato A, Cimaz R, Catelli L, Meroni P. Anti-Ro-associated sinus bradicardia in newborns. *Circulation* 2000, 102, E88-E89.

[116] Hu K, Qu Y, Butjdir M. Functional basis of sinus bradycardia in congenital heart block. *Circ Res* 2004, 94, e32-e38.

[117] Brette F, Leroy J, Le Guennec JY, Salle L. Ca2+ currents in cardiac myocytes: old story, new insights. *Prog Biophys Mol Biol* 2006, 91, 1-82.

[118] Qu Y, Baroudi G, Yue Y, Boutjdir M. Novel molecular mechanism involving α_{1D} (Cav 1.3) L-Type calcium channel in autoimmune-associated sinus bradycardia. *Circulation* 2005, 111, 3034-3041.

[119] Schwartz PJ, Stramba-Badiale M, Segantini A, Austoni P, Bosi G, Giorgetti R, Grancini F, Marni ED, Perticone F, Rosti D, Salice P. Prolongation of the QT interval and the sudden infant death sindrome. *N Eng J Med* 1998, 338, 1709-1714.

[120] Esscher E, Michaelsson M. Q-T interval in congenital complete heart block. *Pediatr Cardiol* 1983, 4, 121-124.

[121] Gascho JA, Schieken R. Congenital complete heart block and long Q-T syndrome requiring ventricular pacing for control of refractory ventricular tachycardia and fibrillation. *J Electroardiol* 1979, 12, 331-335.
[122] Pearl W. Stokes-Adams attacks in congenital heart block. *Pediatr Cardiol* 1988, 9, 125-126.
[123] Duke C, Stuart G, Simpson JM. Ventricular tachycardia secondary to prolongation of the QT interval in a fetus with autoimmune mediated congenital heart block. *Cardiol Young* 2005, 15, 319-321.
[124] Cimaz C, Stramba-Badiale M, Brucato A, Catelli L, Panzeri P, Meroni PL. QT interval prolongation in asymptomatic anti-SSA/Ro-positive infants without congenital heart block. *Arthritis Rheum* 2000, 43, 1049-1053.
[125] Cimaz R, Meroni PL, Brucato A, Fesstovà V, Panzeri P, Goulene K, Stramba-Badiale M. Concomitant disappearance of electrocardiographic abnormalities and of acquired maternal autoantibodies during the first year of life in infants who had QT interval prolongation and anti-SSA/Ro positivity without congenital heart block at birth. *Arthritis Rheum* 2003, 48, 266-268.
[126] Gordon PA, Khamashta MA, Hughes GRV, Rosenthal E. Increase in the heart rate-corrected QT interval in children of anti-Ro-positive mothers, with a further increase in those with siblings with congenital heart block. *Arthritis Rheum* 2001, 44, 242-246.
[127] Witchel HJ, Hancox JC. Familial and acquired long QT syndrome and the cardiac rapid delayed rectifier potassium current. *Clin Exp Pharmacol Physiol* 2000, 27, 753-766.
[128] Lee LA, Pickrell MB, Reichlin M. Development of complete heart block in an adult patient with Sjogren's syndrome and anti-Ro/SSA autoantibodies. *Arthritis Rheum* 1996, 39, 1427-1429.
[129] James TN, Rupe CE, Monto RW. Pathology of the cardiac conduction system in systemic lupus erythematosus. *Ann Intern Med* 1965, 63, 402-410.
[130] Moffit GR. Complete atrioventricular dissociation with Stoke-Adams attacks due to disseminated lupus erythematosus: report of a case. *Ann Intern Med* 1965, 63, 508-511.
[131] Bharati S, de la Fuente DJ, Kallen RJ, Freij Y, Lev M. Conduction system in systemic lupus erythematosus with atrioventricular block. *Am J Cardiol* 1975, 35, 299-304.
[132] Wray R, Iveson M. Complete heart block and systemic lupus erythematosus. *Br Heart J* 1975, 37, 982-983.
[133] Meyniel D, Beaufils M, Bouchoucha S, Mayaud C, Akoun G. Bloc auricolo-ventriculaire complet au cors d'une poussée évolutive de lupus érythémateux aigu disséminé. *Presse Med* 1982, 11, 3797-3798.
[134] Maier WP, Ramirez HE, Miller SB. Complete heart block as the initial manifestation of systemic lupus erythematosus. *Arch Intern Med* 1987, 147, 170-171.
[135] Bilazarian SD, Taylor AJ, Brezinski D, Hochberg MC, Guarnieri T, Provost TT. High-grade atrioventricular heart block in an adult with systemic lupus erythematosus: the association of nuclear RNP (U1 RNP) antibodies, a case report, and review of the literature. *Arthritis Rheum*1989, 32, 170-1174.
[136] Martinez-Costa X, Ordi J, Barbera J, Selva A, Bosch J, Vilardell M. High grade atrioventricular heart block in 2 adults with systemic lupus erythmatosus. *J Rheumatol* 1991, 18, 1926-1928.
[137] Mevorach D, Raz E, Shalev O, Steiner I, Ben-Chetrit E. Complete heart block and seizures in an adult with systemic lupus erythematosus. A possible pathophysiologic

role for anti-SS-A/Ro and anti-SS-B/La autoantibodies. *Arthritis Rheum* 1993, 36, 259-262.

[138] Comin-Colet J, Sanchez-Corral MA, Alegre-Sancho JJ, Valverde J, Lopez-Gomez D, Sabate X, Juan-Mas A, Esplugas E. Complete heart block in an adult with systemic lupus erythematosus and recent onset of hydroxychloroquine therapy. *Lupus* 2001, 10, 59-62.

[139] Edwards CS, Mootoo R, Bhanji A. High grade heart block in association with SLE. *Ann Rheum Dis* 2004, 63, 606.

[140] Behan WM, Aitchison M, Behan PO. Pathogenesis of heart block in a fatal case of dermatomyositis. *Br Heart J* 1986, 56, 479-482.

[141] Logar D, Kveder T, Rozman B, Dobovisek J. Possible association between anti-Ro antibodies and myocarditis or cardiac conduction defects in adults with systemic lupus eryhematosus. *Ann Rheum Dis* 1990, 9, 627-629.

[142] Behan WMA, Behan PO, Gairns J. Cardiac damage in polymyositis associated with antibodies to tissue ribonucleoproteins. *Br Heart J* 1987, 57, 176-180.

[143] O'Neill TW, Mahmoud A, Tooke A, Thomas RD, Maddison PJ. Is there a relationship between subclinical myocardial abnormalities, conduction defects and Ro/La antibodies in adults with systemic lupus erythematosus? *Clin Exp Rheumatol* 1993, 11, 409-412.

[144] Gordon PA, Rosenthal E, Khamashta MA, Hughes GR. Absence of conduction defects in the electrocardiograms [correction of echocardiograms] of mothers with children with congenital heart block. *J Rheumatol* 2001, 28, 366-369.

[145] Lodde BM, Sankar V, Kok MR, Leakan RA, Tak PP, Pillemer SR. Adult heart block is associated with disease activity in primary Sjogren's syndrome. *Scand J Rheumatol* 2005, 34, 383-386.

[146] Lazzerini PE, Acampa M, Guideri F, Capecchi PL, Campanella V, Morozzi G, Galeazzi M, Marcolongo R, Laghi Pasini F. Prolongation of the corrected QT interval in adult patients with anti-Ro/SSA-positive connective tissue diseases. *Arthritis Rheum* 2004, 50, 1248-1252.

[147] Huikuri HV, Castellanos A, Myerburg RJ. Sudden death due to cardiac arrhythmias. *N Eng J Med* 2001, 345, 1473-1482.

[148] Costedoat-Chalumeau N, Amoura Z, Hulot JS, et al. Letter in response to "Prolongation of the corrected QT interval in adult patients with anti-Ro/SSA-positive connective tissue diseases" by Lazzerini et al. in Arthritis Rheum 2004; 50: 1248-1252. *Arthritis Rheum* 2005; 52:676-7; author reply 677-678.

[149] Pineau CA, Huynh T, Bernatsky S, St.Pierre Y, Joseph L, Clarke AE. Prolongation of the corrected QT interval in anti-Ro/SSA positive adults with systemic lupus erithematosus. American College of Rheumatology, San Diego (USA) 12-17 november 2005, program number 1213 [Abstract].

[150] Helming H, Brendorp B, Kober L, Sahebzadah N, Torp-Petersen C. QTc interval in the assessment of cardiac risk. *Card Electrophysiol Rev* 2002; 6: 289-294.

[151] Chen CY, Wang FL, Lin CC. Chronic hydroxychloroquine use associated with QT prolongation and refractory ventricular arrhythmia. *Clin Toxicol* 2006, 44, 173-175.

[152] Guideri F, Acampa M, Rechichi S, Capecchi PL, Lazzerini PE, Galeazzi M, Auteri A, Laghi Pasini F. Effects of acute administration of iloprost on the cardiac autonomic nervous system and ventricular repolarisation in patients with systemic sclerosis. *Ann Rheum Dis* 2006, 65, 836-837.

In: Progress in Cardiac Arrhythmia Research
Editor: Ira R. Tarkowicz, pp. 109-124

ISBN: 1-60021-796-6

Chapter 5

Development and Evaluation of a High-Fidelity Simulator Prototype for Electrophysiology

Roberto De Ponti*[*], *Raffaella Marazzi, Fabrizio Caravati and Jorge A. Salerno-Uriarte

Department of Cardiovascular Sciences, University of Insubria, Ospedale di Circolo e Fondazione Macchi, Varese, Italy

Abstract

Background: Advances in clinical electrophysiology should go hand in hand with training of young physicians, so that their theoretical knowledge is complemented by practicing of manual skills. Generally in medicine, training is based on the master-apprentice model. Although the use of simulators for medical training has been already reported, no prior experience on development and use of simulators for electrophysiologic procedures is available.

Methods: Development of an electrophysiology simulator has been planned starting from the Procedicus VIST, previously realized for simulation and training in endovascular procedures. This hybrid simulator consists of a computer connected to an interface unit (the virtual patient), in which catheters or devices are inserted and manipulated in virtual vessels. Catheters are real in their proximal part and simulated in their distal part. Implementation of this system for electrophysiology includes: 1) integration with computed tomography of a normal heart; 2) increase of the number of vascular accesses to place the catheters necessary for an electrophysiology study and consequent adaptation of the simulation software; 3) developing of different modules that simulate electrophysiology procedures with highest priority given to development of the basic catheter placement and trans-septal catheterization modules. Early evaluation of the prototype by a panel of international experts was planned to

* Correspondence concerning this article should be addressed to Dr. Roberto De Ponti, MD, Department of Cardiovascular Sciences, University of Insubria Ospedale di Circolo e Fondazione Macchi, Viale Borri, 57. IT-21100 Varese, Italy. Phone: +39-0332-278934; Mobile: +39-338-6593175; Fax: +39-0332-393309; E-mail: rdeponti@alice.it.

get necessary feedback on simulation quality. Evaluators are required to attribute a score to the different characteristics of the simulation in a 1-5 scale (5 highest).

Results: In the prototype, catheter placement in the coronary sinus and His bundle area and recording of the intracavitary signals from these sites is possible. A complete trans-septal catheterization procedure can be simulated realistically, including complications. For each procedure a report is automatically generated by the system, which provides essential data to evaluate objectively the trainee performance. For each of the characteristics of the trans-septal simulation evaluated by the international panel, the mean score was > 4.0, ranging from 4.0 to 4.4; > 90% of the evaluators agreed that this simulator could be useful for training purposes. Development of other modules to simulate arrhythmia ablation and three-dimensional mapping procedures has been already planned.

Conclusions: Simulation of electrophysiologic procedures is feasible in a realistic and high fidelity prototype. So far, complete simulation has been obtained for basic catheter placement and trans-septal catheterization. The quality of the simulation has been considered satisfactory by an international panel of electrophysiologists. The clinical impact of virtual training will be assessed in prospective randomized studies.

...for distinction sake, a deceiving by words is commonly called a lye, and a deceiving by actions, gestures, or behavior is called simulation....

Robert South, 1697

Introduction

Rationale for Simulator Training

The advances in catheter ablation of cardiac arrhythmias have led to the achievement of a satisfactory success rate in the treatment of complex arrhythmias (such as atrial fibrillation, atypical atrial flutter and ventricular tachycardia associated with organic heart disease) and to offer catheter ablation as the first-line therapy for arrhythmias with a substrate more simple to approach, such as typical atrial flutter, atrioventricular nodal reentrant tachycardia and accessory pathway-mediated arrhythmias [1-4]. Over the last twenty years, these results have been made possible by progressive improvements in technology and by increased operator experience.

In spite of the increased experience and of sophisticated technologies now available, most training in clinical electrophysiology, as well as in other medical disciplines that include invasive procedures, continues in the traditional way, based on the master-apprentice model. In this model, the trainee is exposed to the procedure with the supervision of an experienced physician and he/she is given more independence as time and experience progress. Although this model is time tested, being in use in one form or another since ancient times, several authors express their opinion against continuation of this model and assess that there is room for improvement and even replacement of this training method [5,6]. In fact, traditional training is a relatively static system with the risk of providing an unstructured experience, because of time constraints and random admission of patients, which may prevent trainees from being exposed to the wide range of possible difficulties determined by the combination of different elements. Moreover, the learning process is individual and different trainees require a different amount of time to learn and safely replicate the same procedure. This is against the idea of perpetuating a training model, which usually has a fixed, and pre-determined time period, determined by the learning ability of the "average trainee". In addition, the importance of maintaining the skills acquired during training should not be underestimated, especially in the case of complex procedures, not very often performed in a case mix of some centres. Even in high-volume centres, experienced operators may find it difficult to maintain high-quality performance due to time constraints and the strong commitment to train younger physicians. Finally, both during and at the end of training, it may be difficult [6] to objectively evaluate the performance of the person in training and decide if or when he/she is able to act as the first operator in a given procedure. This difficulty mainly relies on the subjective nature of evaluation and the attitude of evaluators, while it may be hard to judge objectively a supervised performance, in which continuous and, in some cases, subliminal feedback is provided by the mentor to the trainee.

On the other hand, the quality of medical training in interventional procedures is crucial to avoid medical errors, which have been blamed for 44,000 to 98,000 deaths [7] per year only in the United States, being the eighth leading cause of death, exceeding that caused by traffic accidents. Although *"to err is human"* [7], many medical errors are caused by human factors associated with interventional catheter-based or image-guided procedures [8] and, therefore, they are thought to be preventable by appropriate initial training and verification of skills maintenance over time. This is essential to optimize patient safety, achieve and maintain high quality of patient care and decrease the time and costs for management of procedure related complications and the legal expenses.

In trying to assess the usefulness of a simulator-based training, a promising example comes from flight simulators to train pilots and crews. Although medicine and air transportation are obviously different fields, there are some analogies, as, for example, the fact that in both cases a given procedure is made of a sequence of actions, which should be correctly and timely executed and that in both cases the human factors may play a major role in determining errors, possibly resulting in heavy casualties. Flight simulators have been introduced and developed from the beginning in aviation history and now they are a full-size cockpit replica of a given aircraft model, mounted on hydraulic actuators. They are used not only for training of the candidate pilots, but they are also of crucial importance to train all pilots for emergencies (e.g.: loss of flight control surfaces, complete engine failures and loss of pressurization) that, although of rare occurrence, may be at the base of several accidents. Currently, training on a flight simulator is an essential element for individual pilots and flight crews, and it has been instrumental in reducing errors [9].

Use of Simulators in Medicine

In the wide spectrum of medical practice, basically three different types of simulation can be developed for learning and training purpose. The first is represented by an interactive computer program, which presents different clinical scenarios and guides a process of interactive learning through assessment, evaluation, decision-making and error correction, which usually results in a stronger learning environment than the one of passive learning. This can be used to train individual physician or medical team. The second type is a physical simulator, in which physical objects are substituted for a given human apparatus or operative field. Although this type allows interaction with the trainee to reproduce a given medical procedure and is usually very cheap, it provides a low-fidelity simulation, being not very lifelike. The third type is a hybrid high-fidelity simulator, in which a dedicated computer is combined with a life size mannequin, representing the virtual patient. Especially in catheter-based procedures, this type of simulator, in addition to allowing interaction with the trainee, is able to realistically reproduce a given procedure providing a tactile feed-back to the trainee and to generate a final report to objectively evaluate the trainee performance.

In surgery and interventional procedures, the possibility to develop a simulator which precisely reproduces reality mainly depends on the technology available and the type of procedure to reproduce. However, the original idea that only a simulator that looked and felt like a real patient could substitute for the clinical in-vivo training was wrong. In fact, training on a low-fidelity virtual reality model, as the laparoscopic box trainer, resulted in fewer intraoperative errors been made when performing laparoscopic cholecistectomy by residents who had been trained on this tool, as compared to residents who had not benefit of simulation training [10,11]. On the other hand, the quality standard required for simulation depends on the type of the procedures and on the trainee level. In fact, it has been demonstrated that fidelity is less important at a relatively junior level. In a group of last year medical students, the use of simulator training significantly improved the performance in endoscopic urology with the task of removing a ureteral stone, as compared to the control group, who received only a video-assisted didactic training [12]. Interestingly, there was no statistically significant difference between simulator training using a low-fidelity simulator (basically, an inverted coffee cup for the bladder with two embedded straws for the ureters, of the cost of Canadian $ 20) and the training with a computer-based high-fidelity simulator, whose cost was Canadian $ 3,700. Moreover, the fidelity of the simulation should be correlated to the complexity of the procedure and the possibility of immediate risk for the patient. In complex procedures with a high risk of immediate procedure-related complications for the patient, the quality of the simulator should be necessarily high, especially if the simulator is not intended for exclusive use of novice, but could serve also for senior physician to rehearse a particularly difficult and rare procedure, before doing the actual procedure [5].

Certainly, open surgical procedures are more difficult to simulate [13] than image-based or catheter-based procedure, such as laparoscopy [14,15], urologic endoscopy [12], gastrointestinal endoscopy [16] and endovascular procedures [17]. As demonstrated by the use of a laparoscopic simulator, which resulted in a detectable benefit for learners in the clinical settings [14,15], there is, so far, stronger evidence that virtual reality training is more useful for minimally invasive surgery than for more traditional open procedures. Particularly in the field of endovascular procedures, a high-fidelity simulator for carotid stenting proved very effective in preliminarily assessing baseline physician experience in endovascular procedures and in improving the operators' performance, although in this study the untrained physicians benefit more from simulator training as compared to individuals with previous endovascular experience [17]. Since this simulator realistically reproduces the approach on an actual patient and it is able to distinguish correct from incorrect procedures so that an objective evaluation of every trainee performance can be given in order to improve and shorten the learning process, in 2004 a Food and Drug Administration panel recommended the use of virtual reality simulation as an important component of a training package for carotid artery stenting [18].

Simulator for Electrophysiology Training: Is It Really Needed?

Over the last 20 years, the electrophysiologic scenario has drastically changed and in modern interventional electrophysiology theoretical knowledge of the mechanism and of the elements of differential diagnosis of cardiac arrhythmias should be complemented with manual skills, necessary to maneuver guide-wires, long sheaths and catheters. In some cases, counterintuitive movements are required and in most of the cases a two dimensional fluoroscopic image is the only guidance to assess the positioning of a given tool inside a heart chamber. This requires the operator to develop a particular sensitivity to safely perform both apparently simple procedures, such as basic catheter placement, and more complex procedures, such as trans-septal catheterization and left atrial ablation for atrial fibrillation. The latter procedures require a specific expertise, since a complex sequence of actions has to be correctly and timely performed, with the risk of immediately developing life-threatening complications in case of incorrect procedure execution. Obviously, it takes time to master in this practice with a long period of apprenticeship, during which the patient is exposed to a risk of complications higher than average. Moreover, comprehension and correct application of all theoretical fundamentals for a proper diagnosis and a successful treatment of cardiac arrhythmias should be tested in the real life, while the operator is involved in long-lasting and tiring procedures, in order to avoid the "learning by burning" process, which is an approach no longer acceptable in routine cases.

All these issues render the training in interventional electrophysiology long and demanding, as widely recognized by the guidelines for specialized training in electrophysiology, endorsed by the Heart Rhythm Society [19]. These guidelines recommend the fourth year of the cardiology training to be dedicated in clinical cardiac electrophysiology, but they also report that it is common for trainees to extend this period to 24 months for an additional training to gain more expertise, due to complexity of the field and the growing amount of information and new procedures. Moreover, these guidelines do not establish the optimal number of procedures to be performed during training, but they only give the minimum number of procedures to complete interventional electrophysiology training. This includes 150 electrophysiologic studies, 75 catheter ablation and 10 trans-septal catheterization procedures, while no numeric guidelines have been established yet for atrial fibrillation ablation, but participation in 30-50 mentored procedures is anticipated. At the same time, this document recognizes that trainees who wish to become skilled in some of the more complex electrophysiology procedures would benefit from a longer period of training or post-training mentored practice. The fact that, due to the rapid evolution of new mapping technologies, it is unlike that the trainee is exposed to all mapping technologies is also underlined. Finally, expertise in all theoretical and practical aspects must be ensured by the electrophysiology program director, who should keep adequate records of each individual training experience and performance in various procedures.

Based on all these considerations, the use of a simulator in interventional electrophysiology could respond to the following needs: 1) increased patient safety, avoiding exposure to the early learning curve of each trainee; 2) shortening of the training time, with the possibility of intensive training on simulator with a higher number of procedures being performed in a shorter time than those possible in real patients even in high volume centres; 3) adequate and complete case and procedure mix, with exposure of the trainee to a wide range of possible procedures, from the most simple (as the basic catheter placement) to the toughest (as trans-septal catheterization and atrial fibrillation ablation in the left atrium); 4) possibility of the training director to objectively evaluate trainee performance before going to the real patient. Although training on simulator cannot be the substitute for years of clinical practice, a considerable role in the early training stage and in some particular procedures can be expected.

In this chapter, the results of the first steps in the development of a high-fidelity simulator for electrophysiology procedures are reported. Although the project is still ongoing and only a part has been completed, the preliminary data are quite promising and encouraging.

Method to Develop and Evaluate a Simulator for Electrophysiology

Choosing the Type of Simulator

For all the above considerations a simulator for electrophysiology should allow interaction between the trainee and the virtual patient and, at the same time, a high-fidelity simulation is needed both for the complexity and precision required in electrophysiology procedures. For this reason, the option of developing a physical simulator was originally ruled out and a hybrid model, in which a computer with a dedicated software is combined with an interface device, acting as the virtual patient, was chosen. The Procedicus Vascular Interventional System Trainer (VIST) by Mentice AB, Gothenburg, Sweden (figure 1) was considered as the base to develop the electrophysiology simulator in cooperation with Biosense-Webster, Inc., Diamond Bar, CA, USA. So far, this device has been developed for endovascular procedures, mainly for carotid artery stenting [20], although versions for coronary angiography and stenting and for over-the-wire delivery of the coronary sinus lead in biventricular pacing exist.

The Procedicus VIST is a multimedia device. The computer is a dual 2.8 GHz processor Pentium IV desktop personal computer running Microsoft Windows XP professional with 1 GB RAM, a 40 GB hard disk drive, a GeForce FX5200 128 MB graphic card and two 17-inch flat panel monitors. The computer runs a dedicated software, which contains a three-dimensional representation of the human arterial system and is coupled to an interface device, whose external aspect resembles a patient lying on the bed, as shown in figure 1. All guide-wires, catheters and other devices selected on the computer and introduced in an arterial access on the mannequin are visualized on one of the two flat panel monitor as a virtual fluoroscopy image, when the fluoroscopy or cine-loop pedal is pressed. The second monitor has a touch screen and is used for utilities, such as selection of the type and shape of the device to be inserted and of the fluoroscopic projection. Following the virtual fluoroscopy, a preselected tool can be advanced and manipulated in the virtual vessels. Also dye injection through the tool lumen can be simulated by injecting a flow of air from a syringe connected to the system. Every tool inserted in the device is real in its proximal part, while the distal part, including the different shapes, dimensions and type of guide-wires or catheters, is totally simulated. The movements of a given tool, as it appears on the virtual fluoroscopy, are the results of interaction between the software and the force and rotations applied by the operator to the tool inserted in a dedicated cart connected to a given access on the virtual patient. In fact, the forces applied to the clinical tools are sensed by strain gage sensors, fitted between a cart base and a suspended mechanism that becomes locked to the tool. The resolution of the force measurement system is 0.025 N, with a span of the force measurement of ±2.5 N. The tool diameters are measured with an infrared optical sensor that gives a resolution of 0.02 mm and has a precision of about ±15%. The tool rotation is measured by an optical encoder that gives a resolution of 7.9 to 31.4 milliradiants. Therefore, the combination of real clinical tools in the operator's hand and tactile and visual feedback obtained on the virtual patient results in a very realistic and high quality simulation of carotid angiography. Finally, in order to assess the quality of each performance and the improvement of the trainee's performance over time [20], the system generates a per-procedure report, which lists static metrics, such as procedure time, fluoroscopy time, contrast volume, cine-loop recordings, and dynamic metrics, including all the pre-defined catheter handling errors. Catheter handling errors can be also notified to the operator in real-time during the procedure by a flashing red triangle with error description appearing on the fluoroscopic screen.

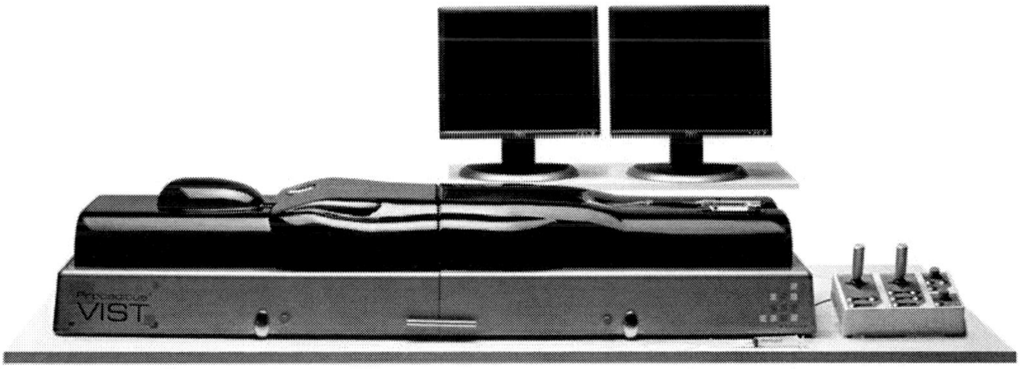

Figure 1. The interface device representing the virtual patient of the Procedicus Vascular Interventional System Trainer, used for simulation of endovascular procedures.

Modification of the Procedicus VIST for Electrophysiology Simulation

For the purpose of electrophysiology training, the software of the Procedics VIST had to include also the venous system and access to all four heart chamber. The heart model was obtained by processing a dynamic acquisition of computed tomography scan of a normal human heart. Heartbeat was simulated in an endless loop at 80 beats per minute.

The peripheral accesses were implemented by adding: 1) two venous accesses from the right femoral vein; 2) one venous access to the left subclavian vein; 3) one arterial access from the left femoral artery. From the superior and inferior vena cava, it should be possible to enter the right atrium and ventricle, the coronary sinus and the left atrium, after trans-septal puncture. It should be also possible to enter the left ventricle with a retrograde trans-aortic approach.

It was planned also to split the screen used to visualize fluoroscopy in two panels: the left panel should visualize, as in the previous version, real time virtual fluoroscopy in different projections, while the right one should be customized to show in a sweeping mode surface electrocardiogram, intracavitary recordings and a pressure line.

Different clinical tools should be included in the electrophysiology version, such as: 1) diagnostic tetrapolar and decapolar catheters; 2) ablation steerable catheters and 3) trans-septal assembly, which includes a long guide-wire, the trans-septal sheath and dilator and the Brockenbrough needle.

Planning the Simulation Modules

The main advantage of building a computer-based simulator is the possibility to develop a modular program, in which different modules, each one representing a given type of procedure, can be separately (concurrently or sequentially) developed. Due to the complexity and the variety of electrophysiology procedures, five different modules were planned: 1) basic catheter positioning; 2) standard supraventricular arrhythmia ablation; 3) trans-septal catheterization; 4) ablation of complex arrhythmia (excluding atrial fibrillation) guided by three-dimensional mapping; 5) atrial fibrillation ablation in the left atrium.

Since the possibility of concurrent development of all modules was considered unlikely and a step-by-step development from more simple to more complex modules was thought to be easier, priority was given to the basic catheter positioning and the trans-septal catheterization modules. Particularly, priority to the last one was established also on the urgent need for specific training in this procedure, whose increase over the last few years is correlated to the unparalleled increase of left atrial ablation for atrial fibrillation [21]. For the basic module a 6 F tetrapolar (Avail, Biosense-Webster, Inc., USA) catheter with Cournand and Josephson shape and 5F decapolar catheter (Supra CS, Biosense-Webster, Inc., USA) were chosen. For the trans-septal module the tools were as follows: a 0.032'' 150 cm long guide-wire, a 6F pig-tail catheter, an 8F trans-septal assembly (Preface Multipurpose, Biosense-Webster, USA), an 18 gauge Brockenbrough needle with two different curves (Medtronic, Inc, USA)

Evaluation of the Simulation Quality

In different centres all over the world, the way to perform some electrophysiologic procedures, especially the more complex ones, may have minor, but not negligible, variants. Moreover, the concept of high-fidelity simulation is very subjective and the perception of the simulation quality may vary among different electrophysiologists. For these reasons, it was initially decided that the prototype had to be evaluated by an international panel of electrophysiologists to assess the quality of simulation and its adaptability to the procedure variants. Although early evaluation has the limitation of receiving the feedback on an incomplete version of the simulator, it was considered essential to identify major limitations or poor quality features at an early stage, so that they can be timely corrected during further development. To this purpose, a detailed feedback was asked to an international panel of electrophysiologists, who were required to test the first prototype with the two initial modules and complete a questionnaire. This questionnaire consisted mainly of nine questions. They are reported in Table 1 and they mainly focus on the characteristics of the trans-septal module. In questions 3 and 9, the evaluators could respond yes or no, whereas in all the other questions a score from 1-5 (5 highest) had to be given. For each of the evaluated characteristics, an average score higher than 3.5 was considered satisfactory. Each evaluator could perform as many procedures as he deemed necessary to give an appropriate feedback of the system. No compensation was provided to the panel for this service.

Table 1. Questionnaire for evaluation of the simulator prototype

1. DOES THE **ANATOMY** OF THE SIMULATOR APPROPRIATELY REPRESENT THE TRUE ANATOMY OF THE RIGHT ATRIUM AND THE FOSSA OVALIS?
2. DOES THE **WORKFLOW** (FLOW OF TASKS) ENCOUNTERED WITH THE SIMULATOR CORRECTLY REPRESENT THE WORKFLOW THAT YOU ENCOUNTER IN A REAL CASE? (E.G. CAN YOU INJECT, INTRODUCE A WIRE, ETC?)
3. ARE YOU SATISFIED WITH THE SIMULATOR **TOOLS/COMPONENTS** REPRESENTING 'REAL LIFE' TOOLS THAT YOU USE IN YOUR TRANS-SEPTAL CASES?
4. DO YOU AGREE THAT THE **SITE OF PUNCTURE** AND THE EXCHANGE OF TOOLS (AT THE SITE OF PUNCTURE) SIMULATE A REAL-LIFE PROCEDURE?
5. DOES THE INSERTION OF THE SHEATH IN THE RIGHT ATRIUM PROVIDE YOU WITH GOOD ENOUGH FORCE FEEDBACK TO SIMULATE THE '**JUMP**' OVER THE UPPER RIDGE OF THE FOSSA OVALIS?
6. DOES THE SIMULATOR PROVIDE YOU WITH ENOUGH INFORMATION TO ALLOW YOU TO REALIZE THAT YOU HAVE **CROSSED** OVER TO THE **LEFT SIDE**?
7. IS THE **INFORMATION** RECEIVED FROM THE SIMULATOR (PARAMETERS, IMAGES, ETC) PROVIDED TO YOU AT THE RIGHT TIME DURING THE SIMULATED PROCEDURE?
8. PLEASE RATE YOUR **OVERALL SATISFACTION** WITH THE SIMULATOR'S PERFORMANCE
9. WOULD YOU RECOMMEND THIS SIMULATOR AS A **TRAINING TOOL** FOR TRANS - SEPTAL PUNCTURE?

Results: The Prototype

Basic Module

This module allows insertion through a venous femoral or subclavian access, manipulation and positioning of tetrapolar/decapolar catheters in the coronary sinus and His bundle area (figure 2 A-B). A real time sweeping surface ECG tracing appears on the top of the right hand side of the screen; the real time sweeping tracings of the coronary sinus and His bundle electrograms appear only when the catheters are correctly placed. Alternatively, the coronary sinus can be cannulated also using the inferior vena cava approach. Each catheter can be continuously tracked on fluoroscopy from the insertion site to the site of correct positioning, using the "tip-follow-up"_option or by manually moving the virtual table using the dedicated joystick. Standard (antero-posterior, 30° right anterior oblique, 30° left anterior oblique views) and any other customized fluoroscopic projection can be used. The fluoroscopic image can be shown as positive or negative and three-dimensional anatomy of the heart and vessels together with the marker of His bundle position can be optionally superimposed. Fluoroscopy time and procedure time are visualized on-line.

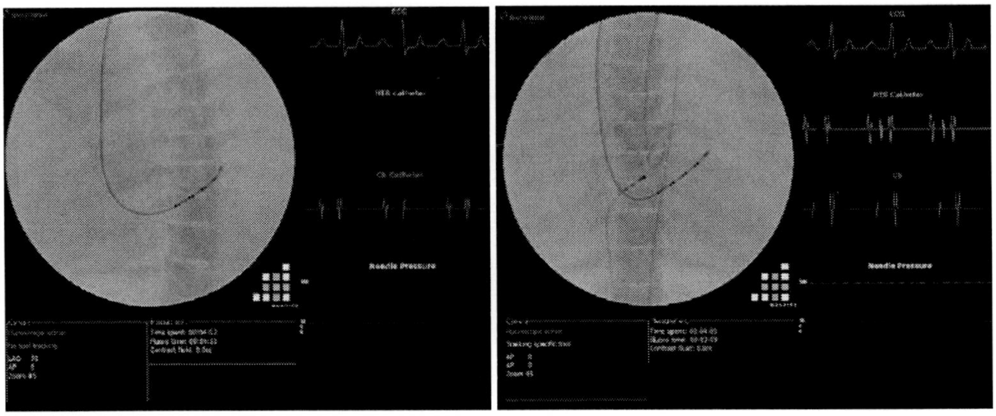

A B

Figure 2. A-B. Display of the main screen of the prototype of the electrophysiology simulator, showing basic catheter placement. In this as in the following figures, the right side of the screen shows real time fluoroscopy including some metrics, such as fluoroscopy time, procedure time and current fluoroscopic projection; the left side of the screen displays sweeping surface and intracavitary recordings, from top to bottom, surface electrocardiogram, His bundle electrogram recording, coronary sinus recording and pressure recording from the Brockenbrough needle lumen. A. Using the left subclavian approach, the 5 F decapolar catheter has been positioned in the coronary sinus, as confirmed in this 30° left anterior oblique fluoroscopic view; signal recorded in the coronary sinus is shown in the third line (in red). B. In this antero-posterior fluoroscopic view, the 6 F tetrapolar catheter is positioned in the His bundle area and the His bundle electrogram is now displayed in the second line (in pale blue). A pig-tail catheter can be optionally positioned in the aortic root, in order to identify the aortic valve plane before trans-septal catheterization is performed.

Trans-Septal Module

The trans-septal catheterization procedure can be performed starting from basic catheter positioning in the coronary sinus and His bundle area, or having these catheters already positioned. Optionally, a pigtail catheter can be positioned in the aortic root, using the left femoral arterial access. The on-line recording of the pressure measured through the Brockenbrough needle lumen is shown in real time on the monitor. Dye injection is possible through the lumen of the needle, dilator or trans-septal sheath.

The whole procedure can be simulated. First the 0.032'' guide-wire is advanced to the superior vena cava (figure 3 A) and the trans-septal sheath is advanced over the wire (figure 3 B). After guide-wire removal and flush of the dilator lumen, the Brockenbrough needle is inserted. Afterwards, the trans-septal assembly is withdrawn from the superior vena cava to the right atrium, while the needle indicator is rotated to 4-4.5 o'clock. During this phase, a right atrial pressure is recorded from the needle lumen and displayed on the monitor; similarly, needle rotation can be continuously monitored on the screen (figure 4 A). Upon engagement of the fossa ovalis, the tip of the trans-septal assembly suddenly moves leftward, with the typical

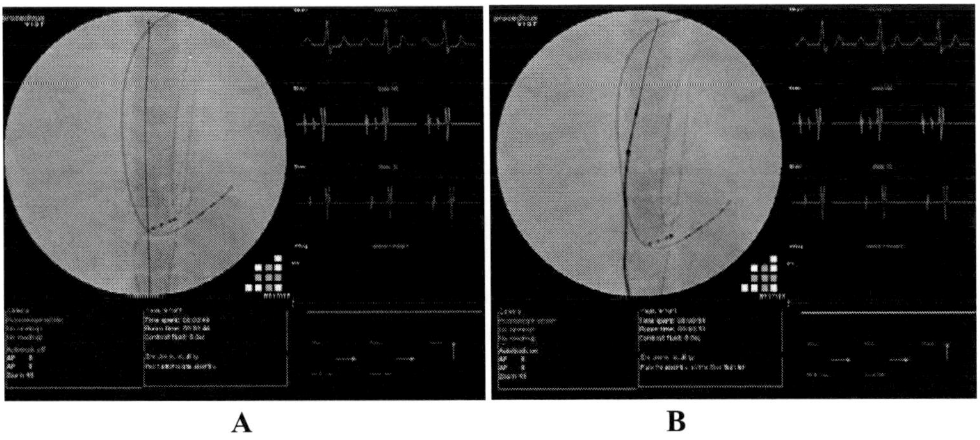

Figure 3. A-B. Display of the main screen of the simulator prototype, during the initial phase of trans-septal catheterization procedure, when all the other catheters have been already positioned. A. A 0.032'' long guide-wire has been advanced from the right femoral vein to the superior vena cava. B. The trans-septal sheath and dilator are advanced to the superior vena cava over the wire.

"jump" observed during the real procedure. Correct positioning and orientation of the assembly tip can be checked in different fluoroscopic projections, as shown in figure 4 A-C. At this point, before atrial septal puncture, "tattoo" of the fossa ovalis by dye injection can be optionally made. Afterwards, the needle is protruded and the whole assembly advanced to intent the fossa ovalis. When fossa perforation occurs, a left atrial pressure appears, as shown in figure 5. The correct positioning of the needle in the left atrium can be also checked by dye injection through the needle lumen. Throughout the procedure, every injection must be preceded by proper aspiration and flush of the lumen. Both the dilator and the trans-septal sheath can be advanced in the left atrium and further check by dye injection is possible.

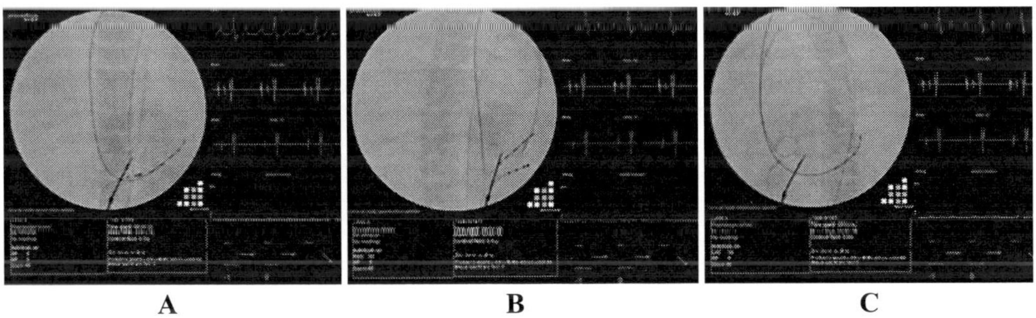

Figure 4. A-C. Display of the main screen of the simulator prototype, during trans-septal electrophysiologic procedure, when, after withdrawal from the superior vena cava, the assembly tip engages the fossa ovalis. A. In the antero-posterior view, the tip of the assembly engages and intents the fossa ovalis; the needle is still inside the dilator lumen and a right atrial pressure is recorded (fourth line, in yellow). In the next procedural step, the needle will be protruded, as the operator fully inserts it in the dilator. In the right inferior corner of the screen, from left to right the three green arrows indicate the orientation of the trans-septal sheath and dilator (both at 3 o'clock) and of the Brockenbrough needle (at 4 o'clock). B and C. Display of the same catheter positioning in 30° right and left anterior oblique projection, respectively.

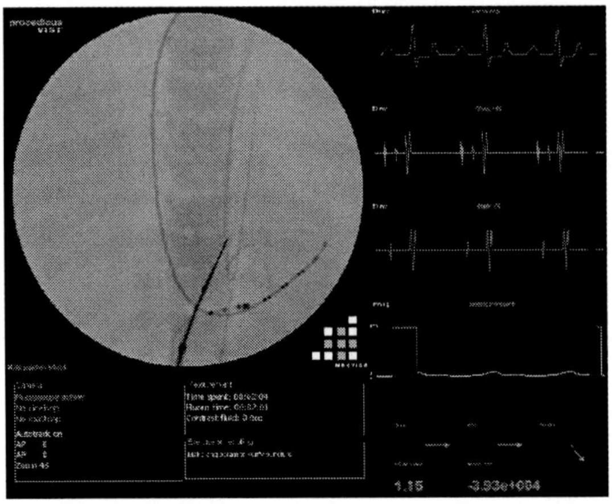

Figure 5. Display of the main screen of the simulator prototype upon atrial septal puncture. In antero-posterior view, the needle was protruded and the atrial septum has just been punctured. The pressure line shows now a left atrial pressure recording (fourth tracing on the right hand side).

In the prototype, two types of anatomy of the fossa ovalis can be selected without the trainee being notified: a normal fossa and a "hard" fossa, more resistant to puncture and, therefore, requiring more pressure to be penetrated. In the next step of development, not only more variants of fossa ovalis anatomy will be included, but at least ten different heart anatomies will also be included. These will be selected among a library of true cases, who underwent the procedure in our laboratory and had a pre-procedure computed tomography scan with the purpose of evaluating the left atrium and pulmonary veins.

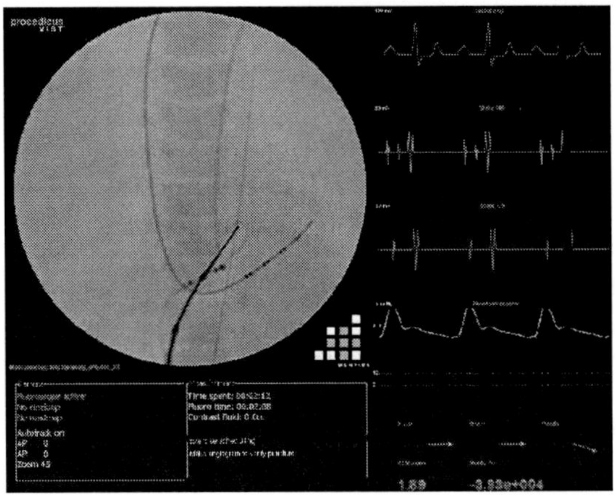

Figure 6. Display of the main screen of the simulator prototype during inadvertent puncture of the aortic root. The trans-septal assembly had been incorrectly withdrawn with needle rotation at roughly 3 o'clock (see the arrow), had missed the fossa ovalis and positioned in the anterior atrial septum. The operator, not having realized the incorrect position of the assembly both in antero-posterior and oblique projections, protruded the needle and advanced the assembly producing needle puncture of the aortic root, as assessed by the arterial pressure recorded through the needle lumen (fourth tracing on the right hand side).

Simulation of major complications is also possible. If the assembly is incorrectly withdrawn from the superior vena cava with the needle rotated at 3 o'clock, the fossa ovalis is not engaged and the assembly tip points anteriorly, towards the aortic root. At this point, if the operator does not realize this incorrect positioning and the needle is protruded and the whole assembly advanced, the aortic root is punctured, as shown in figure 6. In this case, aortic pressure is recorded and the dye injected from the needle lumen visualizes the ascending aorta. Puncture of the atrial free wall is also possible with disappearance of the atrial pressure and visualization of the pericardial space by dye injection. Finally, the system requires proper aspiration and flush of the lumen before every dye injection. In case this is not performed once the needle or the dilator are in the left atrium, this action is considered as a major complication, since occurrence of air embolism is possible at this point.

The system allows creating a "course" for each participant to the training session. This is an archive of all the procedures performed by every trainee, with every procedure summary reporting static metrics, such as fluoroscopy and procedure time, amount of contrast used, and handling errors, such as incorrect rotation of the assembly and needle, injecting without aspiration, distance of the puncture from the centre of the fossa ovalis and excessive insertion of the needle/assembly in the left atrium. Keeping consistent records of all the procedures performed independently by a trainee after initial tutoring may provide data to objectively evaluate the performance, avoiding the risk that the individual performance is influenced, even subliminally, by the presence of an expert electrophysiology. In this way, the decision of promoting a trainee to act as the first operator in a real procedure can be taken on objective and solid data. Similarly, a recurrent error, made repeatedly by a trainee, can be identified and corrected before the real procedure.

The reliability and the software stability have been intensively tested during a two-day session. During this trial, ninety-three procedure where consecutively performed with no system failure and only the need for tool recalibration (a routine operation) after the fifty-second procedure.

Table 2. Average and range values of the score attributed to each of the characteristics of the trans-septal simulation by the international panel of electrophysiologists

Characteristic to be evaluated	Score (range) - all participants	Score (range) - expert EP	Score (range) - other EP
Q1-RA and FO anatomy	4.2 (1-5)	3.9 (1-5)	4.3 (2-5)
Q2-Workflow	4.4 (2-5)	4.4 (2-5)	4.4 (2-5)
Q4-Site of AS puncture	4.3 (2-5)	4.2 (2-5)	4.3 (2-5)
Q5-Force feed-back/"jump" in the FO	4.1 (1-5)	4.0 (1-5)	4.1 (1-5)
Q6-Cross-over to LA	4.0 (1-5)	3.8 (1-5)	4.1 (2-5)
Q7-Information timing	4.4 (3-5)	4.6 (4-5)	4.3 (3-5)
Q8-Overall satisfaction	4.3 (2-5)	4.1 (2-5)	4.4 (2-5)

Abbreviations: AS= atrial septum, EP= electrophysiologists, FO= fossa ovalis, LA= left atrium, RA= right atrium, Q= question (question numbers refer to Table 1.)

Evaluation by the International Panel of Electrophysiologists

The international panel of electrophysiologists consisted of 33 individuals from 14 countries and 4 continents. On average, 2.8 procedures per evaluator were performed. Among these 33 physicians, 9 were considered experts according to the yearly number of procedures performed and the years of experience.

Table 2 shows the average and range values for each of the seven characteristics requiring a score with data subanalysis according to the experience of the evaluators. For each characteristic and for each group of evaluators, the average score was well above the pre-defined cut-off limit of 3.5, suggesting that the quality of simulation was generally considered satisfactory. As expected, the overall satisfaction was lower in the group of experts as compared to other electrophysiologists. The major difference between the two groups of evaluators concerned mainly the anatomy of the fossa ovalis and right atrium and the crossover of the assembly to the left atrium, since the group of experts considered this part of the simulation less satisfactory than the other electrophysiologists. Conversely, the group of experts was on average more satisfied than the group of other electrophysiologists about the timing and flow of information received by the simulator during the procedure.

Finally, 26/33 of the evaluators (78.8%) were satisfied with the tools used in the simulator to reproduce "real life" tools and 31/33 (93.4%) agreed that this simulator module could be used for training in trans-septal catheterization.

Conclusion

The complex field of electrophysiology is becoming more complex over time with the introduction of new and particular procedures that, on one hand, can increase the success rate in the management of complex arrhythmias, while, on the other, render the training period more demanding and prolonged. In this scenario, the training model of master-apprentice has several limitations and does not necessarily allow objective evaluation of the trainee performance.

As in other medical disciplines, the use of simulators in electrophysiology training has a solid rationale. For the complexity of electrophysiology a high-quality hybrid simulator seems necessary and a step-by-step approach with development of a modular structure for different procedures is definitely needed. The first step in the development of this simulator has led to realization of a prototype. Although incomplete, this early version gives the possibility to realistically simulate basic catheter placement and trans-septal catheterization. Although there is room for improvement, especially for the anatomy and tactile feedback during advancing of the trans-septal assembly to the left atrium, third party evaluation achieved satisfactory results. This is encouraging for further development of this prototype.

In the future, a key-issue is to demonstrate whether the skills obtained by the trainee in the virtual reality training can be transposed into clinical practice. To this purpose, prospective randomized and controlled studies using the trans-septal simulation module are in the start-up phase and will involve both novice and beginners in this procedure. Their primary objective is to assess the difference in performance in the clinical practice of conventional training versus simulator training. Secondary objectives are time required for training and the confidence of the trainee in the procedure.

References

[1] Natale A, Newby KH, Pisanò E, Leonelli F, Fanelli R, Potenza D, Beheiry S, Tommassoni G. Prospective randomized comparison of antiarrhythmic therapy versus first-line radiofrequency ablation in patients with atrial flutter. *J Am Coll Cardiol* 2000; 35: 1898-1904.

[2] Cheng CH, Sanders GD, Hlatky MA, Heidenreich P, McDonald KM, Lee BK, Larson MS, Owens DK. Cost-effectiveness of radiofrequency ablation for supraventricular tachycardia. *Ann Intern Med* 2000; 133: 864-76.

[3] Blomstrom-Lundqvist C, Scheinman MM, Aliot EM, Alpert JS, Calkins H, Camm AJ, Campbell WB, Haines DE, Kuck KH, Lerman BB, Miller DD, Shaeffer W, Stevenson WG, Tomaselli GF, Antman EM, Smith SC Jr, Faxon DP, Fuster V, Gibbons RJ, Gregoratos G, Hiratzka LF, Hunt SA, Jacobs AK, Russell RO Jr, Priori SG, Blanc JJ, Budaj A, Burgos EF, Cowie M, Deckers JW, Garcia MA, Klein WW, Lekakis J, Lindahl B, Mazzotta G, Morais JC, Oto A, Smiseth O, Trappe HJ, European Society of Cardiology Committee, NASPE-Heart Rhythm Society. ACC/AHA/ESC guidelines for the management of patients with supraventricular arrhythmias-executive summary. A report of the American College of Cardiology/America Heart Association and the European Society of Cardiology Committee for practice guidelines developed in collaboration with NASPE-Hart Rhythm Society. *J Am Coll Cardiol* 2003; 42: 1493-531.

[4] Da Costa A, Thevenin J, Roche F, Romeyer-Bouchard C, Abdellaoui L, Messier M, Denis L, Faure E, Gonthier R, Kruszynski G Pages JM, Bonijoly S, Lamaison D, Defaye P, Barthelemy JC, Gouttard T, Isaaz K, Loire-Ardeche-Drome-Isere-Puy-de-Dome Trial of Atrial Flutter Investigators. Results from the Loire-Ardeche-Drome-Isere-Puy-de-Dome (LAPID) trial on atrial flutter, a multicentric prospective randomized study comparing amiodarone and radiofrequency ablation after the first episode of symptomatic atrial flutter. *Circulation* 2006; 114: 1670-72.

[5] Gallagher AG, Cates CU. Virtual reality training for the operating room and cardiac catheterisation laboratory. *Lancet* 2004; 364: 1538-40.

[6] Patel AA, Gould DA. Simulators in interventional radiology training and evaluation: a paradigm shift is on the horizon. *J Vasc Interv Radiol* 2006; 17: S163-73.

[7] Kohn JT, Corrigan JM, Donaldson MS. *To err is human: building a safer health system.* Washington DC, Institute of Medicine, 1999.

[8] Cuschieri A. The dawn of a new century: reflections on surgical issues. *Surg Endosc* 2000; 14: 1-4.

[9] Helmreich RL. Managing human error in aviation. *Sci Am* 1997; 276: 62-7.

[10] Seymour NE, Gallagher AG, Roman SA, O'Brien MK, Bansal VK, Andersen DK, Satava RM. Virtual reality training improves operating room performance: results of a randomized, double-blinded study. *Ann Surg* 2002; 236: 458-63.

[11] Grantcharov TP, Kristiansen VB, Bendix J, Bardram L, Rosenberg J, Funch-Jensen P. Randomized clinical trial of virtual reality simulation for laparoscopic skills training. *Br J Surg* 2004; 91: 146-50.

[12] Matsumoto ED, Hamstra SJ, Radomski SB, Cusimano MD. The effect of bench model fidelity on endourological skills: a randomized controlled study. *J Urol* 2002; 167: 1243-47.

[13]Seymour NE, Rotnes JS. Challenges to the development of complex virtual reality surgical simulations. *Surg Endosc* 2006; 20: 1774-1777.

[14]Fried GM, Feldman LS, Vassiliou MC, Fraser SA, Stanbridge D, Ghitulescu G, Andrew CG._Proving the value of simulation in laparoscopic surgery. *Ann Surg* 2004; 240: 518-28.

[15]Scott DJ, Bergen PC, Rege RV, Laycock R, Tesfay ST, Valentine RJ, Euhus DM, Jeyarajah DR, Thompson WM, Jones DB. Laparoscopic training on bench models: better and more cost effective than operating room experience? *J Am Coll Surg* 2000; 191: 272-83.

[16]Ritter EM, McClusky III DA, Lederman AB, Gallagher AG, Smith CD. Objective psychomotor skills assessment of experienced and novice flexible endoscopists with a virtual reality simulator. *J Gastrointest Surg* 2003; 7: 871-78.

[17]Hsu HJ, Younan D, Pandalai S, Gellespie BT, Jain RA, Schippert DW, Narins CR, Khanna A, Surowiec SM, Davies MG, Shortell C, Rhodes JM, Waldman DL, Green RM, Illig KA. Use of computer simulation for determining endovascular skill levels in a carotid stenting model. *J Vasc Surg* 2004; 40: 1118-25.

[18]Gallagher AG, Cates CU. Approval of virtual reality training for carotid stenting: what this means for procedural-based medicine. *J Am Med Ass* 2004; 292: 3024-26.

[19]Naccarelli GV, Conti JB, DiMarco JP, Tracy CM. Task force 6: training in specialized electrophysiology, cardiac pacing and arrhythmia management. *J Am Coll Cardiol* 2006; 47: 904-10.

[20]Patel AD, Gallagher AG, Nicholson WJ, Cates CU. Learning curves and reliability measures for virtual reality simulation in the performance assessment of carotid angiography. *J Am Coll Cardiol* 2006; 47: 1796-802.

[21]De Ponti R, Cappato R, Curnis A, Della Bella P, Padeletti L, Raviele A, Santini M, Salerno-Uriarte JA. Trans-septal catheterization in the electrophysiology laboratory: data from a multicentre survey spanning 12 years. *J Am Coll Cardiol* 2006; 47: 1037-42.

In: Progress in Cardiac Arrhythmia Research
Editor: Ira R. Tarkowicz, pp. 125-139
ISBN: 1-60021-796-6

Chapter 5

NIP-141/NIP-142: A Novel Mixed Channel Blocker for Treatment of Atrial Fibrillation

Norio Hashimoto[1,*] *and Hikaru Tanaka*[2]
[1]Biological Research Laboratories, Nissan Chemical Industries, Ltd., Saitama, Japan;
[2]Department of Pharmacology, Toho University Faculty of Pharmaceutical Sciences, Chiba, Japan.

Abstract

Atrial fibrillation (AF) is the most common cardiac arrhythmia in the adult population and is associated with increased cardiovascular morbidity and mortality, and stroke. Currently available antiarrhythmic drugs are moderately effective in restoring normal sinus rhythm in patients with AF. However, excessive delay of ventricular repolarization (excessive QT prolongation) by these agents may be associated with increased risk for proarrhythmia (early afterdepolarization leading to *torsades de pointes* arrhythmia). Therefore, selective blockers of cardiac ion channels that are exclusively present in the atria are highly desirable, as it is expected to be devoid of any ventricular proarrhythmia.

NIP-142 and the hydrochloride salt (NIP-141) are novel benzopyrane derivatives which block potassium, calcium and sodium channels and shows atrial selective action potential duration prolonging profile. These compounds preferentially block the ultrarapid delayed rectifier potassium current (I_{Kur}) and the acetylcholine-activated potassium current (I_{KACh}). Because I_{Kur} and I_{KACh} have been shown to be expressed more abundantly in atrial than in ventricular myocyte, the atiral specific repolarization prolonging effects of NIP141 and NIP-142 are thought to be due to the blocking of these potassium currents. In canine models, NIP-142 was shown to terminate the microreentry type of AF induced by vagal nerve stimulation and the macroreentry type of atrial flutter induced by an intercaval crush. These effects of NIP-142 have been thought to be due to the prolongation of atrial effective refractory period (ERP), because this compound prolonged atrial ERP without affecting intraatrial and interatrial

* E-mail address: hashimotot@nissanchem.co.jp. TEL: 81-480-92-2513; FAX: 81-480-90-1014. Correspondence concerning this article should be addressed to Norio Hashimoto, Biological Research Laboratories, Nissan Chemical Industries, Ltd. 1470 Shiraoka, Minamisaitama, Saitama 349-0294, Japan

conduction time in these models. The ERP prolongation by NIP-142 was greater in the atrium than in the ventricle. NIP-142 also terminated the focal activity type of AF induced by aconitine. In addition, NIP-141 restored the atrial ERP shortening and the loss of rate adaptation induced by short-term rapid atrial pacing in anesthetized dogs. Although clinical trials are required to provide evidence of efficacy and safety, the novel mixed channel blocker NIP-141/142 would be a useful drug for treatment of several type of AF with a low risk of proarrhythmia.

Introduction

Atrial fibrillation (AF) is the most commonly encountered arrhythmia in clinical practice, with an overall prevalence of about 1% of the population [1-3]. The prevalence of AF is strongly age-dependent, affecting approximately 5% of individuals older than 65 years and approximately 8% of those older than 80 years [4,5]. This disease is associated with increase in mortality and morbidity, and adversely affects quality of life [6,7]. One of the most debilitating consequences of the disease is the accompanying risk of stroke, which occurs in an estimated 60,000 patient with AF per year [3]. Pharmacological approaches for AF treatment have centered on ion channel blockers. However, currently available antiarrhythmic drugs have been only modestly successful in terminating or preventing AF and are not tolerated by many patients. Thus, a considerable unmet medical need for safer and more effective agents exists.

"Multiple reentry" appears to play a major role in AF pathophysiology [8]. An effective way to prevent or terminate multiple reentry is to prolong effective refractory period (ERP). The ERP can be prolonged by drugs that inhibit K^+ channels. Currently available drugs that prolong ERP have in common their action of blocking the rapid component of the delayed rectifier potassium current (I_{Kr}) [9]. Clinical studies have shown that these drugs can terminate AF in about 30% of cases [10,11]. However, the benefit of these drugs (I_{Kr} blocker) is limited because their ventricular action (prolonged ventricular ERP and QT interval) often is associated with increased risk of torsades de pointes (TdP) arrhythmia [12,13]. Therefore, the pharmaceutical industry has focused on "atrial specific drugs" in the search for safe drugs that terminate or prevent AF [14-16].

Potential Targets for Atrial Specific ERP Prolongation

Although most potassium currents are present in both atrium and ventricle, the ultrarapid delayed rectifier potassium current (I_{Kur}) and the acetylcholine-dependent potassium current (I_{KACh}) have been reportedly shown to be expressed more abundantly in atrial than ventricular myocytes [17-20]. Thus, these two potassium currents are potential targets for atrial specific drugs.

Pathohpysiological l Role of I_{Kur} in AF

I_{Kur}, which is composed of Kv1.5 (KCNA5) in human, is a major component of the repolarization phase of the action potential (AP), and its inhibition is known to prolong the action potential duration (APD). In animal models, I_{Kur} blockers prolonged atrial effective refractory period (ERP) and showed atrial anti-arrhythmic efficacy without affecting ventricular repolarization and QT interval [21-24]. In recent years, the pharmaceutical industry has developed some I_{Kur} blocking compounds (RSD1235, AVE0118 and AZD7009) for treatment of AF. These drugs are now in phase II or phase III of clinical development and have good efficacy in treating AF with a low risk of proarrhythmia in human [25,26,88].

It was demonstrated that the action of I_{Kr} blocker was reduced in patients with long-lasting AF [27]. Courtemanche et al demonstrated on a mathematical basis that the effects of I_{Kr} blockade on the APD was reduced in remodeled atrial cells, in contrast, I_{Kur} is mostly activated when the atrial APD is short, with consecutively less activation with long atrial refractoriness [28]. In fact, Wettwer et al also demonstrated that I_{Kur} blockers (4-aminopyridine at low concentration and AVE0118) shortened APD of human trabeculae from patients with sinus rhythm but prolongs APD of that from AF patients [18]. Thus, the effects of an I_{Kur} blocker may enhanced in remodeled atria (as shown in long-lasting AF patients), although this current is reportedly downregulated in remodeled atria [29,30].

I_{Kur} blockade is also expected to enhance L-type calcium current activation, increase systolic calcium influx and enhance atrial contractility, because this current increases in the plateau potential of atrial AP. Indeed, 4-aminopyridine at low concentration, which selectively blocks I_{Kur} channel [31], significantly increased force of contraction in human atrial trabeculae in a concentration-dependent manner [18]. In addition, an I_{Kur} blocker AVE0118 fully restores atrial contractility after conversion in goat model of AF [32]. It became clear that the loss of atrial contractile function and the low blood flow velocity in left atrial appendage after cardioversion of AF to sinus rhythm contributes to the thromboembolic risk associated with AF [33]. However, positive inotropic drugs such as dobutamine and isoprenaline are of questionable benefit because of their low efficacy and proarrhythmic side effects [34,35]. Thus, I_{Kur} blockade might be a potential approach to increase atrial contractility without proarrhythmic side effects in patients after cardioversion of AF.

Pathohpysiological Role of I_{KACh} in AF

The cardiac I_{KACh}, which is composed of two homologous proteins GIRK1 and GIRK4 [36,37], is the inward rectifier potassium current. This current is normally small but activated by acetylcholine secreted from the vagal nerve or adenosine, via muscarinic M2 receptor and adenosine A1 receptor, respectively. Vagal nerve activation, acetylcholine administration or adenosine administration shortens atrial ERP, increases atrial ERP dispersion and promotes AF [38-40], possibly via I_{KACh} activation. A recent report with GIRK4 knockout mice showed that I_{KACh} channel plays a crucial role in the generation of AF [41]. More recently, we reported that selective I_{KACh} blockers terminated AF induced by vagal nerve stimulation or aconitine in dog model with atrial selective ERP prolongation [42,43].

Although enhancement of I_{KACh} could be responsible for the initiation of paroxysmal AF in humans [44,45], the pathophysiological role of I_{KACh} in persistent AF patients remains unclear. Dobrev et al showed that the activation of I_{KACh} by muscarinic receptor stimulation is smaller than in atria from AF patients compared to that in SR [46,47]. Bosch et al also reported that the total acetylcholine-induced current in atrial cardiomyocytes from AF patients is larger than in those from SR patients. This increase was due to an increased density of I_{K1}; the density of I_{KACh} was rather decreased in AF patients.[48]. In addition, reduced muscarinic receptor-related activation of I_{KACh} in AF patients could be explained by decreased expression of the channel subunits [46,49,50]. These results suggest that the I_{KACh} channel is downregulated in persistent AF patients. However, recent studies suggest that a consititutively active component of I_{KACh} exists and that it may be upregulated in persistent AF patients. Tertiapin, a selective I_{KACh} blocking peptide, concentration-dependently inhibited the whole cell I_{KACh} in AF patients with a higher potency than in patients with SR [51]. Although the muscarinic-receptor-activated component of I_{KACh} was larger in patients with SR, the basal outward rectifying potassium current was larger in persistent AF patients. Single channel analysis revealed the presence of constitutive active I_{KACh} channels in persisitent AF patients, but not in patients with SR [51] Such tertiapin-sensitive current component contributing to basal inward current was also detected in dog left atria and pulmonary veins and the component was increased in atrial tachycardia-remodeled preparation [52]. In addition, tertiapin increased atrial APD and suppressed atrial tachyarrhythmia in canine atrial tachycardia-remodeled preparation [53]. These results suggest that the receptor-independent constitutively active I_{KACh} is upregulated in persistent AF parients. Like I_{Kur} blocker, the effect of I_{KACh} blocker is also enhanced in persistent AF patients.

Eletrophysiological Effects of a Novel Atrial Specific Drug, NIP-141/142

NIP-142, (*3R*,4S**)-4-cyclopropylamino-3,4-dihydro-2,2-dimethyl-6-(4-methoxyphenylacethylamino)-7-nitro-2*H*-1-benzopyran-3-ol (Figure 1) and the hydrochloride salt of (NIP-141) are synthesized benzopyrane derivatives by Nissan Chemical Industries Ltd. (Funabashi, Japan) .

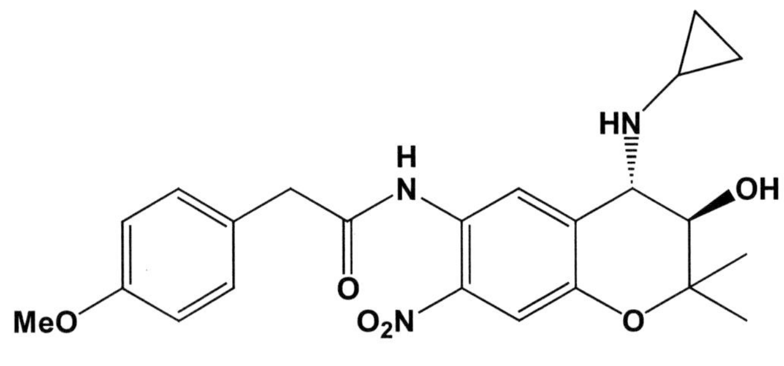

Figure 1. Chemical structure of NIP-142, (*3R*,4S**)-4-cyclopropylamino-3,4-dihydro-2,2-dimethyl-6-(4-methoxyphenylacethylamino)-7-nitro-2*H*-1-benzopyran-3-ol.

Effect of NIP-142 on Membrane Currents

Effects of NIP-142 on various outward (repolarizing) membrane currents have been studied by voltage clamp analysis (Table 1). The delayed rectifier potassium current is composed of three components, the rapid component I_{Kr}, the slow component I_{Ks}, and the ultrarapid component I_{Kur}. Effect on I_{Kr} and I_{Ks} was examined with HEK293 cells expressing the human ether-a-go go (hERG) channel or the KCNQ1/KCNE1 channel, respectively [54]. NIP-142 concentration-dependently inhibited both channel currents at 10 and 100 μM. EC_{50} values for inhibition of the hERG channel current and the KCNQ1/KCNE1 channel were 44 μM and 12 μM, respectively. Effect on the I_{Kur} was examined in both HEK293 cells and *Xenopus* oocytes expressing the humanKv1.5 channel. NIP-142 concentration-dependently inhibited the Kv1.5 channel current. EC_{50} value for inhibition of the Kv1.5 channel tail current in HEK293 cells and *Xenopus* oocytes was 4.8 μM and about 100 μM, respectively. The potency was higher in HEK293 cells than in *Xenopus* oocytes, which is a phenomenon commonly observed with many organic compounds. The inhibition of I_{Kur} by NIP-142 was frequency-independent and larger at the end than at the beginning of the depolarization pulse. A cross-over of the tail current was observed when compared in the absence and presence of NIP-142. These results suggest that NIP-142 has inhibitory effect on the Kv1.5 channel through interaction with both open and closed states of the channel [55]. The molecular identity of the transient outward current is considered to vary among experimental animal species. In the case of the mouse, it is considered to be the sum of Kv4.2 and Kv4.3 channel currents. The potency of NIP-142 on the mouse Kv4.2 and Kv4.3 currents expressed in *Xenopus* oocytes were found to be very low, EC_{50} values being higher than 100 μM. In isolated guinea-pig ventricular myocytes, NIP-142 inhibited the inward rectifier potassium current: about 40% inhibition was observed with 10 μM NIP-142. Effects on the acetylcholine-activated potassium current (I_{KACh}) was examined in HEK293 cells [54] and *Xenopus* oocytes [56] expressing the GIRK1/GIRK4 channel. Concentration-dependent inhibition of the current was observed in both cells: the EC_{50} value for inhibition of the GIRK1/GIRK4 current in HEK293 cells and *Xenopus* oocytes was 0.64 μM and about 10 μM, respectively. The inhibition was independent on the voltage and frequency of the voltage clamp pulse. Concerning inward (depolarizing) currents, NIP-142 concentration-dependently inhibited the L-type and T-type calcium current in isolated guinea-pig ventricular myocytes: the inhibition of the peak inward current by 10 μM NIP-142 was about 50% and 25% for the L-type and T-type calcium current, respectively. NIP-142 (10 μM) had no effect on the hyperpolariztion-activated inward current (Ih) in isolated rabbit sino-atrial node cells.

Effect of NIP-142 on the Refractory Period and the Action Potential of Isolated Atrial and Ventricular Myocardium

Effect of NIP-142 on the refractory period was performed in isolated guinea-pig atrial and ventricular tissue preparations. The shortest stimulation interval resulting in a postextrasystolic potentiation was used as an index of the myocardial refractory period. NIP-142 (10 and 100 μM) concentration-dependently prolonged the refractory period in the atrium but not in the ventricle. The action potential was measured with standard glass microelectrode techniques. NIP-142 concentration-dependently prolonged APD only in the atrium. No significant changes in other action potential parameters, such as resting membrane potential, action potential amplitude and maximum rate of rise, were observed. Thus, the atria-specific increase in refractory period by NIP-142 could be largely explained by the effects on the APD [56].

The atria-specific nature of NIP-142 is different from that of classical class III antiarrhythmic drugs, such as E-4031, which prolong APD both in the atria and ventricle mainly through blockade of I_{Kr} [57]. This suggests that inhibition of I_{Kr}, which largely contributes to repolarization in both atrial and ventricular myocardium, may not be the mechanism of action for NIP-142. There is some evidence that I_{Kur} and Ito, which were inhibited by high concentration NIP-142 [55,58,59], are more abundantly present in the atrium than in the ventricle of human hearts [17,60,62]. There is a report suggesting presence of the Kv1.5 protein in guinea-pig atrium [63], but the presence of I_{Kur} and Ito has not been confirmed in the guinea-pig atrium. In any case, inhibition of neither I_{Kur} nor Ito could explain the prolongation of refractory period and APD by NIP-142 because 100 μM 4-aminopyridine, which blocks I_{Kur} [64,65], prolonged APD only in the ventricle and 1 mM 4-aminopyridine, which blocks I_{Kur} and Ito [64], prolonged APD both in the atria and ventricle [56]. These results with guinea pig myocardium cannot rule out the contribution of Ito blockade to the antiarrhythmic activity of NIP-142 because the density of the current is much smaller than in human atria and atria from other experimental animal species such as the dog and rabbit. The shortening of APD in the ventricle may be explained by its inhibitory effect on calcium channels [58]. That the ventricular refractory period was not changed by NIP-142 may indicate lack of arrythmogenic activity of the drug.

The atria-specific prolongation of APD by NIP-142 was mimicked by the I_{KACh} blocker tertiapin [66,67]. I_{KACh} is considered to be more abundant in atrial muscle than in ventricular muscle [38] and to play an important role in the repolarization of atrial myocytes [69]. The atria-specific prolongation of APD by tertiapin indicates that I_{KACh} contributes to atrial repolarization under basal condition. Stimulation of the muscarinic receptor in the mammalian atria results in shortening of the action potential duration through activation of I_{KACh}. NIP-142 (100 μM) completely reversed the carbachol-induced shortening of APD in the canine [70] and guinea-pig [54] atrium. Such reversal was also observed when NIP-142 was applied after the action potential was shortened with adenosine, which also activates I_{KACh} independently of muscarinic receptors. Thus, I_{KACh} is a strong candidate for the main target of NIP-142.

One of the major problems with existing antiarrhythmic drug acting through prolongation of refractory period and APD is "reverse use-dependence", thus the effect of a drug being weakened under higher stimulation frequency. Such effect is observed both in vivo and in vitro [71] and is considered to underlie ineffectiveness of the drug under high frequency atrial fibrillation. In the guinea-pig atria, 1 μM E-4031 prolonged APD when applied at pacing frequencies less than 1 Hz, but not at frequencies higher than 2 Hz. In contrast, the prolonging effect of NIP-142 on atrial APD was unaffected by stimulation frequency [56] suggesting that the potency of the drug may be maintained under atrial fibrillation.

Lack of Effect on the Muscarinic Receptor and Gi Protein

Blockade of muscarinic receptors by NIP-142 could be excluded by lack of effect on carbachol-induced negative inotropy in the ventricle. Preliminary ligand binding experiments also supports this view. NIP-142 also reversed adenosine-induced shortening of the atrial action potential suggesting that it has inhibitory effect on common mechanisms downstream of the two receptors including the Gi protein and the G-protein coupled potassium channel. Whether NIP-142 has any effect on the Gi protein was examined in contractile force experiments with isolated guinea-pig myocardial tissue preparations. In mammalian atria, muscarinic-receptor stimulation is known to produce negative inotropy through inhibition of adenylate cyclase and activation of the G-protein coupled potassium channel [72]. Both NIP-142 and tertiapin inhibited the carbachol-induced negative inotropy in the atrium showing the effectiveness of these agents in myocardial tissue preparations. Muscarinic-receptor stimulation of the ventricular myocardium produces negative inotropy only when the cAMP pathway has been pre-stimulated [73] by activation of adenylate cyclase [74,75]. Carbachol had no effect on ventricular contractile force in the absence of adenylate cyclase-stimulation, but showed concentration-dependent negative inotropy when applied after preactivation of adenylate cyclase by 0.5 mM forskolin. This carbachol-induced negative inotropy was not observed in the presence of atropine or when the cAMP mediated pathway was directly preactivated by dibutyryl cAMP, which indicates that this negative inotropy is produced by Gi protein-mediated inhibition of adenylate cyclase. That both NIP-142 and tertiapin had no effect on this negative inotropy indicates that these agents have no effect on agonist binding to muscarinic receptors and Gi protein function. This suggests that NIP-142 is unlikely to produce non-specific response through perturbation of various muscarinic receptor and Gi protein-mediated regulatory mechanisms.

Effect of NIP-142 in AF Models

In animal studies, NIP-142 terminated various types of AF models, as shown in Table 2. Nagasawa et al reported that intravenous injection of NIP-142 (3 mg/kg) terminated vagal nerve stimulation-induced AF after increase in fibrillation cycle length and prevented reinitiation of AF [70]. This model is known as a microreentry type of AF model. NIP-142 (3 mg/kg, i.v.) also terminated macroreentry type of atrial flutter induced after placement of an intercaval crush without affecting atirial flutter cycle length [70]. These antiarrhythmic effects were achieved by the atrial ERP prolongation, because NIP-142 prolonged about 10% of atrial ERP without affecting intraatrial and interatrial conduction time in these models. Recently, we reported that NIP-141 (10 mg/kg, i.v.) also terminated focal activity type of AF induced by aconitine [76]. The mechanism of AF termination in this model remains unclear, but it is probably due to the blockade of I_{KACh} or sodium channel site 2 receptor, because an I_{KACh} blocker tertiapin and sodium channel binding site 2 receptor blocker phenytoin was effective in this model [42,76].

Nagasawa et al reported that the ERP prolongation by NIP-142 was greater in the presence of vagal nerve stimulation than in the control state [70]. We also noticed NIP-142 (3 mg/kg, i.v.) prolonged about 20 ms prolongation of atrial ERP with vagal nerve stimulation, but had no significant atrial ERP prolongation without vagal nerve stimulation up to 10 mg/kg [76]. These results suggest that the atrial ERP prolongation of NIP-142 is mainly due to the inhibition of I_{KACh}.

The pathophysiology of AF patient is highly complex. The development of AF leads to functional changes in atria that perpetuate the arrhythmia by a process known as electrical remodeling [79]. The features of electrical remodeling are shortening of the atrial ERP and the loss of rate adaptation [80,81]. NIP-141 restored the atrial ERP shortening and the loss of rate adaptation induced by short-term atrial rapid pacing in anesthetized dogs. Because several studies have shown that the some L type calcium channel blockers prevent atrial ERP shortening and loss of rate adaptation caused by rapid pacing [82-84], it is likely that the prevention of atrial ERP shortening and loss of rate adaptation by NIP-141 is due to blockade of L-type calcium channel. L-type calcium channel blocker verapamil restored the shortening of atrial ERP in relatively short-term (less than 24 hr) [82,83], but not relatively long-term (1 week to 6 weeks) [85] rapid atrial pacing. In contrast, some researchers found that T-type calcium channel blockers can prevent atrial ERP shortening by rapid atrial pacing [83,85]. As previously described, NIP-141 blocks not only L-type but also T-type calcium channel in guinea pig ventricular muscle cells [58]. Thus, it is likely that this compound can prevent atrial remodeling by long-term AF.

Table 1. Inhibitory Effects of NIP-142 on membrane currents

channel	host cell	effect of NIP-142(IC_{50})	reference
Kv1.5	HEK293	4.8 μM	55
	Xenopus oocyte	100 μM	55
GIRK1/GIRK4	HEK293	0.64 μM	54
	Xenopus oocyte	10 μM	56
hERG	HEK293	44 μM	54
KCNQ1/KCNE1	HEK293	12 μM	-
Kv4.3, Kv4.2	*Xenopus* oocyte	>100 μM	-

Table 2. Effects of NIP-142 on atrial fibrillation (AF) and atrial flutter (AFL) models

model	effective dose of NIP-142	reference
vagally-induced AF model	3 mg/kg	70
intercaval crush-induced AFL model	3 mg/kg	70
aconitine-induced AF model	10 mg/kg	76
atrial rapid pacing model	2.5 mg/kg/10 min + 2 mg/kg/hr	76

Lack of Proarrhythmic Risk of NIP-142

NIP-142 (1-10 mg/kg, i.v.) had no significant prolongation in ventricular ERP in pentobarbital anesthetized dog [76]. Nagasawa et al also showed that NIP-142-induced prolongation of atrial ERP was greater than that of ventricular ERP [70]. Because ventricular ERP or QT duration is not suitable surrogate for drug-induced TdP [77,78], we also evaluate the proarrhythmic risk of NIP-142 in methoxamine-sensitized rabbit model in vivo. Intravenous infusion of NIP-142 (30 mg/kg/30 min) induced no ventricular arrhythmia in 8 rabbits. In contrast, an I_{Kr} blocker clofilinum (15 mg/kg/30 min) induced TdP in six of 8 rabbits. These results suggest that NIP-142 has little effects on ventricular repolarization and has a low risk of proarrhythmia.

Conclusion

Drugs with multiple targets appear to be effective against various types of arrhythmia and to have low risk of proarrhythmia. Amiodarone is the current golden standard for the treatment and prevention of AF [87]. This drug is a mixed channel blocker which blocks potassium, sodium and calcium current including I_{Kur} and I_{KACh} [61,68] which are expressed more abundantly in atrial than ventricular myocytes. Like amiodarone, NIP-141/142 is a mixed channel blocker with potassium, sodium and calcium channel blocking profile. This compound preferentially blocks I_{Kur} and I_{KACh} and has atrial-selective ERP prolonging effect. Thus, NIP-141/142 is expected to a useful drug for treatment and prevention of AF with a low risk of proarrhythmia.

References

[1] Fuster, V., Ryden, L.E., Asinger, R.W., Cannom, D.S., Crijns, H.J., Frye R.L., Halperin, J.L., Kay, G.N., Klein, W.W., Levy, S., McNamara, R.L., Prystowsky, E.N., Wann, L.S., Wyse, D.G., Gibbons, R.J., Antman, E.M., Alpert, J.S., Faxon, D.P., Fuster, V., Gregoratos, G., Hiratzka, L.F., Jacobs, A.K., Russell, R.O., Smith, S.C. Jr, Klein, W.W., Alonso-Garcia, A., Blomstorm-Lundqvist, C., de Backer, G., Flather, M., Hradec, J., Oto, A., Parkhomenko, A., Silber, S., Torbichi, A. (2001). American College of Cardiology (ACC)/American Heart Association (AHA)/European Society of Cardiology (ESC) guidelines for management of patients with atrial fibrillation: executive summary report of the ACC/AHA Task Force on practice guidelines and the ESC Committee for practice guidelines and policy conferences (committee to develop guidelines for the management of patients with atrial fibrillation) developed in collaboration with the North American Society of Pacing and Electrophysiology. *Circulation,* **104**, 2118-2150.

[2] Singer, D.E., Albers, G.W., Dalen, J.E., Go, A.S., Halperin, J.L., Manning, W.J. (2004). Antithrombic therapy in atrial fibrillation: the Seventh ACCP Conference on Antithrombolic and Thrombolytic Therapy. *Chest,* **126**, 429S-456S.

[3] Go, A.S., Hylek, E.M., Phillips, K.A., Chang, Y., Henault, L.E., Selby, J.V., Singer, D.E. (2001). Prevalence of diagnosed atrial fibrillation in adults: national implications for rhythm management and stroke prevention: the anticoagulation and risk factors in atrial fibrillation (ATRA) study. *JAMA,* **285**, 2370-2375.

[4] Kannel, W.B., Wolf, P.A., Benjamin, E.J., Levy D. (1998). Prevalence, incidence, prognosis, and predisposing conditions for atrial fibrillation: population-based estimates. *Am J Cardiol,* **82**, 2N-9N.

[5] Furberg, C.D., Pasty, B.M., Manolio, T.A., Gardin, J.M., Smith, V.E., Rautaharju, P.M. (1994). Prevalence of atrial fibrillation in elderly subjects (the Cardiovascular Health Study). *Am J Cardiol,* **74**, 236-241.

[6] Benjamin, E.J., Wolf, P.A., D'Agostino, R.B., Silbershatz, H., Kannel, W.B., Levy D. (1998). Impact of atrial fibrillation on the risk of death: the Framingham Heart Study. *Circulation,* **98**, 946-952.

[7] Gronefeld, G.C., Lilienthal, J., Kuck, K.H., Hohnloser, S.H. : Pharmacological Intervention in Atrial Fibrillation (PIAF) Study Investors. (2003). Impact of rate versus rhythm control on quality of life in patients with persistent atrial fibrillation: results from a prospective randomized study. *Eur Heart J,* **24**, 1430-1436.

[8] Wolf, P.A., Mitchell, J.B., Baker, C.S., Kannel, W.B. and D'Agostino, R.B. (1998). Impact of atrial fibrillation on mortality, stroke, and medical costs. *Arch Intern Med,* **158**, 229-234.

[9] Guerra, P.G., Talajic, M., Roy, D., Dubuc M., Thibault B., Nattel S. (1998). Is there a feature for antiarrhythmic drug therapy? *Drugs,* **56**, 767-781.

[10] Ellenbogen, K.A., Stambler, B.S., Wood, M.A., Sager, P.T., Wesley, R.C. Jr., Meissner, M.C., Zoble, R.G., Wakefield, L.K., Perry, K.T., Vanderlugt, J.T. (1996). Efficacy of intravenous ibutilide for rapid termination of atrial fibrillation and atrial flutter: a dose-response study. *J Am Coll Cardiol,* **28**, 130-136.

[11]Falk, R.H., Pollak, A., Singh, S.N., Friedrich, T. (1997). Intravenous dofetilide, a class III antiarrhythmic agent, for the termination of sustained atrial fibrillation or flutter. Intravenous dofetilide investigators. (1997). *J Am Coll Cardiol,* **29**, 385-390.

[12]Waldo, A.L., Camm, A.J., deRuyter, H., Friedman, P.L., MacNeil, D.J., Pauls, J.F., Pitt, B., Pratt, C.M., Schwartz, P.J., Veltri, E.P. (1996). Effects of d-sotalol of mortality in patients with left ventricular dysfunction after recent and remote myocardial infarction. The SWORD Investigators. Survival with oral d-sotalol. *Lancet,* **9019**, 7-12.

[13]Torp-Pederson, C., Moller, M., Bloch-Thomsen, P.E., Kober, L., Sandoe, E., Egstrup, K., Anger, E., Carlsen, J., Videbeak, J., Marchant, B., Camm A.J. (1999). Dofetilide in patients with congestive heart failure and left ventricular dysfunction. Danish Investigations of arrhythmia and mortality on dofetilide study group. *N Engl J Med,* **341**, 857-865.

[14]Goldstein, R.N., Stambler, B.S. (2005). New antiarrhythmic drugs for prevention of atrial fibrillation. *Prog Cardiovasc Dis* **48**, 12-28.

[15]Vos, M.A. (2004). Atrial-apecific drugs: the way to treat atrial fibrillation? *J Cardiovasc Electrophysiol,* **15**, 1451-1452.

[16]Knobloch, K., Brendel, J., Rosenstein, B., Bleich, M., Busch, A.E., Wirth, K.J. (2004). Atrial-selective antiarrhythmic action of novel I_{Kur} vs. I_{Kr}, I_{Ks} and I_{KACh} class Ic drugs and beta blockers in pigs. *Med Sci Monit,* **10**, BR221-BR228.

[17]Wang, Z., Fermini B., Nattel S. (1993). Sustained depolarization-induced outward current in human atrial myocytes. Evidence for a novel delayed rectifier K^+ current similar to Kv1.5 cloned channel current. *Circ Res,* **73**, 1061-1076.

[18]Wettwer, E., Hala, O., Christ T., Heubach, J.F., Dobrev, D., Knaut M., Varro, A., Ravens, U. (2004). Role of I_{Kur} in controlling action potential shape and contractility in the human atrium: influence of chronic atrial fibrillation. *Circulation,* **110**, 2299-2306.

[19]Mcmorn S.O., Harrison S.M., Zang, W.J., Yu, X.J., Boyett, M.R. (1993). A direct negative inotropic effect of acetylcholine on rat ventricular myocytes. *Am J Physiol,* **265**, H1393-H1400.

[20]Dobrzynski H., Marples D.D., Musa, H., Yamanushi T.T., Henderson, Z., Takagishi, Y., Hanjo, H., Kodama, I., Boyett, M.R. (2001). Distribution of the muscarinic K^+ channel proteins Kir3.1 and Kir3.4 in the ventricle, atrium, and sinus node of the heart. *J Histochem Cytochem,* **49**, 1221-1234.

[21]Blaauw, Y., Gogelein, R.G., Tieleman, A., van Hunnik, U., Schotten, U., Allessie, M.A. (2004). "Early" class III drugs for the treatment of atrial fibrillation: Efficacy and atrial selectivity of AVE0118 in remodeled atria of the goat. *Circulation,* **110**, 1717-1724.

[22]Nattel, S., Matthews, C., De Blasio, E., Han, W., Li, D., Yue, L. (2000). Dose-dependence of 4-aminopyridine plasma concentrations and electrophysiological effects in dogs: Potential relevance to ionic mechanisms in vivo. *Circulation,* **101**, 1179-1184.

[23]Wirth, K.J., Paehler, T., Rosenstein, B., Knobloch, K., Maier, T., Frenzel, J., Brendel, J., Busch, A.E., Bleich, M. (2003). Atrial effects of the novel K^+-channel-blocker AVE0118 in anaesthetized pigs. *Cardiovasc Res,* **60**, 298-306.

[24]Carlsson, L., Chartier, D., Nattel, S. (2006). Characterization of the in vivo and in vitro electrophysiological effects of the novel antiarrhythmic agent AZD7009 in atrial and ventricular tissue of the dog. *J Cardiovasc Pharmacol,* **47**, 123-132.

[25]Roy, D., Rowe, B.H., Stiell, G., Coutu, B., Ip, J.H., Phaneuf, D., Lee, J., Vidaillet, H., Dickinson, G., Grant, S., Ezrin, A.M., Beatch, G.N: CRAFT Investors. (2004). A randomized, controlled trial of RSD1235, a novel anti-arrhythmic agent, in the treatment of recent onset atrial fibrillation. *J Am Coll Cardiol,* **44**, 2355-2361.

[26]van Gelder, I.C., Almgren, O., Walfridsson, H., Kulakowski, P., Ronazeki, A., Dedek, V., Malm, A., Crijins, H. (2005). Facilitation of DC cardioversion of atrial fibrillation/flutter and reduced immediate relapse with intravenous AZD7009. *Circulation, S II,* 112(17).

[27]Tse, H.F., Lau, C.P. (2002). Electrophysiologic actions of *dl*-sotalol in patients with persistent atrial fibrillation. *J Am Coll Cardiol,* **40**, 2150-2155.

[28]Coutremanche, M., Ramirez, R.J., Nattel, S. (1999). Ionic target for drug therapy and atrial fibrillation-induced electrical remodeling: insight from a mathematical model. *Cardiovasc Res,* **42**, 477-489.

[29]van Wagoner, D.R., Pond, A.L., McCarthy, P.M., Trimmer, J.S., Nerbonne, J.M. (1997). Outward K^+ current densities and Kv1.5 expression are reduced in chronic human atrial fibrillation. *Cir Res,* **80**, 772-781.

[30]Bosch, R.F., Nattel, S. (2002). Cellular electrophysiology of atrial fibrillation. *Cardiovasc Res,* **54**, 259-269.

[31]Amos, G.J., Wettwer, E., Metzger, F., Li, Q., Himmel, H.M., Ravens, U. (1996). Differences between outward current of human atrial and subendocardial ventricular myocytes. *J Physiol (Lond),* **491**, 31-50.

[32]de Haan, S., Greiser, M., Harks, E., Blaauw, Y., van Hunnik, A., Verheule, S., Allessie, M., Schotten, U. (2006). AVE0118, blocker of the transient outward current (I_{to}) and ultrarapid delayed rectifier current (I_{Kur}), fully restores atrial contractility after cardioversion of atrial fibrillation in the goat. *Circulation,* **114**, 1234-1242.

[33]Black, I.W., Fatkin, D., Sagar, K.B., Khandheria, B.K., Leung, D.Y., Galloway, J.M., Feneley, M.P., Walsh, W.F., Grimm, R.A., Stollberger, C., et al. (1994). Exclusion of atrial thrumbus by transesophageal echocardiography does not preclude embolism after cardioversion of atrial fibrillation: multicenter study. *Circulation,* **89**, 2509-2513.

[34]Kamalesh M., Copeland, T.B., Sawada, S. (2000). Effects of inotropic stimulation on left atrial appendage function in atrial myopathy of chronic atrial fibrillation. *Echocardiography,* **17**, 313-318.

[35]Sanders, P., Morton, J.B., Kistler, P.M., Vohra, J.K., Kalman, J.M., Sparks, P.B. (2003). Reversal atrial mechanical dysfunction after cardioversion of atrial fibrillation: implications for the mechanism of tachycardia-mediated atrial cardiomypathy. *Circulation,* **108**, 1976-1984.

[36]Kubo, Y., Reuveny, E., Slesinger, P.A., Jan, Y.N., Jan, L.Y. (1993). Primary structure and functional expression of a rat G-protein-coupled muscarinic potassium channel. *Proc Natl Acad Sci USA,* **90**, 802-806.

[37]Krapivinsky, G., Gordon E.A., Wickman, K., Velimirovic, B., Krapivinsky, L., Clapham, D.E. (1995). The G-protein-gated atrial K^+ channel I_{KACh} is a heteromultimer of two inwardly rectifying K^+-channel proteins. *Nature,* **374**, 135-141.

[38]Allessie, M.A., Lammers, W.J., Bonke, I.M., Hollen, J. (1984). Intra-atrial reentry as a mechanism for atrial flutter induced by acethylcholine and rapid pacing in dogs. *Circulation,* **70**, 123-135.

[39]Liu L, Nattel, S. (1997). Differing sympathetic and vagal effects on atrial fibrillation: role of refractoriness and heterogeneity. *Am J Physiol,* **273**, H805-H816.

[40]Kabell, G., Buchanan, L.V., Gibson J.K., Belardinelli, L. (1994). Effects of adenosine on atrial refractoriness and arrhythmia. *Cardiovasc Res,* **28**, 1385-1389.

[41]Kovoor, P., Wickman, K., Maguire, C.T., Pu, W., Gehrmann, J., Berul, C.I., Clapham, D.E. (2001). Evaluation of the role of I_{KACh} in atrial fibrillation using a mouse knockout model. *J Am Coll Cardiol,* **37**, 2136-2143.

[42]Hashimoto, N., Yamashita, T., Tsuruzoe, N. (2006). Tertiapin, a selective I_{KACh} blocker, terminates atrial fibrillation with selective atrial effective refractory period prolongation. (2006). *Phamcol Res,* **54**, 136-141.

[43]Hashimoto, N., Matsuda, T., Matsumoto, R., Yamashita, T., Ishiwata, N, Tsuruzoe, N. (2005). A novel I_{KACh} channel blocker, NIP-151, terminates atrial fibrillation with atrial specific effective refractory period prolongation. *Circulation,* **112**, AbsII-191.

[44]Leclercq, J.F., Attuel P., Coumel, P. (1996). Role of the autonomic nerve system in atrial arrhythmigenesis. In: Waldo, A.L., Toboul, P. editors. *Atrial flutter: advanced in mechanism and management.* Armonk, NY: Futura Publishing Company, Inc.; 293-302.

[45]Chen Y.J., Chen, S.A., Tai, C.T., Wen, Z.C., Feng, A.N., Ding, Y.A., Cheng, M.S. (1998). Role of atrial electrophysiology and autonomic nervous system in patients with supraventricular tachycardia and paroxysmal atrial fibrillation. *J Am Coll Cardiol,* **32**, 732-738.

[46]Dobrev, D., Graf, E., Wettwer, E., Himmel, H.M., Hala, O., Doerfel C., Christ, T., Schuler, S., Ravens, U. (2001). Molecular basis of downregulation of G-protein-coupled inward rectifying K^+ current (I_{KACh}) in chronic human atrial fibrillation: decrease in GIRK4 mRNA correlates with reduced I_{KACh} and muscarinic receptor-mediated shortening of action potentials. *Circulation,* **104**, 2551-2557.

[47]Dobrev, D., Wetter, E., Kortner, A., Knaut, M., Schuler, S., Ravens, U. (2002). Human inward rectifier potassium channels in chronic and postoperative atrial fibrillation. *Cardiovasc Res,* **54**, 397-404.

[48]Bosch, R.F., Zeng, X., Grammer, J.B., Propovc, K., Mewis, C., Kuhlkamp, V. (1999). Ionic mechanisms of electrical remodeling in human atrial fibrillation. *Cardiovasc Res,* **44**, 121-131.

[49]Brundel, B.J., Van Gelder, I.C., Henning, R.H., Tieleman, R.G., Tuinenburg, A.E., Wietses, M., Grandjean, J.G. Van Glist, W.H., Crijns, H.J. (2001). Alterations in potassium channel gene expression in atria of patients with persistent and paroxysmal atrial fibrillation: differential regulation of protein and mRNA levels for K^+ channels. *J Am Coll Cardiol,* **37**, 926-932.

[50]Brundel, B.J., van Gelder, I.C., Henning, R.H., Tiel,man, R.G., Tuinenburg, A.E., Wietses, M., Grndjean, J.G.m Van Glist, W.H., Crijns, H.J. (2001). Ion channel remodeling is related to intraoperative atrial effective refractory periods in patients with paroxysmal and persistent atrial fibrillation. *Circulation,* **103**, 684-690.

[51]Dobrev, D., Friedrich, A., Voigt, N., Jost, N., Wettwer, E., Christ, T., Knaut, M., Ravens, U. (2005). The G protein-gated potassium current I_{KACh} is constitutively active in patients with chronic atrial fibrillation. *Circulation,* **112**, 3697-706.

[52]Ehrlich, J.R., Cha, T.J., Zhang, L., Chartier, D., Villeneuve, L., Herert, T.E., Nattel, S. (2004). Characterization of a hyperpolarization-activated time-dependent potassium

current in canine cardiomyocytes from pulmonary vein myocardial sleeves and left atrium. *J Physiol,* **557**, 583-597.

[53]Cha, T.J., Ehrlich, J.R., Chartier, D., Qi, X.Y., Xiao, L., Nattel, S. (2006). Kir3-based inward rectifier potassium current: potential role in atrial tachycardia remodeling effects on atrial repolarization and arrhythmias. *Circulation,* **113**, 1730-1737.

[54]Matsuda, T., Ito, M., Ishimaru, S., Tsuruoka, N., Saito, T., Iida-Tanaka, N., Hashimoto, N., Yamashita, T., Tsuruzoe, N., Tanaka, H., Shigenobu, K. (2006). Blockade by NIP-142, an antiarrhythmic agent, of carbachol-induced atrial action potential shortening and GIRK1/4 channel, *J Pharmacol Sci,* **101**, 303-310.

[55]Matsuda, T., Masumiya, H., Tanaka, N., Yamashita, T., Tsuruzoe, N., Tanaka, Y., Tanaka, H., Shigenobu, K. (2001). Inhibition by a novel anti-arrhythmic agent, NIP-142, of cloned human cardiac K^+ channel Kv1.5 current., *Life Sci,* **68**, 2017-2024.

[56]Matsuda, T., Takeda, K., Ito, M., Yamagishi, R., Tamura, M., Nakamura, H., Tsuruoka, N., Saito, T., Masumiya, H., Suzuki, T., Iida-Tanaka, N., Itokawa, M., Yamashita, T., Tsuruzoe, N., Tanaka, H., Shigenobu, K. (2005). Atria selective prolongation by NIP-142, an antiarrythmic agent, of refractory period and action potential duration in guinea-pig myocardium, *J Pharmacol Sci,* **98**, 33-40.

[57]Sanguinetti, M., Jurkiewicz, N. (1990). Two components of cardiac delayed rectifier K+ current: differential sensitivity to block by class III antiarrhythmic agents, *J Gen Physiol,* **96**, 195-215.

[58]Matsuda, T., Masumiya, H., Saito, T., Tanaka, H., Shigenobu, K. (1999). NIP-142, a novel benzopyran derivative: Electrophysiological study on the mechanisms of bradycardiac effects, *Jpn J Pharmacol,* **79**, 178P.

[59]Seki, A., Hagiwara, N., Kasanuki, H. (2002). Effects of NIP-141 on K currents in human atrial myocytes., *J Cardiovasc Pharmacol,* **39**, 29-38.

[60]Fedida, D., Wible, B., Wang, Z., Fermini, B., Faust, F., Nattel, S., Brown, A.M. (1993) .Identity of a novel delayed rectifier current from human heart with a cloned K^+ channel current., *Circ Res,* **73**, 210-216.

[61]Kobayashi, S., Reien, Y., Ogura, T., Saito, T., Masuda, Y., Nakaya, H. (2001).. Inhibitory effect of bepridil on hKv1.5 channel current: comparison with amiodarone and E-4031. *Eur J Pharmacol,* **430**, 149-57.

[62]Li, G.R., Feng, J., Yue, L., Carrier, M., Nattel, S. (1996). Evidence for two components of delayed rectifier K^+ current in human ventricular myocytes., *Circ Res,* **78**, 689-696.

[63]Dobrzynski, H., Rothery, S., Marples, D.D., Coppen, S.R., Takagishi, Y., Honjo, H., Tamkun, M.M., Henderson, Z., Kodama, I., Severs, N.J., Boyett, M.R. (2000) Presence of the Kv1.5 K+ channel in the sinoatrial node., *J Histochem Cytochem,* **48**, 769-780.

[64]Bouchard, R., Fedida, D. (1995). Closed- and open-state binding of 4-aminopyridine to the cloned human potassium channel Kv1.5. *J Pharmacol Exp Ther,* **275**, 864-876.

[65]Wang, Z., Fermini, B., Nattel, S., (1995) Effects of flecainaide, quinidine, and 4-aminipyridine on transient outward and ultrarapid delayed rectifier currents in human atrial myocytes, *J Pharmacol Exp Ther,* **272**, 184-196.

[66]Kitamura, H., Yokoyama, M., Akita, H., Matsushita, K., Kurachi, Y., Yamada, M. (2000) .Tertiapin potently and selectively blocks muscarinic K^+ channels in rabbit cardiac myocytes., *J Pharmacol Exp Ther,* **293**, 196-205.

[67]Jin, W., Lu, Z. (1998) A novel high-affinity inhibitor for inward-rectifier K+ channels., *Biochemistry,* **37**, 13291-13299.

[68]Huang, C.X., Zhao, Q.Y., Liang, J.J., Chen, H., Yang, B., Jiang, H., Li, G.S. (2006). Differential densities of muscarinic acetylcholine receptor and I_{KACh} in canine supraventricular tissues and the effect of amiodarone on cholinergic atrial fibrillation and I_{KACh}. *Cardiology,* **106**, 36-43.

[69]Kaibara, M., Nakajima, T., Irisawa, H., Giles, W. (1991). Regulation of spontaneous opening of muscarinic K^+ channels in rabbit atrium., *J Physiol,* **433**, 589-613.

[70]Nagasawa, H., Fujiki, A., Usui, M., Tani, M., Inoue, H., Yamashita, T., Fujikura, N. (1999). Effects of a novel antiarrhythmic agent NIP-142 on vagally-induced canine atrial figrillation., *Jpn. Circ. J.,* **63** (Suppl. 1), 846.

[71]Sugimoto, T. (1999). Epidemiology of atrial fibrillation. In: Hayakawa K. and Kasanuki H., editors. *Atrial Fibrillation, Flutter, and Tachycardia.* In: eds Igaku-Shoin Ltd, Tokyo, 14-18.

[72]Endoh, M. (1999). Muscarinic regulation of Ca^{2+} signaling in mammalian atrial and ventricular myocardium, *Eur. J. Pharmacol.,* **375**, 177-196.

[73]Levy, M. (1971). Sympathetic-parasympathetic interactions in the heart, *Circ. Res.,* **29**, 437-445.

[74]Watanabe, A., Besch, H.J. (1975). Interaction between cyclic adenosine monophosphate and cyclic guanosine monophosphate in guinea pig ventricular myocardium, *Circ. Res.,* **37**, 309-317.

[75]Rardon, D.P., Pappano, A.J. (1986). Carbachol inhibits electrophysiological effects of cyclic AMP in ventricular myocytes, *Am. J. Physiol.,* **251**, H601-H611.

[76]Hashimoto, N., Fujikura, N., Yamashita, T., Tsuruzoe, N. (2007). NIP-141, a Multiple Ion Channel Blocker, Terminates Aconitine-induced Atrial Fibrillation and Prevents the Rapid Pacing-Induced Atrial ERP Shortening in Dogs. Europace, *in press.*

[77]Thomsen, M.B., Volders, P.G., Stengl, M., Spatjens, R.L., Beekman, J.D., Bischoff U., Kall, M.A., Frederiksen, K., Martz, J., Vos, M.A. (2003). Electrophysiological safety of sertindole in dogs with normal and remodeled hearts. *J Pharmacol Exp Ther,* **307**, 776-784.

[78]Thomsen, M.B., Verduyn, S.C., Stengl, M., Beekman, J.D., de Pater, G., van Opstal, J., Volders, P.G., Vos, M.A. (2004). Increased short-term variability of repolarization predicts d-sotalol-induced torsades de pointes in dogs. *Circulation,* **110**, 2453-2459.

[79]Wijffels, M.C., Kirchhof, C.J., Dorland, R., Allessie, M.A. (1995). Atrial fibrillation begets atrial fibrillation: a new study in awake chronically instrumented goats. *Circulation,* **92**, 1954-1968.

[80]Hertervig, E.J., Yuan, S., Carlson, J., Kongstad-Rasmussen, O., Olsson, S.B. (2002). Evidence for electrical remodeling of the atrial myocardium in patients with atrial fibrillation: a study using the monophasic action potential recording technique. *Clin Physiol Funct Imaging,* **22**, 8-12.

[81]Lau, C.P., Tse, H.F. (1997). Electrical remodeling of chronic atrial fibrillation. *Clin Exp Pharmacol Physiol,* **24**, 982-983.

[82]Goette, A., Honeycutt, C., Langberg, J.J. (1996). Electrical remodeling in atrial fibrillation. Time course and mechanism. *Circulation,* **94**, 2968-2974.

[83]Daoud, E.G., Marcovitz, P., Knight, B.P., Goyal, R., Man, K.C., Strickberger, S.A., Armstrong, W.F., Morady, F. (1999). Short-term effect of atrial fibrillation on atrial contractile function in humans. *Circulation,* **99**, 3024-3027.

[84]Ohashi, N., Mitamura, H., Tanimoto, K., Fukuda, Y., Kinebuchi, O., Kurita, Y., Shiroshita-Takeshita, A., Miyoshi, S., Hara, M., Takatsuki, S., Ogawa, S. (2004). A comparison between calcium channel blocking drugs with different potencies for T-and L-type channels in preventing atrial electrical remodeling. *J Cardiovasc Pharmacol,* **44**, 386-392.

[85]Lee, S.H., Yu, W.C., Cheng, J.J., Hung, C.R., Ding, Y.A., Chang, M.S., Chen, S.A. (2000). Effects of verapamil on long-term tachycardia-induced atrial electrical remodeling. *Circuration,* **67**, 340-346.

[86]Fareh, S., Benardeau, A., Thibault, B., Nattel, S. (1999). *The T-type Ca^{2+} channel blocker mibefradil prevents the development of a substrate for atrial fibrillation.* **100**, 2191-2197.

[87]Roy, D., Talajic, M., Dorian, P., Connolly, S., Eisenberg, M.J., Green, M., Kas, T., Lambert, J., Dubuc, M., Gagne, P., Nattel, S., Thibolt, B. (2000). Amiodarone to prevent reoccurrence of atrial fibrillation.canadian trial of atrial fibrillation investigators. *N Eng J Med,* **342**, 913-920.

[88]Crijns, H.J., van Gender, I.C., Walfridsson, H., Kulakowski, P., Ronaszeki, A., Dedek,V., Malm, A., Almgen, O. (2006). Safe and effective conversion of persistent atrial fibrillation to sinus rhythm by intravenous AZD7009. *Heart Rhythm,* **3**, 1321-1331.

In: Progress in Cardiac Arrhythmia Research
Editor: Ira R. Tarkowicz, pp. 141–167
ISBN 1-60021-796-6

Chapter 6

A Combination Algorithm for Automatic QRS Complex Detection in ECG Signals

Carsten Meyer,[*] José Fernández Gavela[†] and Matthew Harris[‡]
Philips Research Laboratories
Weisshausstr. 2, D-52066 Aachen, Germany

Abstract

QRS detection is the crucial first step in every automatic ECG analysis. Subsequent ECG processing, e.g. automatic arrhythmia classification, relies on an accurate QRS detection performance. Much work has been carried out in automatic QRS complex detection, using various methods ranging from filtering and threshold methods, through wavelet methods, to neural networks, and others. Performance is generally good, but each method has situations where it fails. In particular, cardiac arrhythmias continue to present challenges to automatic ECG detection algorithms due to the irregular rhythms and waveforms. In this paper we describe and evaluate an approach to improve QRS detection performance by automatically combining different detection algorithms, here the Pan-Tompkins and wavelet method. The goal is to benefit from the strengths of both algorithms. A key point of the algorithm is to balance the contribution of the individual methods by introducing appropriate parameters. These parameters are estimated in a data-driven way. We provide experimental results on the Massachusetts Institute of Technology-Beth Israel Hospital (MIT-BIH) Arrhythmia Database. It is shown that our combination approach improves overall QRS detection results compared to both individual methods. A set of examples is provided to

*E-mail address: Carsten.Meyer@philips.com
†E-mail address: Jose.FernandezGavela@telefonica.es
‡E-mail address: Matthew.Harris@philips.com

illustrate the results of our combination algorithm. Furthermore, we address the performance of our method specifically during arrhythmic episodes of the patients. We also discuss patient individual optimizations of the combination parameters for further performance improvements.

1. Introduction

The QRS complex is the most prominent feature in the electrocardiogram (ECG) signal, and corresponds to the ventricular excitation. The automatic detection of QRS complexes (and central R-peaks) in an ECG signal is the crucial first step in any automatic ECG analysis. For any subsequent ECG processing and classification, a reliable QRS detection performance is of paramount importance. For example, the determination of peak amplitudes and time intervals in the ECG signal relies heavily on an accurate beat detection. Furthermore, in automatic cardiac arrhythmia classification the QRS complex provides the reference for detection of other ECG waves, and defines the time frame for a subsequent morphological analysis. In [1], for instance, suitable time frames were placed around the R-peaks, and autoregressive modeling was performed on the windowed ECG signal in order to classify cardiac arrhythmias. Similarly, [2] positioned time frames around the QRS complex to calculate the correlation coefficients for arrhythmia classification. Here, the frames only spanned the duration of the QRS complex rather than the whole cardiac cycle.

For automatic QRS complex detection (and more generally automatic ECG signal segmentation), a number of algorithmic techniques have been developed. Many algorithms involve a pre-processor stage where the ECG signal is transformed to accentuate the QRS complex, and a decision stage, where a QRS complex is detected, using thresholding. The most well known such method is the Pan-Tompkins algorithm [3]. Neural networks, trained to be adaptive non-linear predictors of the ECG signal, have been used for QRS complex detection [4,5]. As most of the ECG signal contains non-QRS segments, and the signal in a QRS segment looks very different to the rest of the signal, such neural networks have a large prediction error on QRS segments (and low prediction error elsewhere). Consequently, the prediction error constitutes a feature for QRS complex detection [4,5]. In another method, adaptive filters have been used to give an estimate of the current ECG sample as a weighted sum of previous ECG samples. The weights in the sum are updated according to the changing signal statistics. Sharp changes in the weights and in the errors of the current ECG sample estimate were used as features for QRS complex detection (see e.g. [6]). Other approaches include cross-correlation methods, where a QRS-complex template is aligned to the ECG signal [7,8], and syntactic approaches, where the ECG signal is represented as a piecewise linear approximation, and is analyzed using syntactic rules [9,10]. For an overview of these and other approaches see e.g. [11] and [12].

However, the large variation in the QRS complex waveforms as well as noise continue to present challenges to the algorithms, so that further performance improvements are still an important goal of current research.

Instead of further optimizing any individual QRS detection method, we focus in this paper on *combining* two such state-of-the-art algorithms, namely the Pan-Tompkins [3] and the wavelet algorithm [13–15]. This is motivated first by the general notion that such a combination approach, which can be seen as an example for an "ensemble classifier" [1], may improve upon the performance of the individual classifiers [16]. Second, for the task of QRS complex detection, the large performance gain that can be achieved by the *optimal* combination of the two algorithms - determined on our database in a "cheating experiment" (see section 3.2.) - strongly motivate a combination approach. The goal of our paper is to develop a *data-driven* framework for combining algorithms in automatic QRS complex detection.

In a previous approach, Moraes *et. al.* [17] combined two QRS detection methods, namely an algorithm proposed by Engelse and Zeelenberg [18] and a second one based on the Pan-Tompkins and Ligtenberg-Kunt algorithms [19]. In this approach, classification by the secondary detector is invoked *only* in case the first classifier observes an "undefined" event [17]. In this case the output from the secondary detector is used to determine whether the event is a QRS complex.

Our combination algorithm differs from the approach by Moraes *et. al.* in three aspects: First, in our approach the prediction of *both* algorithms always enter into determining the final decision. Second, we propose a "flexible" (instead of a fixed) combination scheme which is triggered by two parameters allowing to balance the influence of the two individual algorithms. Third, these parameters are estimated in a data-driven way allowing to adapt our combination scheme to individual data sets. In experiments on the MIT-BIH Arrhythmia database we show that our combination approach improves performance over both individual algorithms.

This chapter is an extended version of the article "Combining Algorithms in Automatic Detection of QRS Complexes in ECG Signals" (IEEE Transactions on Information Technology in Biomedicine, Vol. 10, No. 3 (July 2006) [20]). Here, we additionally address the performance of our algorithm on various arrhythmic beat and rhythms types, namely premature ventricular contractions (PVC), atrial premature contractions (APC), atrial fibrillation, ventricular tachycardia, ventricular bi- and trigeminy and supraventricular tachyarrhythmia. The analysis shows that our combination algorithm is particularly successful in reducing QRS complex detection errors in arrhythmic episodes. A set of examples from various arrhythmic passages illustrates the performance of our algorithm. Moreover, we provide results demonstrating that patient-specific optimizations of the combination parameters can provide further performance improvements.

The rest of the paper is organized as follows:
In Section 2. we give a brief description of the Pan-Tompkins and wavelet algorithms used in our combination approach. Section 3. is dedicated to describing our framework for combining the two QRS complex detection methods. This also includes an oracle experiment yielding the best possible combination performance (section 3.2.). Our combination algorithm is described in detail in Section 3.3.. The experimental evaluation of our algorithm is presented in Section 4., including patient-specific optimizations of the combination parameters (Section 4.6.), the evaluation of our algorithm on arrhythmic beats and rhythms (Section 4.7.), and a set of examples (Section 4.8.). Finally, in Sections 5. and 6. we summarize and conclude our study.

[1] By "classification" we mean the binary decision of detecting or not detecting a QRS complex in a given time frame.

2. QRS Complex Detection Methods Used in Our Combination Algorithm

We apply our combination approach to the Pan-Tompkins and wavelet QRS detection algorithms, which are among the best performing algorithms for this task [21]. In this section we briefly describe both methods; for more details we refer the reader to the corresponding original articles.

2.1. Pan-Tompkins Method

The Pan-Tompkins algorithm (PT) [3] is the most well known example of a filter threshold method for QRS complex detection. The ECG signal is first preprocessed to enhance the quality of the filtered signal. This preprocessing consists of a bandpass filter, a differentiator, a squaring operation and a moving window integrator. The bandpass filter suppresses high frequency noise e.g. from muscle contractions and from power-line interference as well as low frequency noise e.g. from baseline wander and T-wave interference; the allowed frequency range is between about 5 and 15 Hz. The differentiator accentuates large slopes from the QRS complex while suppressing low frequency components of the P- and T-waves. The squaring operation makes all data points positive and nonlinearly amplifies large slopes from the QRS complexes. Finally, the integrator carries out a smoothing operation with window length corresponding to the width of the QRS complex, to suppress local maxima of the signal within the QRS complex duration.

The key parameter of the PT decision stage is the threshold θ. QRS complexes are detected in regions where the filtered signal rises above the threshold θ. The actual position of the detected R-peak is chosen at the position of the maximal absolute unfiltered signal in the interval where the filtered signal is above θ. To increase the detection rate, a "search back procedure" is introduced: If no QRS complex is detected within a time interval Δ proportional to the average time between two consecutive R-peaks, QRS complexes are looked for where the filtered signal rises above a second, lower threshold θ_2 (a fixed fraction of θ). To remove wrong QRS complexes detected too close to each other, a "refractory rule" applies, i.e. QRS complexes are not allowed to be within 0.3s (*refractory time*[2]) of each other. The thresholds θ and θ_2 are dynamically updated according to the average amplitude of the R-peaks in the filtered signal as well as the average value of "noisy" (non-QRS) peaks in the filtered signal. For a more detailed description of the algorithm see [3].

Interesting for our combination approach is the threshold parameter θ. By varying this parameter, we can control the sensitivity of the algorithm, and thus the number of detected QRS complexes. Increasing θ results in only very prominent maxima in the filtered signal being found (and thus very likely QRS complexes), and lowering θ means more maxima will be detected, some of which may be noise.

[2]The refractory time should reflect physiologic properties of the muscle cells. However, in our experiments, on noisy excerpts large P-waves between 200 and 300ms from the QRS complex were additionally detected as QRS complexes. Therefore, we used the value 0.3s for the refractory time, providing better results on the database than with 0.2s as used in [3].

2.2. Wavelet Method

The general idea of the wavelet method is to decompose the ECG signal into components of different discrete scales in the time domain, permitting the representation of the temporal characteristics of the signal at different resolutions. QRS complexes are detected by comparing the different scales against adaptive thresholds and aligning over the different scales. In our experiments, we used the wavelet QRS detector described in Li et al. [13], and Mallat and Hwang [14].

The wavelet transform is a decomposition of a signal into a set of basis functions, similar to a Fourier decomposition. In the Fourier decomposition, the wavelet basis functions are dilations and translations of the sine function. Comparably, the wavelet basis functions are dilations (characterized by a parameter a) and translations (characterized by a parameter b) of a prototype function $\psi(t)$, called the mother wavelet. The wavelet transformation $W(a,b)$ of the signal $x(t)$ is thus defined as

$$W(a,b)(x) = \frac{1}{\sqrt{a}} \int_{-\infty}^{+\infty} x(t)\psi\left(\frac{t-b}{a}\right) dt. \tag{1}$$

Examining the components of the wider (more dilated) basis functions (large a) gives information about the lower frequency components of the signal as a function of time (b in the transformed space). Similarly, the components for small a give high frequency information about the signal as a function of time. By choosing $a = 2^j$ and $b = 2^j l$ (called the "dyadic" wavelet transform), the wavelet transformation can be simply implemented with repeated use of finite impulse response filters [15, 21, 22]. We thus obtain a sequence of functions (indexed by j), which are called "scales". Low scales contain high frequency information about the signal, and high scales contain low frequency information about the signal.

In the wavelet QRS detection algorithm from Li *et. al.* [13], we use a quadratic spline wavelet with compact support. The Fourier transform $\Psi(\omega)$ of the mother wavelet $\psi(t)$ is then given by

$$\Psi(\omega) = j\omega \left(\frac{\sin(\omega/4)}{\omega/4}\right)^4. \tag{2}$$

The first four scales of the wavelet transformation are considered. The first scale contains high frequency noise, and the QRS complex. The QRS complex is so prominent, that it is clearly visible on all four scales; however it is most prominent in the second and third scales. The fourth scale contains lower frequency information including T-wave information and baseline drift. The wavelet method for detecting QRS complexes involves identifying clear peaks in each scale, and matching them correctly across the different scales. Specifically, a QRS complex shape is transformed to a maximum-minimum pair by the wavelet transformation. A QRS complex is proposed if a maximum-minimum pair of sufficient size appears in all scales, has a positive Lipschitz regularity exponent, and does not occur too near to another QRS complex (within the *refractory time*). Similar to the PT method, the wavelet algorithm contains a search back routine with lowered thresholds if a significant time has elapsed without detecting any QRS complex. For more details on the wavelet algorithm see Li et al. [13].

The wavelet QRS detection algorithm has been compared with a multitude of other QRS detection algorithms on standard databases, and been shown to have one of the highest sensitivities and positive predictabilities of the algorithms tested [21]. It is also different to the Pan-Tompkins algorithm described in section 2.1., and makes different QRS detection errors. This leads us to expect that a combination with the Pan-Tompkins algorithm could be advantageous.

3. Combination Approach

3.1. Motivation

The PT algorithm is good at detecting clear QRS complexes, but, may sometimes fail to detect wider QRS complexes with smaller amplitude. The implemented wavelet method is better able to detect wider and unusually shaped QRS complexes, but is sometimes prone to missing some normal shaped complexes. By combining the predictions of the two classifiers we aim to obtain an improved QRS complex detection algorithm, combining the strengths of the individual algorithms, while compensating their weaknesses. Our combination approach is an example for an *ensemble* classifier (see e.g. [16]). As discussed in [16], an ensemble classifier can be more accurate than any of its individual members if the individual classifiers are doing better than random guessing, and if they make different (uncorrelated) errors on new data points [23]. This motivates our approach from a theoretical perspective.

The second motivation comes from an empirical validation, by evaluating the *maximal* improvement that can be obtained by combining the base algorithms, assuming the *perfect* decision strategy if both classifiers disagree in their predictions. This will be explained in the next section.

3.2. Oracle Experiment

As stated above, the motivation for combining two QRS complex detection methods is the expected performance gain an ensemble classifier may provide compared to the individual algorithms. Clearly, a combination with 0% error is virtually impossible, since there are cases where both methods make incorrect predictions. Instead, there is a lower bound to the reachable error rate, dictated by the quality of the two QRS complex detection methods. This lower bound gives the *maximal* performance gain the ensemble can provide over the individual algorithms. It can be determined using the *"oracle" method*, which assumes the *perfect* decision strategy.

First, it is reasonable to assume that in case of agreement of the two algorithms whether to predict a QRS complex location or not, this decision is accepted ("majority vote"). At times where both algorithms make the wrong decision, the combination will also be incorrect. Thus there is an intrinsic lower bound to the error rate that can be achieved by the optimal combination, dictated by the accuracy of the two individual algorithms. If instead the two algorithms disagree about the presence of a QRS complex at a given time, in the oracle experiment the idea is to take the *correct* decision, using the cardiologist annotation.

Table 1. Decision rule for combination algorithm. QRS detection denoted '1', no detection '0'. PT: Pan-Tompkins, WVT: wavelet.

PT	WVT	local decision strategy	output of combin. algor.
0	0	accept	0
0	1	locally rerun PT, $\theta' = \alpha \cdot \theta$, $\alpha \in [0,1]$	output of PT rerun
1	0	locally rerun PT, $\theta' = \beta \cdot \theta$, $\beta \in [1,\infty)$	output of PT rerun
1	1	accept	1

Formally, this can be viewed as adding a third classifier to the ensemble performing a *perfect* classification (corresponding to the manual annotation), and accepting the majority vote of the three classifiers. This is a *cheating experiment*, giving the result for the best possible combination of the two individual algorithms. The results of the oracle experiment (discussed in section 4.) demonstrate that the QRS detection performance can be dramatically improved by optimally combining the two individual detection methods. This indicates that the PT and wavelet methods partly contain complementary information about the location of the QRS complexes. This strongly motivates a combination approach.

In the following section, we suggest an automatic decision strategy that does not use the manual annotation.

3.3. Combination Algorithm

In our combination approach, first the two individual algorithms (wavelet and PT) are run in parallel. If both classifiers agree whether to predict a QRS complex location at time t, this decision is accepted. In case of disagreement between the two individual classifiers at time t, the basic idea is to rerun the PT algorithm[3] *locally* (i.e. in a suitable time window around time t), however with adjusted threshold θ'. More specifically, we introduce two parameters $\alpha \in [0;1]$ and $\beta \in [1;\infty)$, which specify the amount of PT threshold reduction and increase, respectively, in the local PT rerun. The parameter α is used to reduce the PT threshold when the PT method does not detect a QRS complex location at time t, however the wavelet algorithm does. Conversely, the factor β is applied to increase the PT threshold when PT detects a QRS complex location at time t, but wavelet doesn't. Intuitively, the parameters α and β test the "confidence" of the PT decision with respect to a threshold change, trying to reproduce the wavelet decision. The result of the local PT rerun with adjusted threshold determines whether or not to accept the QRS complex in the final output. This decision process for our data-driven combination algorithm is displayed in Table 1.

There are several reasons for introducing two parameters α and β. First, a parameterization of the decision strategy allows to adapt the combination algorithm to different data sets, by appropriately selecting parameter values. Second, two separate parameters

[3]The PT method is controlled by few simple thresholds that have a direct and intuitive influence on the detected QRS complex location times. In contrast, changing thresholds in the wavelet method affects the identification of peaks in the different scales, and thus makes correct matching across scales hard to control.

for threshold adjustment allow to independently address QRS complexes missed by PT and wavelet, respectively. Moreover, for suitable parameter values, our combination algorithm can recover both individual algorithms as well as realize other simple combinations of the two classifiers, as shown in Figure 1: By setting $\alpha = 0, \beta \to \infty$, the combination algorithm is equivalent to the wavelet method; setting $\alpha = 1, \beta = 1$ recovers the PT method. Choosing $\alpha = 0, \beta = 1$ leads, for local PT and wavelet predictions on the presence of a QRS complex at time t, to the logical "OR" of the two binary predictions; this is equivalent to the Boolean union of the two sets of QRS complex locations. Finally, setting $\alpha = 1, \beta \to \infty$ locally realizes the logical "AND", i.e. a "consensus" decision, where a QRS complex is detected if and only if it is predicted by both the wavelet and the PT algorithm (equivalent to the Boolean intersection of the QRS complex locations)[4].

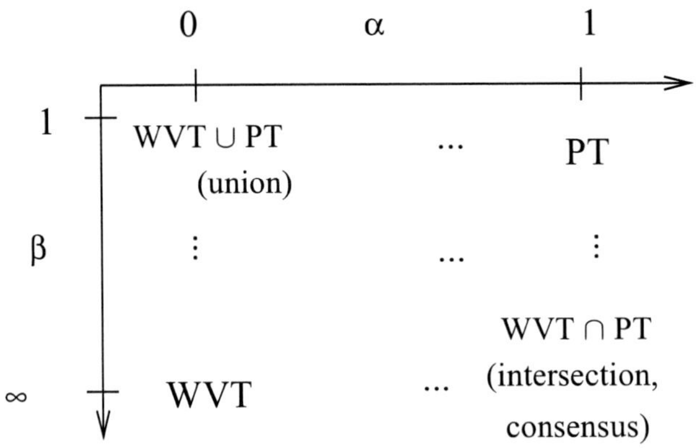

Figure 1. Theoretical "limiting cases" of the combination algorithm in the two-dimensional array of (α, β)-values. WVT: wavelet, PT: Pan-Tompkins method.

From Figure 1 it can be inferred that by increasing α, the QRS complexes predicted only by the wavelet algorithm are increasingly removed. In contrast, increasing β more and more removes the contribution of QRS complexes predicted only by the PT algorithm.

Since our combination algorithm can interpolate between the predictions of both individual algorithms as well as Boolean combinations, we can expect to improve performance over the best individual algorithm, by optimizing the values of the parameters α and β. This will be explained in more detail in section 3.4..

So far, we have assumed a suitably discretized time scale for QRS complex detection, e.g. defined by the sample rate. In practice, a large sample rate may lead the two algorithms to position the same QRS complex at slightly different times t_1 and t_2. We introduce a tolerance interval δ to account for physiological relevance of such small time misplacements. Specifically, we *match* QRS complex locations predicted by the two algorithms at slightly different times t_1 and t_2, i.e. treat them as a single QRS complex, if t_1 and t_2 are within δ of each other ("peak matching"). This generally keeps the combination algorithm from predicting two different QRS complexes within the interval δ, which is especially important

[4]In practice, we cannot apply our combination approach if $\alpha \to 0$, since in this case, the PT algorithm fails. This is as QRS complexes are detected between up and down crossings of the threshold θ. If the threshold is too low, the whole signal is above the threshold, and there are no longer any threshold crossings.

for the Boolean union (see section 4.3.2.). Moreover, the location of a slightly misplaced peak in one method may be corrected in the combination[5]. In all experiments described in section 4., peak matching is performed *before* applying any combination algorithm. The impact of δ is experimentally investigated in section 4.3.2.. Our combination algorithm is summarized in the flow chart of Figure 2.

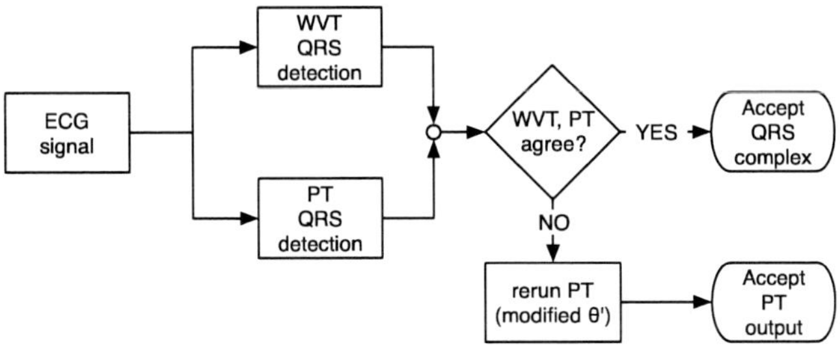

Figure 2. Flow chart of the combination algorithm. Both QRS detection methods — wavelet (WVT) and Pan-Tompkins (PT) — are run in parallel. For each QRS complex detected by either wavelet or PT, it is checked whether the QRS complex is also detected by the other base algorithm within the tolerance interval δ (peak matching). If yes, the QRS complex is accepted (at the time of the larger predicted R-peak). If not, the PT algorithm is rerun locally with modified threshold θ', and the output of the PT rerun determines whether the QRS complex is accepted or not.

Any matched QRS complex (predicted by both the PT and the wavelet method within the tolerance interval δ) is accepted by all investigated combination algorithms, i.e. a QRS complex location is detected at the time of the larger peak. *Unmatched* QRS complexes, i.e. QRS complexes predicted by only one algorithm within δ, are treated as follows: Our data-driven combination algorithm, as explained above, decides on acceptance of the QRS complexes by the (local) PT rerun with adjusted threshold θ' (see Table 1 and Figure 2). In contrast, the "union" algorithm accepts *all* unmatched QRS complexes, while the "intersection" algorithm accepts *no* unmatched QRS complex. Finally, the oracle approach selects the *correct* decision, i.e. does or does not accept the unmatched QRS complex, depending on the cardiologists' annotation.

3.4. Estimation of Parameters α and β

At any particular time where the wavelet and the PT algorithms disagree on the prediction of a QRS complex, appropriate (i.e. locally optimal) values for α and β could in principle recover the correct decision by the combination algorithm. Unfortunately, we do not know the locally optimal values for α and β in advance. Therefore, we need a decision criterion to select suitable parameter values. The simplest approach is to assume *global* (i.e.

[5]The location of the larger of the two R-peaks is selected. In the oracle experiment, if the detected QRS complexes correspond to an annotated QRS complex, the location of the R-peak being closer to the annotated R-peak is chosen.

patient- and time-independent) values for α and β. Here, we estimate both parameters offline in a data-driven way, by minimizing the number of errors (as defined in Section 4.2.) on separate, suitably chosen training data from various patients (Section 4.3.1.). The estimated parameters are then used for any new ECG signal to be segmented, at any position where wavelet and PT disagree on the prediction of a QRS complex. However, other estimation criteria (e.g. unsupervised estimation on patient-specific data) are also conceivable.

In the next section, we discuss our experimental results on the MIT-BIH Arrhythmia database.

4. Experiments

4.1. Database

The MIT-BIH Arrhythmia database was used for development and analysis of our QRS complex detection algorithm. This database contains 48 half-hour excerpts of two-channel ambulatory ECG recordings, obtained from 47 patients of the Beth Israel Hospital (BIH) Arrhythmia Laboratory Boston between 1975 and 1979. These 48 recordings were selected from a background set of 4000 long-term ambulatory ECG recordings collected from a mixed population of inpatients (about 60%) and outpatients (about 40%) at the BIH: 23 recordings were chosen at random from the background set, providing a representative sample of waveforms and artifacts that an arrhythmia detector might encounter in routine clinical use. The remaining 25 recordings were selected from the same set to include a variety of rare but clinically important phenomena (complex ventricular, junctional, and supraventricular arrhythmias and conduction abnormalities) that would not be well-represented in a small random sample.

All recordings were sampled at 360 Hz with 11-bit resolution over a 10mV range. Two or more cardiologists independently annotated each record. Disagreements were resolved to obtain the computer-readable reference annotations for each beat included in the database. The MIT-BIH database contains 110k beats in total (on average about 2280 ± 450 per patient). More information on the database can be found in [24] and in the internet[6]. The algorithms in this paper were run only with the first of the two channels from each excerpt (as the base algorithms were designed for one channel input).

By extracting every third excerpt, we divided the data into training and test sets. The training set (30 excerpts, 66103 QRS complexes) was used to estimate the optimal values of the parameters α and β, while the test set (17 excerpts, 41529 QRS complexes) was used to evaluate the algorithms using the parameter values estimated on the training set[7].

[6] www.physionet.org/physiobank/database/html/mitdbdir/intro.htm

[7] The excerpt 207 was not used neither in the training nor the test set due to periods of ventricular fibrillation producing a large number of automatically detected QRS complexes which are not annotated, yielding a high number of insertions for this patient.

4.2. Error Rates

We will discuss the accuracy of the algorithms in various ways. We will talk about two sorts of errors: false positives (FP - incorrectly detected QRS complexes) and false negatives (FN - missed QRS complexes). We will call the sum of FP and FN the total error (# error). The total error is given in absolute value, and as a percentage of the total number of annotated QRS complexes (% error). A QRS complex is taken to be correctly detected if it is detected within 100ms of the annotation time. The general conclusions of the paper are not affected if this tolerance is reduced.

4.3. Training

The parameters of both individual base algorithms (PT and wavelet) have been optimized independently to yield optimal performance on the MIT-BIH arrhythmia database. In the following, we discuss the estimation of parameters for the combination algorithm.

4.3.1. Estimation of α and β by Minimizing the Training Error

As discussed in section 3.4., a simple way to estimate global (patient- and time-independent) values for the parameters α and β is to minimize the number of errors (i.e. the sum of false positives and false negatives) on separate training data, collected from various representative patients. Since changes of α and β affect different subsets of QRS complex locations, we can optimize the two values independently. Thus, we first set $\beta = 1$ and choose α_{opt} in order to minimize the total number of false positives and false negatives (Figure 3a). As expected, with decreasing α, the number of false negatives decreases and the number of false positives increases, since more and more wavelet QRS complex predictions are considered in addition to the PT predictions. For the sum of false positives and false negatives, we see a shallow minimum around $\alpha = 0.3$ and select an optimal value of $\alpha_{opt} = 0.3$.

Then, using $\alpha_{opt} = 0.3$, we choose β_{opt} to minimize the total number of false positives and false negatives as a function of β (Figure 3 b). Increasing β yields the expected behaviour of decreasing false positives and increasing false negatives, since we increasingly remove PT QRS complex predictions. Here, however, the total number of false positives and false negatives has its (shallow) optimum at $\beta_{opt} = 1$. This is because for most patients, the number of PT false positives is very small. Therefore, there is no gain in further removing PT predictions by setting $\beta > 1$. Thus, we select globally optimized values of $\alpha_{opt} = 0.3$ and $\beta_{opt} = 1.0$.

4.3.2. Influence of "Peak Matching Interval" δ

The peak matching interval δ (introduced in section 3.3.) arises since it does not make sense physiologically to distinguish QRS complex locations t_1 and t_2 if their time difference is smaller than some threshold value δ. Therefore, such QRS complexes are matched, i.e. treated as a single QRS complex (see Section 3.3.). The value of δ may influence the number of detected QRS complexes in any combination algorithm.

a)

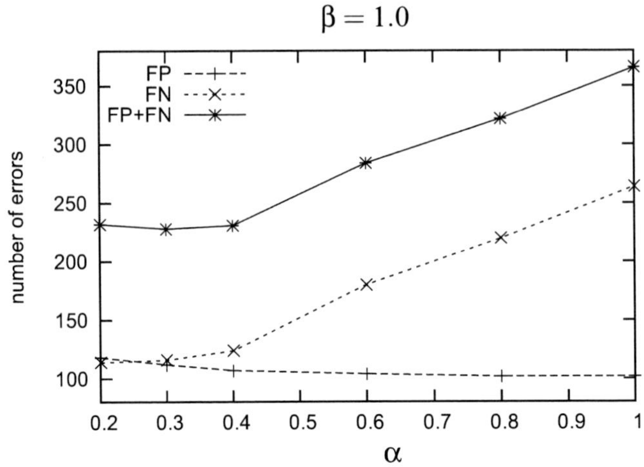

b)

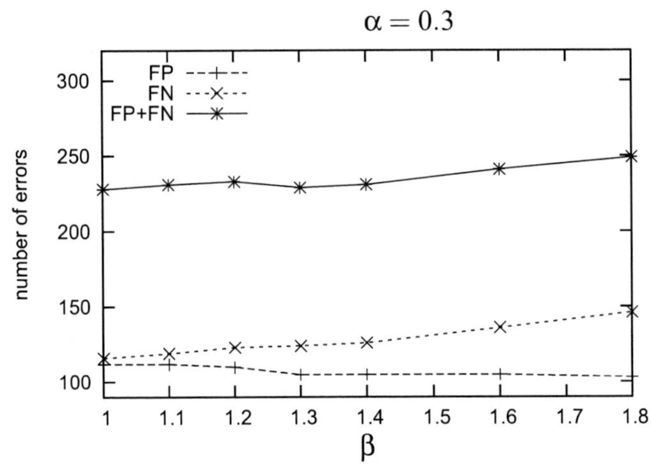

Figure 3. Number of false positives (FP), false negatives (FN) and their sum on the training data as a function of α for $\beta = 1.0$ (a) and as function of β for $\alpha = 0.3$ (b).

Except for the union, however, we observed only a weak dependence of the training error on the value of δ in the investigated interval (see Figure 4). For the union, the error rate increases with decreasing δ: For a smaller peak matching interval, more and more QRS complexes predicted by PT and wavelet at slightly different times will be treated independently (not matched), and the union then accepts them as separate QRS complexes, giving rise to false positives. Our data-driven combination algorithm, however, is able to reject most of these false positives in the PT rerun, so that its error rate is nearly independent of the value of δ in the investigated interval[8]. For analogous reasons, also the training error

[8]This was confirmed on the test set, where $\delta = 120ms$ and $\delta = 240ms$ resulted in similar error rates.

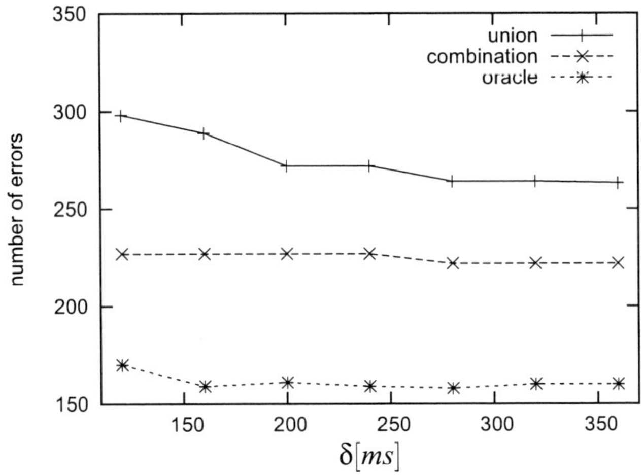

Figure 4. Number of errors on the training set as a function of the peak matching interval δ, for the union, our data-driven combination algorithm ($\alpha = 0.3$, $\beta = 1.0$) and the oracle. The intersection shows only a weak dependence on δ and is not shown due to its large error rate.

for the oracle and intersection show only a small variation with δ in the investigated interval.

Table 2. Training error using original and combination methods.

algorithm	# FP	# FN	# err in 66103	% err
wavelet	166	289	455	0.69
PT	104	269	373	0.56
union	166	106	272	0.41
intersection	78	468	546	0.84
comb. $\alpha = 0.25, \beta = 1.0$	116	113	229	0.35
comb. $\alpha = 0.3, \beta = 1.0$	**111**	**116**	**227**	**0.34**
comb. $\alpha = 0.3, \beta = 1.1$	111	119	230	0.35
comb. $\alpha = 0.4, \beta = 1.0$	106	124	230	0.35
oracle	65	94	159	0.24

4.3.3. Training Results

In Table 2 we compare the training error of our combination algorithm against the union and intersection algorithms as well as the optimal oracle method (see Section 3.). We chose $\delta = 240ms$ in order to have a fair comparison to the union.

On the training set, we obtain better performance for the PT than for the wavelet algorithm (373 versus 455 errors). The union algorithm strongly decreases the error rate (to 272 errors), mostly due to reducing the number of false negatives as a result of combin-

Table 3. Error on the test set using various original and combination methods.

	Test				Test without excerpts 105 and 108			
algorithm	# FP	# FN	# err in 41529	% err	#FP	# FN	# err in 37194	% err
wavelet	310	508	818	1.97	58	314	372	1.0
PT	78	182	260	0.63	25	153	178	0.48
union	198	100	298	0.72	38	77	115	0.31
combination $\alpha = 0.25, \beta = 1.0$	138	103	241	0.58	28	75	103	0.28
combination $\alpha = 0.3, \beta = 1.0$	**134**	**101**	**235**	**0.57**	**28**	**75**	**103**	**0.28**
combination $\alpha = 0.3, \beta = 1.1$	105	111	216	0.52	28	83	111	0.30
combination $\alpha = 0.4, \beta = 1.0$	132	101	233	0.56	27	76	103	0.28
oracle	46	86	132	0.32	14	72	86	0.23

ing the QRS complex predictions of both algorithms. Note that because of peak matching, only the larger peak of the two QRS complexes predicted by both algorithms within the time interval δ is accepted in order to avoid too many false positives; $\delta = 240ms$ is nearly optimal for the union (see Figure 4). Our data-driven combination algorithm significantly decreases the number of false positives compared to the union, leading to 227 training errors for the (globally) optimal values $\alpha = 0.3, \beta = 1.0$. This error rate is hardly affected by modifying α in an interval $[0.25; 0.4]$ and β in an interval $[1.0; 1.1]$. The best error rate that can be achieved by optimally combining the wavelet and PT algorithms, given by the (cheating) oracle method, is 159 errors. In Figure 5, results of our combination algorithm are compared with the PT algorithm for the individual patients.

4.4. Test Results

Results on the test set are shown in Table 3 ($\delta = 240ms$). Again, we obtained fewer errors with the PT method than with the wavelet algorithm on our database. Note that for the patients 105 and 108, the wavelet algorithm produced a large number of extra errors (see below).

The general trends discussed in section 4.3.3. are also observed on the test data. In particular, the union and our combination approach dramatically reduce the number of false negatives compared to the individual algorithms. However, the large number of wavelet errors especially on the excerpts 105 and 108 detriments the union and our combination algorithm. One reason for the large number of wavelet errors is that the wavelet algorithm is often unable to identify the correct location of potential QRS complexes. A misplaced wavelet peak may result in two errors, namely a false negative *and* a false positive error (if it is more than 100ms from the annotated position). On the other hand, peak matching with sufficiently large δ (see Section 4.3.2.) removes such an error pair, if there is a nearby, more pronounced PT peak that is matched with the wavelet peak[9]. Although (nearly) optimizing the peak matching interval δ for the union, the large number of wavelet false positives in particular on patients 105 and 108 detriments the union, so that it performs worse than PT on the (complete) test set. In contrast, our data-driven combination algorithm allows to reduce this effect and limit the number of false positives by accepting only a subset of the wavelet QRS complex predictions, controlled by the parameter α. (In addition, false positives predicted by PT can be removed by increasing β). Thus, our combination approach outperforms both the union and the PT algorithm on the test set.

The negative effect of the wavelet false positives on the performance of the union (and our combination algorithm) can be seen by removing excerpts 105 and 108 from the test data. Then, both the union and our combination algorithm clearly outperform the PT method, by strongly decreasing the number of PT false negatives while inserting only a small number of additional false positives, compared to PT. Our data-driven combination method (slightly) improves upon the union, by further reducing the number of false positives. However, recall that the performance of the union has been nearly optimized by setting $\delta = 240ms$. In contrast, our combination algorithm nearly gave the same results when using $\delta = 120ms$ instead of $\delta = 240ms$.

Again, the results for our combination algorithm are hardly affected by variations of the (global) value for α within the interval $[0.25; 0.4]$. On the test set, however, slightly increasing β has a larger effect on the error rate than observed on the training set, since the (relative) number of PT false positives is larger on the test set than on the training set (especially for patients 105 and 108).

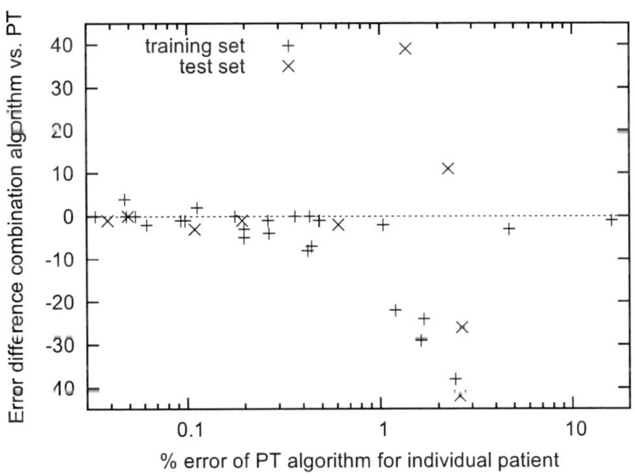

Figure 5. (Absolute) error reduction by our combination algorithm ($\alpha = 0.3$, $\beta = 1.0$) as compared to the PT algorithm, as a function of the PT error rate (in %, logarithmic scale) for the individual patients of the MIT-BIH database. 13 patients (5 training, 8 test) have zero error on both the PT and combination algorithm and are not shown.

[9]This is an explanation for the union having less false positive errors than the wavelet algorithm.

4.5. Patient Analysis

Combining our training and test results (including patient 207), we arrive at an error rate of 0.70% for our data-driven combination approach ($\alpha = 0.3$, $\beta = 1.0$), compared to 0.85% for the PT algorithm, 1.36% for wavelet and 0.83% for the union. Note that patient 207 exhibits periods of ventricular fibrillation with a large number of peaks which are not annotated, producing an extremely large number of insertions for this patient. Excluding patient 207, our combination algorithm yields an error rate of 0.43% compared to 0.59% for PT and 1.18% for wavelet.

Figure 5 shows the (absolute) error reduction by our combination algorithm compared to the PT method for the individual patients, as a function of the patients' PT error rate. For 24 patients, our combination approach reduces the number of PT errors (on the average by 9.5 errors per patient); 20 patients yield identical results, and for four patients (105, 108, 111, 232) our data-driven combination increases the number of errors compared to PT. This is mostly due to the large number of wavelet false positives (see above), especially for the patients 105 and 108 (showing the largest error increase with our algorithm). For these patients, by using a larger, patient-specific value for α, the number of false positives can be strongly reduced, as will be explained in the following section.

On the other hand, for those patients for which the wavelet algorithm was better than PT, our combination approach was able to outperform the wavelet result (patients 210 and 221) or produce the same or a similar result (at most one error difference, 11 patients). In this set, only for patients 101, 207 and 217 our combination algorithm was worse than wavelet (but still better than PT).

Therefore, we conclude that for most patients of the MIT-BIH arrhythmia database, our combination algorithm outperformed or performed comparably to the better of the two base algorithms.

4.6. Patient-Specific Optimization

So far, we have used *global* values for the parameters α and β, which were estimated once on separate training data and then kept fixed for all patients. In this section, we investigate *patient-specific* values for α and β, which are chosen manually *a posteriori* for individual patients ("cheating"). The goal is to demonstrate the potential of such a patient-specific optimization. Results are shown in table 4.

For example, using $\alpha = 0.8$ instead of $\alpha = 0.3$ for patient 108, we observe 18 false positives instead of 55, corresponding to 31 errors (instead of 63). Similarly, applying the same parameter setting to patient 111, the 4 false positives inserted as result of wavelet detections could be removed, recovering the optimal PT result for this patient. Conversely, setting $\beta = 5.0$ instead of $\beta = 1.0$ for patient 101, some errors inserted due to wrong PT detections could be removed, improving the combination result. Finally, for patient 104, setting $\alpha = 0.8$ and $\beta = 2.0$ further improves the combination result, increasing the gain already achieved by the combination method with globally optimal parameters.

In these experiments, we have modified the parameters α and β *a posteriori* ("cheating"), to illustrate the performance gain that can be achieved by using patient-specific combination parameters. Appropriate strategies to choose (or estimate) the parameters individ-

Table 4. Patient-specific parameters α and β. Shown are the results for the base algorithms and the combination with globally optimal parameters $\alpha = 0.3$ and $\beta = 1.0$ as well as with manually chosen parameters α and β.

algorithm	# FP	# FN	# err
	Patient 108		
wavelet	77	52	129
PT	14	10	24
comb. $\alpha = 0.3, \beta = 1.0$	55	8	63
comb. $\alpha = 0.8, \beta = 1.0$	18	13	31
	Patient 111		
wavelet	40	10	50
PT	0	1	1
comb. $\alpha = 0.3, \beta = 1.0$	4	1	5
comb. $\alpha = 0.8, \beta = 1.0$	0	1	1
	Patient 101		
wavelet	2	1	3
PT	5	4	9
comb. $\alpha = 0.3, \beta = 1.0$	5	3	8
comb. $\alpha = 0.3, \beta = 5.0$	3	3	6
	Patient 104		
wavelet	76	36	112
PT	78	25	103
comb. $\alpha = 0.3, \beta = 1.0$	77	23	100
comb. $\alpha = 0.8, \beta = 2.0$	73	22	95

ually for each patient (e.g. by unsupervised adaptation) remain to be investigated in future work.

4.7. Results on Arrhythmic Passages

In this section we analyze the results of our combination algorithm specifically on arrhythmic beats and episodes. Due to the small number of patients showing some of the arrhythmia types, we discuss the results on the full data set (i.e. combining training and test data).

In a first analysis, we analyze the error rates of the QRS detection algorithms for specific *beat* types, namely for QRS complexes which are annotated in the database as being either a premature ventricular contraction (PVC, about 6.5% of all beats) or an atrial premature contraction (APC, about 2.3% of all beats); all other beats are ignored. PVCs and APCs are among the most common arrhythmic beat types. Evaluation results are shown in Table 5.

Regarding PVC, the combination algorithm significantly outperformed both the wavelet and the PT method. Again this is due to strongly reducing the number of false negatives,

Table 5. Error specifically for beats labeled as premature ventricular contraction (PVC, about 6.5% of all beats) or atrial premature contraction (APC, about 2.3% of all beats) on all patients of the MIT-BIH arrhythmia database.

	Premature ventricular contraction (PVC)			
algorithm	# FP	# FN	# err in 7127	% err
wavelet	14	317	331	4.64
PT	7	217	224	3.14
combination, $\alpha = 0.3, \beta = 1.0$	7	68	75	1.05
	Atrial premature contraction (APC)			
algorithm	# FP	# FN	# err in 2544	% err
wavelet	2	5	7	0.28
PT	1	1	2	0.08
combination, $\alpha = 0.3, \beta = 1.0$	2	1	3	0.12

without increasing the number of false positives. Regarding the individual patients for the PVC beats, we observed strong improvements over the better of the two base algorithms especially for patients 106, 203, 208, 210 and 221 (at least 5 errors less compared to the base algorithm which performed better for the individual patient). For the other patients, the combination method achieved at least the performance of the better of the two base algorithms. Only patients 107 (plus 2 errors) and 228 (plus 1 error) were slightly degraded. Thus, the combination method is able to “switch” between both base algorithms: If the wavelet method turns out to be better for an individual patient or a specific passage within the patients’ signal, the combination algorithm often reproduces the wavelet detections. In contrast, if the PT algorithm achieves a better performance for a patient or a specific passage, the combination method mostly accepts the PT detections (see also the examples in Section 4.8.).

Regarding APC, at very low error rates the combination algorithm made one error more than the PT algorithm inspired by a wavelet false positive. Here, the number of errors is however too small to draw statistical conclusions.

In a second analysis, we calculated the error rates for specific *rhythm* types. Here, the ECG signal is divided into episodes of specific arrhythmias, where the type as well as the start and end point of each episode are annotated in the database. Specifically, we considered all arrhythmia types exhibited by at least 5 patients in the MIT-BIH arrhythmia database. These are atrial fibrillation (115 episodes from 8 patients, 9.0% of the total recording time), ventricular tachycardia (61 episodes from 13 patients, 0.2% of the total recording time), ventricular bigeminy (221 episodes from 12 patients, 2.9% of the total recording time), ventricular trigeminy (83 episodes from 12 patients, 1.3% of the total recording time), and supraventricular tachyarrhythmia (26 episodes from 7 patients, 0.2% of the total recording time). Results were collected for all episodes of a given type and all patients in the MIT-BIH arrhythmia database; see Table 6.

For the considered types of arrhythmic episodes, the same trends were observed as for

Table 6. Error on selected types of arrhythmic episodes on all patients of the MIT-BIH arrhythmia database.

	Atrial fibrillation			
algorithm	# FP	# FN	# err in 11937	% err
wavelet	24	150	174	1.46
PT	10	146	156	1.31
combination, $\alpha = 0.3, \beta = 1.0$	14	53	67	0.56
	Ventricular tachycardia			
algorithm	#FP	# FN	# err in 399	% err
wavelet	1	26	27	6.77
PT	0	15	15	3.76
combination, $\alpha = 0.3, \beta = 1.0$	0	9	9	2.26
	Ventricular bigeminy			
algorithm	# FP	# FN	# err in 3288	% err
wavelet	6	69	75	2.28
PT	3	20	23	0.70
combination, $\alpha = 0.3, \beta = 1.0$	3	8	11	0.34
	Ventricular trigeminy			
algorithm	#FP	# FN	# err in 1360	% err
wavelet	2	44	46	3.38
PT	0	17	17	1.25
combination, $\alpha = 0.3, \beta = 1.0$	0	7	7	0.52
	Supraventricular tachyarrhythmia			
algorithm	# FP	# FN	# err in 467	% err
wavelet	1	0	1	0.21
PT	1	0	1	0.21
combination, $\alpha = 0.3, \beta = 1.0$	1	0	1	0.21

arrhythmic beats: Overall, the combination algorithm significantly outperformed both base algorithms, by strongly reducing the number of false positives, while only moderately (or even not at all) increasing the number of false negatives. For the individual patients, the combination algorithm performed again at least as well as the better of the two base algorithms. Moreover, for some patients additional improvements over the best base algorithm were observed (e.g. for patient 106 regarding ventricular bigeminy and patient 208 regarding ventricular trigeminy). For supraventricular tachyarrhythmia, we observed only one error, which was done by both wavelet and PT and thus also by the combination algorithm.

These results suggest that the combination algorithm performs particularly well on arrhythmic beat types like PVC and rhythm types like atrial fibrillation, ventricular tachycardia, ventricular bi- and trigeminy, significantly outperforming QRS detection performance compared to both base algorithms (wavelet and PT).

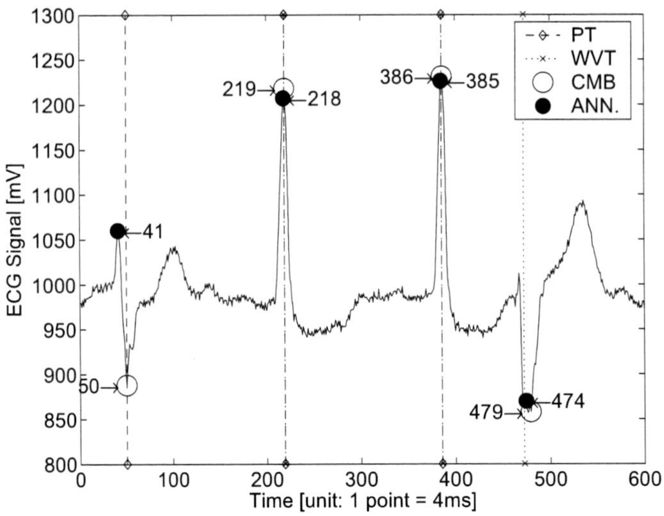

Figure 6. Example for automatic QRS complex detection, patient 210. QRS complexes detected by the PT method ("PT") are marked with a dashed line, those detected by wavelet ("WVT") with a dotted line; dashed-dotted lines refer to QRS complexes predicted by both algorithms. Predictions of the combination algorithm ("CMB") are marked with an open circle, and the manual annotations ("ANN") with a filled circle (for both, the corresponding time point is indicated next to the symbol). This episode is manually annotated as 'ventricular trigeminy'. The peaks at 218 and 385 are manually annotated as normal beats, those at 41 and 474 as PVCs.

4.8. Examples

In this section we discuss various examples for the corrections made using our data-driven combination algorithm. In Figures 6 and 7, the combination algorithm correctly accepts all peaks detected by either PT or wavelet, and thus corrects a false negative from the PT and one from the wavelet method. Figure 6 (patient 210) is manually annotated as "ventricular trigeminy". In Figure 7 (patient 208) the rhythm changes from a normal sinus rhythm to ventricular trigeminy (before the peak at point 516). Here, the QRS complex at time point 82 (manually annotated as fusion between a ventricular and a normal beat, visible in the second channel) is missed by both PT and wavelet and thus also by the combination algorithm. In Figure 8 (patient 203), manually labeled as ventricular tachycardia with a rhythm change to atrial fibrillation (after the peak at time point 206), the QRS complex at time point 206 is missed by PT, but detected by the combination algorithm due to a corresponding wavelet detection. The proposed wavelet peak at time point 22 is improved by a peak matching correction, triggered by a corresponding PT peak at time point 50.

Figures 9 (patient 106) and 10 (patient 203) present examples where in one episode the combination approach improves upon the PT algorithm, whereas in another episode from the same patient the combination algorithm improves upon the wavelet method. In Figure 9 a), the combination accepts all PT QRS detections, correcting for two wavelet false negatives. In Figure 9 b), the combination method corrects the PT false negative at time

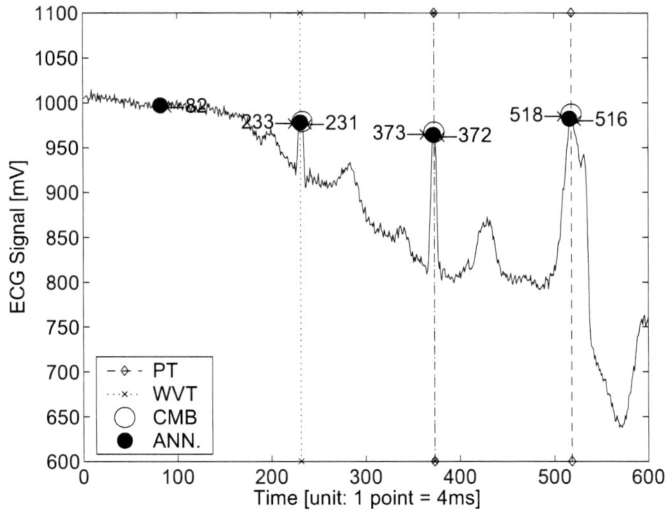

Figure 7. Example for automatic QRS complex detection, patient 208 (the symbols are explained in Figure 6). This episode is manually annotated as 'normal sinus rhythm' with a rhythm change to 'ventricular trigeminy' (before the peak at time point 516). In the manual annotation, there is also a QRS complex at time point 82 (fusion of ventricular and normal beat); this peak is visible in the second channel. The peaks at 231 and 372 are labeled as normal beats, the peak at 516 as PVC.

point 157 and improves the PT prediction at time point 50 by peak matching, both triggered by wavelet predictions. Finally, in Figure 10 a), the combination algorithm accepts all QRS complexes predicted by wavelet, thus correcting for two peaks missed by PT. The peak at time point 338, however, is missed by both PT and wavelet and thus by the combination algorithm. In the episode in Figure 10 b), the combination method correctly accepts all QRS complexes predicted by PT and thus corrects for two peaks missed by wavelet.

5. Summary and Discussion

We developed a framework for combining state-of-the-art algorithms for detection of QRS complexes in ECG signals, namely the Pan-Tompkins (PT) and the wavelet algorithms. The basic idea is to run both algorithms in parallel. When both methods disagree whether to predict a QRS complex in a particular time window, we applied a data-driven strategy for deciding whether or not to accept the candidate QRS complex. More precisely, in cases of disagreement we suggest to locally rerun the PT method with a modified threshold, accepting the result of the local rerun as the final decision. The local decisions can formally be seen as the majority vote of a (three-component) ensemble classifier, where the third classifier corresponds to one of the first two classifiers, however with modified threshold. We introduced two parameters α and β to control the threshold adjustment, which are both estimated on training data. By varying α and β we can, in theory, interpolate between the predictions of the individual algorithms and Boolean combinations like union and intersection.

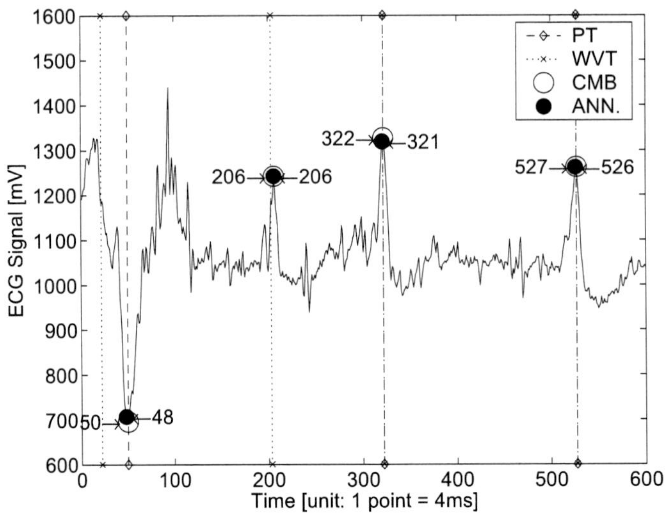

Figure 8. Example for automatic QRS complex detection, patient 203 (the symbols are explained in Figure 6). This episode is manually annotated as 'ventricular tachycardia' with a rhythm change to 'atrial fibrillation' (after the peak at time point 206). The QRS complex at time point 48 is manually annotated as PVC, those at 206, 321 and 526 as normal beats.

In experiments on the MIT-BIH arrhythmia database we showed that our combination algorithm outperformed both base algorithms as well as the union (and intersection) of the two methods. In particular, the combination method strongly improved QRS detection performance on arrhythmic beat types like premature ventricular contractions and on common rhythm types like atrial fibrillation, ventricular tachycardia, ventricular bigeminy and ventricular trigeminy. This improvement in QRS detection performance can mostly be attributed to strongly reducing the number of missed QRS complexes compared to the base algorithms, from combining the predictions of both methods. On the other hand, the number of false positives is only moderately increased, since our data-driven approach only *selectively* accepts QRS complexes for which the two algorithms disagree, controlled by the (optimized) parameters α and β. This is especially important for noisy patients, in order to reject a potentially large number of false positives in any of the base algorithms. As illustrated in various examples, the data-driven selection of QRS complexes from the base algorithms may lead the combination method in certain episodes to accept mainly QRS predictions from the PT algorithm, while in other episodes from the same patient it may basically follow the wavelet QRS predictions. This is particularly beneficial in arrhythmic passages, due to the variations in QRS morphology and frequency. Thus, for most of the patients of the MIT-BIH arrhythmia database, our combination algorithm performed at least as well as the better of the two base algorithms. An issue for further work is to verify our results on other databases as well as for improved base algorithms. Moreover, it might be interesting to investigate how the parameters of the individual algorithms (refractory period, thresholds etc.) should be chosen in order to result in an optimal performance of the combination algorithm.

An easy way to specify the parameters α and β of the combination algorithm is to use

a)

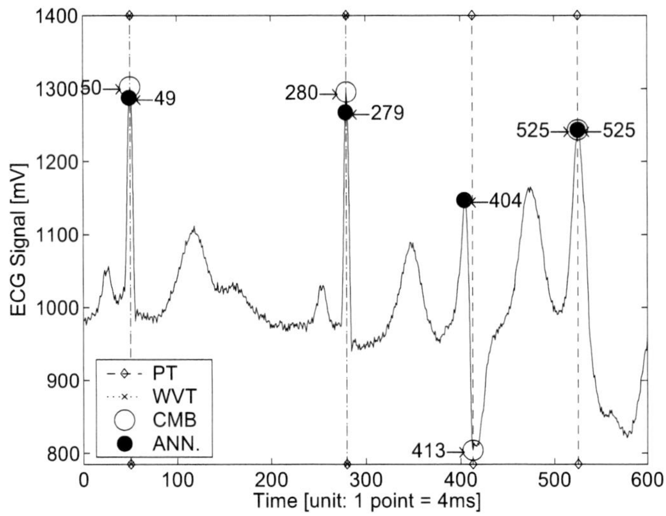

b)

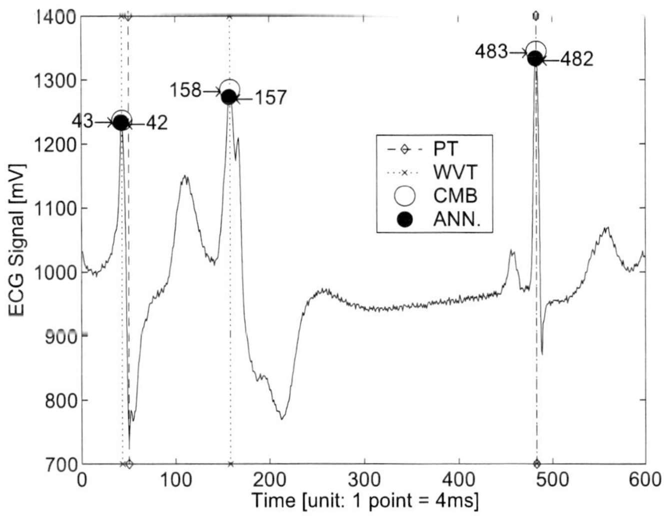

Figure 9. Example for automatic QRS complex detection, patient 106 (the symbols are explained in Figure 6). The episode in a) is manually annotated as 'normal sinus rhythm' (beats at time points 49 and 279 are annotated as normal beats, those at time points 404 and 525 as PVCs), the episode in b) as 'normal sinus rhythm' with a rhythm change to 'ventricular bigeminy' (after the last peak; peaks at time points 42 and 157 are annotated as PVCs, the peak at 482 as normal beat).

global (patient- and time-independent) values for α and β, estimated on separate, representative training data. However, for some patients, one base algorithm may generate many more errors (false positives or false negatives) than the other base method, which may dete-

a)

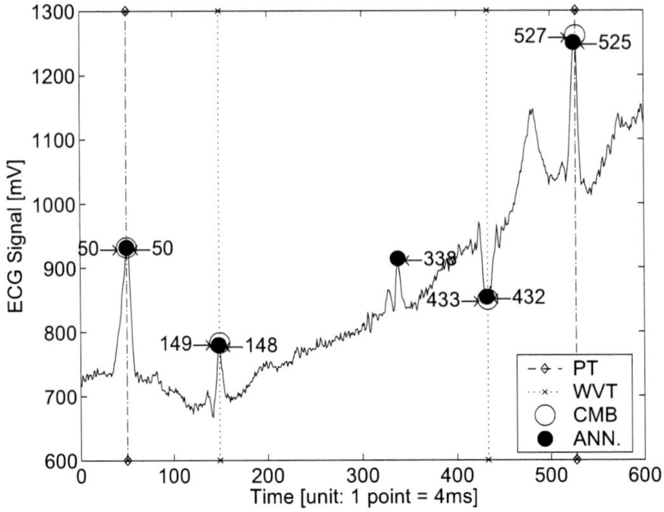

b)

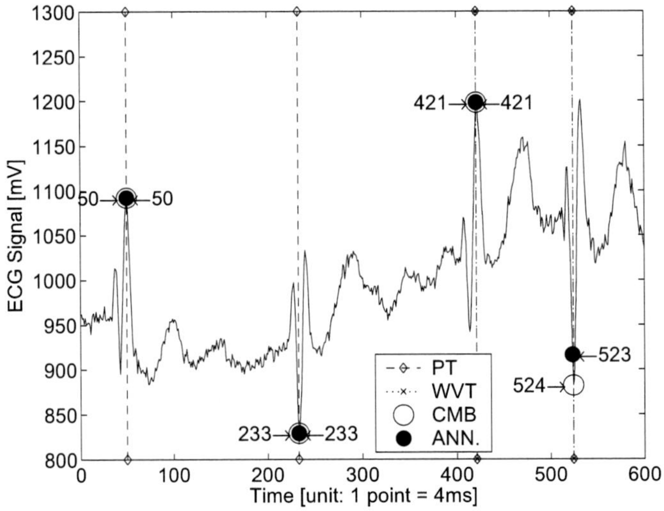

Figure 10. Example for automatic QRS complex detection, patient 203 (the symbols are explained in Figure 6). The episode in a) is manually annotated as 'atrial fibrillation' (beats at time points 50, 148, 338 and 525 are annotated as normal beats, that at time point 432 as PVC), the episode in b) as 'atrial fibrillation' (all QRS complexes manually annotated as normal beats).

riorate the performance of the combination algorithm for these patients. This motivates to introduce *patient specific* values for α or β, in order to remove at least a fraction of these errors in the combination algorithm. Varying α and β *a posteriori*, we have demonstrated the performance gain from such patient-specific combination parameters for several patients.

This led the combination method also for these specific patients to provide an error rate close to or even better than the better of the two base algorithms. Suitable strategies to estimate and optimize patient-specific values for α and β however remain to be investigated in future work. A possible approach is to start with the global values for α and β for each new patient, and to *adapt* the parameters in an unsupervised way according to an appropriate criterion. Another approach would be to cluster the patient data (or appropriately windowed data episodes) in order to estimate α and β individually for each cluster on respective training data. Then, for each new patient, the data would have to be classified into the appropriate cluster, and the estimated cluster values for α and β would be used.

We developed our combination algorithm to combine the wavelet and PT methods for automatic detection of QRS complexes. Our general framework, however, can be adopted to other algorithms and other contexts as well, provided a suitable parameter can be identified for one of the two algorithms which allows to modify the predictions of this algorithm in a continuous way. The parameters α and β then merely serve to "interpolate" between the individual algorithms and their union and intersection, as we discussed in detail. Performance improvements can be expected if a (sufficiently large) set of cases exists where both algorithms disagree in their prediction, and if the predictions are uncorrelated within this set.

Moreover, while we were focussing on a single ECG channel, our approach can also be applied to two ECG leads, combining e.g. PT predictions from channel 1 with PT predictions (or other algorithms) from channel 2.

6. Conclusion

Combining two state-of-the art algorithms for QRS complex detection in a data-driven approach has been shown to significantly improve performance over the individual base algorithms. This was achieved by strongly reducing the number of false negatives due to combining the predictions of both base algorithms, while only moderately increasing the number of false positives due to only *selectively* accepting additional peaks. In particular, the performance gain was demonstrated for arrhythmic beat and rhythm types. This can be attributed to the variations in morphology and frequency of QRS complexes which may be difficult to be handled by a single algorithm. Moreover, our data-driven combination approach provides a flexible way for adapting the combined classifier to individual data sets or conditions (e.g. patients or patient groups).

References

[1] D. Ge, N. Srinivasan, and S. M. Krishnan, "Cardiac arrhythmia classification using autoregressive modeling", *Biomed. Eng. Online.*, 13. Nov. 2002, vol. 1:5.

[2] C. C. Chiu, T. H. Lin, and B. Y. Liau, "Using correlation coefficient in ECG waveform for arrhythmia detection", *Biomed. Eng. Appl. Basis Comm.*, 2005, vol. 17, pp. 147-152.

[3] J. Pan and W. L. Tompkins, "A Real-Time QRS Detection Algorithm", *IEEE Trans. Biomed. Eng.*, 1985, vol. 32, pp. 230-236.

[4] Q. Xue, Y. H. Hu and W. J. Tompkins, "Neural-network-based adaptive matched filtering for QRS detection", *IEEE Trans. Biomed. Eng.*, 1992, vol. 39, pp. 317-329.

[5] Y. H. Hu, W. J. Tompkins, J. L. Urrusti and V. X. Afonso, "Applications of artificial neural networks for ECG signal detection and classification", *J. Electrocardiology*, 1993, vol. 26, pp. 67-73.

[6] A. Krykos, E. Giakoumakis, G. Carayannis, "Time Recursive Prediction Techniques on QRS Detection Problem", *Proc. 9th Annu. Conf. IEEE Engineering in Medicine and Biology Society, Boston, MA*, 1987, pp. 1885-1886.

[7] S. Abboud and D. Sadeh, "The use of cross-correlation function for the alignment of ECG waveforms and rejection of extrasystoles", *Computers and Biomedical Research*, 1993, vol. 16,pp. 273-286.

[8] T. Last, C. D. Nugent, and F. J. Owens, "Multi-component based cross correlation beat detection in electrocardiogram analysis", *Biomed. Eng. Online.*, 23. July 2004, vol. 3:26.

[9] S. L. Horowitz, "A syntactic algorithm for peak detection in waveforms with applications to cardiology", *Communications of the ACM*, 1975, vol. 18, pp. 281-285.

[10] G. Belforte, R. De Mori and F. Ferraris, "A contribution to the automatic processing of electrocardiograms using syntactic methods", *IEEE Trans. Biomed. Eng*, 1979, vol. 26, pp. 125-136.

[11] C. D. Nugent, J. A. C. Webb, G. T. H. Wright, and N. D. Black, "Electrocardiogram 1: Pre-processing prior to classification", Automedica, 1998, vol. 16, pp. 263-282.

[12] B. U. Köhler, C. Henning and R. Orgelmeister, "The principles of software QRS detection", *IEEE Eng. Med. Biol. Mag.*, 2002, vol. 21, pp. 42-57.

[13] C. Li, C. Zheng and C. Tai, "Detection of ECG Characteristic Points Using Wavelet Transforms", *IEEE Trans. Biomed. Eng.*, 1995, vol. 42, pp. 21-28.

[14] S. Mallat and W.L. Hwang, "Singularity Detection and Processing with Wavelets", *IEEE Trans. Inform. Theory*, 1992, vol. 38, pp. 617-643.

[15] J.P. Martinez, S Olmos and P. Laguna, "Evaluation of a wavelet based ECG waveform detector on the QT database", *Proc. IEEE Computers in Cardiology*, 2000, vol. 27, pp. 81-84.

[16] T. G. Dietterich, "Ensemble Methods in Machine Learning", *Lecture Notes in Computer Science*, 2000, vol. 1857, pp. 1-15.

[17] J. C. T. B. Moraes, M. M Freitas, F. N. Vilani and E. V. Costa, "A QRS Complex Detection Algorithm Using Electrocardiogram Leads", *Proc. IEEE Computers in Cardiology*, 2002, vol. 29, pp. 205-208.

[18] W. A. H. Engelse and C. Zeelenberg, "A Single Scan Algorithm for QRS Detection and Feature Extraction", *Proc. IEEE Computers in Cardiology*, 1979, pp. 37-42.

[19] A. Ligtenberg and M. Kunt, "A Robust-Digital QRS Detection Algorithm for Arrhythmia Monitoring", *Computers and Biomedical Research* 1983, vol. 16, pp. 273-286.

[20] C. Meyer, J. Fernández Gavela and M. Harris, "Combining Algorithms in Automatic Detection of QRS Complexes in ECG Signals", *IEEE Trans. Info. Techn. in Biomedicine*, 2006, vol. 10, no. 3, pp. 468-475.

[21] J.P. Martinez, R. Almeida, S Olmos, A.P. Rocha and P. Laguna, "A Wavelet Based ECG Delineator: Evaluation on Standard Databases", *EEE Trans. Biomed. Eng.*, 2004, vol. 51, pp. 570-581.

[22] S. Mallat, "Zero-crossings of a wavelet transform", *IEEE Trans. Inform. Theory*, 1991, vol. 37, pp. 1019-1033.

[23] L. Hansen and P. Salomon, "Neural network ensembles", *IEEE Trans. Pattern Analysis and Machine Intelligence*, 1990, vol. 12, pp. 993-1001.

[24] R. Mark and G. Moody, "MIT-BIH Arrhythmia data base directory", *Cambridge: Massachusetts Institute of Technology*, 1988.

In: Progress in Cardiac Arrhythmia Research
Editor: Ira R. Tarkowicz, pp. 169-182
ISBN: 1-60021-796-6

Chapter 7

Differential Effect of I_{Kr} and I_{Ks} Block on Action Potential in Isolated Rabbit Heart

Samar Al Makdessi*, Hicham Sweidan and Ralph F. Bosch**
University of Tübingen, Institute of Physiology, Tübingen, Germany.
**University of Tübingen, Department of Cardiology, Tübingen, Germany

Abstract

The fast (I_{Kr}) and the slow (I_{Ks}) components of the delayed rectifier potassium current are important targets for class III antiarrhythmic drugs that exert their antiarrhythmic potential by prolongation of repolarization. In the present study, we analyzed the effects of blocking I_{Kr} and I_{Ks} on action potential repolarization in isolated perfused rabbit heart. Dofetilide (10^{-8} to 10^{-5} M) was used as I_{Kr} blocker, and chromanol 293B (293B) (10^{-7} to $3x10^{-5}$ M) to block I_{Ks}. Epicardial monophasic action potentials were recorded by means of contact electrodes and the action potential duration (APD) was measured at 20% (APD_{20}), 50% (APD_{50}) and 90% (APD_{90}) repolarization.

Dofetilide exhibited a dose-dependent prolongation of APD_{90}, and, to a lesser extent of APD_{50} at all cycle lengths (1000, 750, 600, 500, 400, and 333 ms) with an IC_{50} of 4.7 nM (APD_{90}). Under basal conditions, the application of 293B resulted in a mild APD prolongation which was significant only for APD_{20} (20.7 ± 12.2%, $p<0.05$ at a cycle length of 500 ms, IC_{50}: 7.0 µM). APD_{90} was not prolongated at concentrations up to $3x10^{-5}$ M.

The delay in repolarization observed with dofetilide displayed a clear reverse rate-dependence whereas the effects of 293B were similar at all frequencies tested.

Under β-adrenergic stimulation with isoproterenol (10^{-8}M, 15 min), dofetilide exerted only a small, temporal prolongation of APD_{90} (14.1 ± 12.6%, $p<0.05$), while a much more pronounced effect was observed with 293B over the complete registration period (34.7 ± 17.9%, $p<0.05$). Both substances exhibited no significant effect on APD_{50} and APD_{20} under β-adrenergic stimulation.

* E-mail address: makdessi-sweidan@uni-tuebingen.de. Phone: +49-7071-2976061; Correspondence concerning this article should be addressed to Dr. Samar Al Makdessi, Institue of Physiology, Gmelinstr. 5, D-72076 Tübingen, Germany.

Conclusions: Dofetilide showed a potent and dose-dependent APD prolongation which was associated with a reverse rate-dependence, while 293B effect was rate-independent and less pronounced under basal conditions.

With an increase in adrenergic tone, the effect of I_{Ks} block increased substantially and the APD prolongation was stronger compared to I_{Kr} block. These properties of I_{Ks} block make this channel an interesting target for novel antiarrhythmic agents with a potentially advantageous profile over currently available drugs.

Keywords: Dofetilide, Chromanol 293B, Isoproterenol, Isolated rabbit heart, Reverse rate-dependence.

Introduction

Among the multiple K currents which contribute to repolarization in the mammalian heart, the delayed rectifier current was found to play a major role and constitutes an important target for antiarrhythmic drugs (Colatsky et al., 1990), particularly class III agents.

Two components of the delayed rectifier current have been identified, one rapid, I_{Kr}, and one slow, I_{Ks} (Sanguinetti & Jurkiewicz, 1990). These two components markedly differ in their kinetics. It has been found in rabbit ventricle that I_{Kr} is activated by depolarization, increases progressively and initiates phase 3 repolarization, whereas I_{Ks}, which possesses a slow deactivation rate accumulates when heart rate increases (Jurkiewicz & Sanguinetti, 1993; Nattel & Singh, 1999; Seebohm et al., 2001). I_{Kr} was estimated to contribute more to I_K during resting ventricular action potential than does I_{Ks} (Varró et al., 2000; Lengyel et al., 2001).

Dofetilide is a prototype of a highly selective I_{Kr} antagonist (Sanguinetti & Jurkiewicz, 1990; Jurkiewicz & Sanguinetti, 1993). It increases APD as well as the effective refractory period (Kovàcs et al., 2003) without influencing conduction velocity. It has no effect on other ionic currents such as I_{Ca}, I_{Na} or I_{Ks} and possesses no β-blocking activity (Kalus & Mauro, 2000). A major draw back of dofetilide and other I_{Kr} blockers is the reverse rate-dependence: their effect is reduced at rapid heart rate while it prolongs APD excessively at slow rates.

I_{Ks} blockers, such as chromanol 293B (293B) have the advantage of a rate-independent action on a cellular level (Bosch et al., 1998). Moreover, their effect could increase at high frequencies due to I_{Ks} accumulation in the activated open state (Jurkiewicz & Sanguinetti, 1993). Various experimental models have been used for the investigation of I_{Kr} and I_{Ks} blockade: isolated myocytes (Sanguinetti et al., 1991; Bosch et al., 1998; Fujisawa et al., 2000, Jost et al., 2005), isolated papillary muscle of guinea pig (Tande et al., 1990; Schreieck et al., 1997; Varró et al., 2000, Gogelein et al., 2000) or rabbit (Lengyel et al., 2001), isolated guinea pig lefr atrium (Kovàcs et al., 2003), rabbit perfused left ventricukar wedge prepraration (Chen et al., 2006), dog ventricular preparations (Burashnikov & Anzelevitch, 2000; Varró et al., 2000; Biliczki et al., 2002), and intact dog (Bauer et al., 2002). The interest in using the isolated paced Langendorff-perfused rabbit heart for the investigation of new antiarrhythmic drugs increased considerably in the last years (Valentin et al., 2004; Lawrence et al., 2006). This model was found to be able to provide detailed informations on the drug-induced electrophysiological effects as well as to predict a compound's arrhythmogenic potential in human within clinically relevant concentration ranges (Chen et al., 2006). The greatest advantage in using the isolated perfused rabbit heart is that the kinetiks of I_{Kr} and I_{Ks}

activation and deactivation was found to be similar in rabbit, dog and humans. This may allow the extrapolation of the results obtained on the rabbit heart to the human heart (Lengyel et al., 2001; Jost et al., 2005).

The present study aimed to compare the effects of dofetilide and 293B on the APD in isolated Langendorff-perfused rabbit hearts, and to investigate the frequency dependence of the effects as well as the influence of β-adrenergic stimulation with isoproterenol.

Material and Methods

All the procedures used were in accordance with §4 of the German animal welfare legislation and guidlines on animal care of the University of Tübingen. New Zealand rabbits of both sex weighing 3.44 ± 0.53 kg (n=38) were sacrified by cervical dislocation. The hearts were rapidly excised and canulated onto a Langendorff perfusion system. The hearts were perfused retrogradly via the aorta under constant pressure (68 mmHg) with a modified Krebs-Henseleit solution maintained at 37°C and continuously gased with carbogen. The composition of the perfusion fluid was (in mmol/l): NaCl, 118, KCl, 4.7, $CaCl_2$, 2.5, $MgSO_4$, 1.6, $NaHCO_3$, 24.9, $NaHPO_4$, 1.2, Glucose, 5.5, Na Pyruvate, 2.0, Na_2 EDTA, 0.5.

ECG was continuously monitored by means of three silver electrodes, two of them being immersed in the heart chamber at equidistant location from the heart and connected to a recorder (Mingograph 7, Siemens-Elema, Germany), and the third being clipped to the canula. Epicardial monophasic action potentials (MAP) were recorded by means of a contact catheter (Biotronic, Berlin, Germany) placed at the upper part of the left ventricle and connected to an amplifier (Siemens AG, Germany) which was connected to an analog recorder (Mingograph 7, Siemens-Elema, Germany). Recordings were done at a paper speed of 200 mm/sec.

The hearts were allowed to equilibrate 20-30 minutes, until stable recordings were obtained. Coronary flow was 80.62 ± 20.57 ml/min. In the first group of experiments, the atrio-ventricular node was ablated using a high temperature cautery after excision of the right atrium, in order to be able to pace the ventricles at the desired cycle lengths. Heart rate declined from 139.17 ± 18.47 to 50.53 ± 7.98 beats/min. Then, the hearts were paced by means of an external pulse generator (Siemens-Elema, Germany) with a pacing electrode installed into the right ventricular cavity. Control MAP were recorded at 1000, 750, 600, 500, 400, and 333 ms, after an equilibration period of 60 beats at each pacing rate. Then either dofetilide (made available by Pfizer, Sandwich, England) or 293B (made available by Aventis GmbH, Frankfurt, Germany) were added. Each concentration was equilibrated for 10 minutes after which MAP were recorded at the above-mentioned pacing rates. In the second group of experiments, Isoproterenol (Sigma, Deisenhofen, Germany) (10^{-8} mol/l), freshly prepared and stabilized with ascorbic acid, 10^{1} mol/l) was perfused for 8 minutes. Hearts were left to beat spontaneously. Then either dofetilide (10^{-7} mol/l) or 293B ($3x10^{-5}$ mol/l) was added. MAP were recorded every minute during 15 minutes. Action potential duration (APD) recorded was measured by the method proposed by Franz (Franz et al., 1986).

Statistical Analysis

Results are expressed as mean ± SEM. Experimental groups were statistically compared by means of the Student t-test. The paired t-test was used to estimate the differences within the same group, whereas the unpaired t-test compared the block of I_{Kr} to that of I_{Ks}. A two-way ANOVA was used when multiple comparisons were needed. $P<0.05$ was considered as the significance level.

Results

1. Dose-Dependent Effects of Dofetilide and 293B on APD

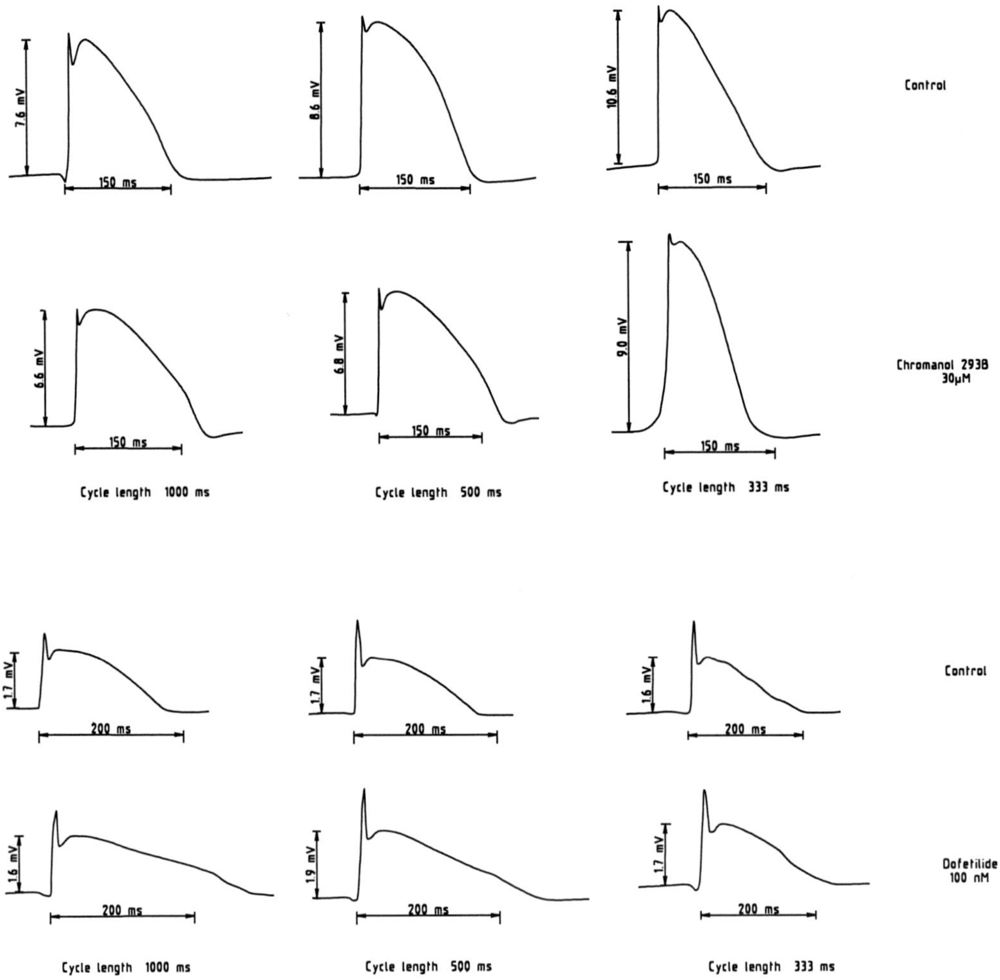

Figure 1. Epicardial monophasic action potentials recorded in isolated Langendorff-perfused rabbit heart in the presence of Dofetilide (100 nM) and Chromanol 293B (293B, 30 μM) at 1000, 500 and 333ms cycle length.

An example of the MAP recorded under control conditions and after I_{Kr} and I_{Ks} block is illustrated in Figure 1. Table 1 gives the control values of each of APD_{20}, APD_{50}, and APD_{90} recorded at cycle lengths ranging from 1000 to 333 ms in group 1 (dofetilide) and group 2 (293B) before pharmacological intervention. For all phases of repolarization, a clear shortening of APD was observed with an increased stimulation frequency. Addition of dofetilide, at concentrations ranging between 10^{-9} and 10^{-6} mol/l resulted in a dose-dependent prolongation of both APD_{90} and APD_{50} at all stimulation rates, the effect APD_{90} on being the most pronounced (Figure 2). IC_{50} for dofetilide was 4.7 nM. No effect was observed on APD_{20} at any stimulation rate.

Table 1. Changes of action potential durations recorded at 20% (APD_{20}), 50% (APD_{50}) and 90% (APD_{90}) repolarization according to the cycle length under basal conditions. Group 1 and 2 refer to the groups on which dofetilide and chromanol 293B will be applied respectively. Data are expressed as mean ± SEM

Cycle length (ms)		1000	750	600	500	400	333
APD_{20}	Group 1	72.5 ± 16.0	72.9 ± 17.8	74.0 ± 17.8	71.1 ± 13.8	69.6 ± 20.5	63.0 ± 17.0**
	Group 2	75.2 ± 17.1	78.± 18.8	80.2 ± 18.5	78.4 ± 17.7	74.8 ± 17.6	70.9 ± 18.5
APD_{50}	Group 1	121.9 ±24.0	124.± 23.6	124.4 ± 24.0	118.4 ± 19.9	111.1 + 21.8	102.3 + 20.7**
	Group 2	128.6 ± 24.0	131.± 27.1	132.6 ± 25.7	129.6 ± 25.3	122.9 ± 22.9	115.8 ± 22.4*
APD_{90}	Group 1	175.6 ± 26.9	175.± 26.1	177.2 ± 27.7	169.8 ± 22.9	159.2 ± 20.1	150.8 ± 21.0***
	Group 2	180.5 ± 24.3	184.± 25.0	183.5 ± 22.9	179.0 ± 20.6	167.9 ± 18.0**	159.5 ± 19.5***

*$p<0.05$, **$p<0.01$ and ***$p<0.001$ vs the values obtained at 1000 ms, n=12 for both groups.

At all investigated pacing rates, concentrations of 293B up to $3x10^{-5}$ mol/l only slightly increased APD_{90} as well as APD_{50} values which were not different from control values. For example, at 500 ms, the application of 30 µmol/l 293B prolonged APD_{90} by 12.5 ± 20.7 ms, whereas the prolongation at 333 ms was 10.0 ± 22.8 ms (p=ns vs control for both). In contrast to later phases of repolarization, exhibited a dose-dependent prolongation at pacing intervals between 1000 and 400 ms (Figure 2). The IC_{50} of 293B at 500 mswas 7.0 µmol/l.

2. Rate-Dependent Effects of I_{Kr} and I_{Ks} Block on the APD

Figure 3 shows the effects of inceasing the pacing rate on the APD_{90} obtained after perfusing dofetilide (100 nmol/l) and 293B (30µmol/l). Block of I_{Ks} currents by 293B was associated with a minor, rate-independent effect on APD_{90}: 2.5 ± 11.3% (from 190.5 ± 24.3 to 195.2 ± 24.9 ms) increase at 1000 ms and 9.0 ± 12.3% (from 159.5 ± 19.5 to 173.9 ± 31.6 ms) at 333 ms (p=ns for both). In contrast, the APD prolongation with dofetilide showed a strong reverse rate-dependence and was most pronounced at slow rates: 39.2 ± 21.05% from 175.6 ± 26.9 to 237.6 ± 30.4 ms) at 1000 ms. At this rate, I_{Kr} block resulted in a significantly higher prolongation of APD_{90} ($p<0.05$) compared to I_{Ks} block. The effect decreased progressively as the stimulation rate increased to reach a value of 17.5 ± 17.5% at 333 ms, the rate at which no significant difference remained between I_{Kr} and I_{Ks} block.

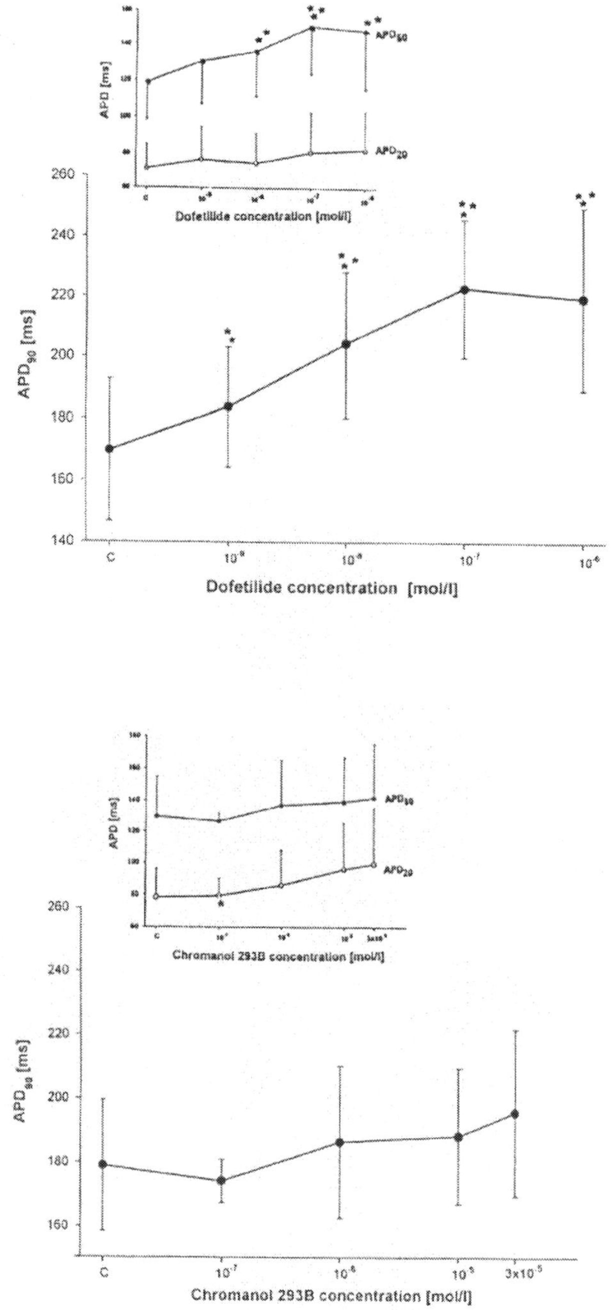

Figure 2. Dose-dependent effects of Dofetilide and Chromanol 293B (293B) on action potential duration at 20% (APD_{20}), 50% (APD_{50}) and 90% (APD_{90}) repolarization. Cycle length: 500 ms. IC_{50}: 4.7 nM (Dofetilide) and 7.0 μM (293B). Data are expressed as mean ±SEM. *p<0.0 5, **p<0.01 and ***p<0.001 vs control. n=12 for both substances.

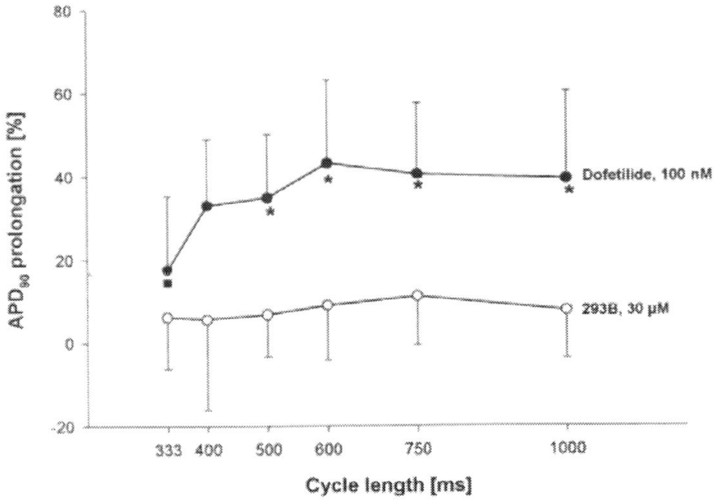

Figure 3. Rate-dependent effect of Dofetilide (100 nM) and Chromanol 293B (293B, 30 μM) on APD_{90} prolongation (expressed as percentage). Data are expressed as mean±SEM. *$p<0.05$ Dofetilide vs 293B, ▪ $p<0.0$ 5 333ms vs 1000ms.

A comparison between I_{Kr} and I_{Ks} block on APD_{20}, APD_{50} and APD_{90} at pacing intervals of 1000, 500, and 333 ms is illustrated in Figure 4 in which the absolute elongations (in ms) are considered. 293B showed no frequency dependence of its effects on any of the APDs. At the longest cycle length (1000 ms), the effect of I_{Ks} blockade was significantly different from that of I_{Kr} blockade on both APD_{50} and APD_{90}. At 500 ms cycle length, only APD_{50} prolongation was significantly different between dofetilide and 293B, whereas no significant difference remained as the cycle length was shortened to 333 ms. On the other hand, one can remark the reverse rate-dependence of Dofetilide: The prolongation of APD_{90} diminishes significantly ($p<0.05$) when increasing heart rate (1000 vs 333 ms cycle length).

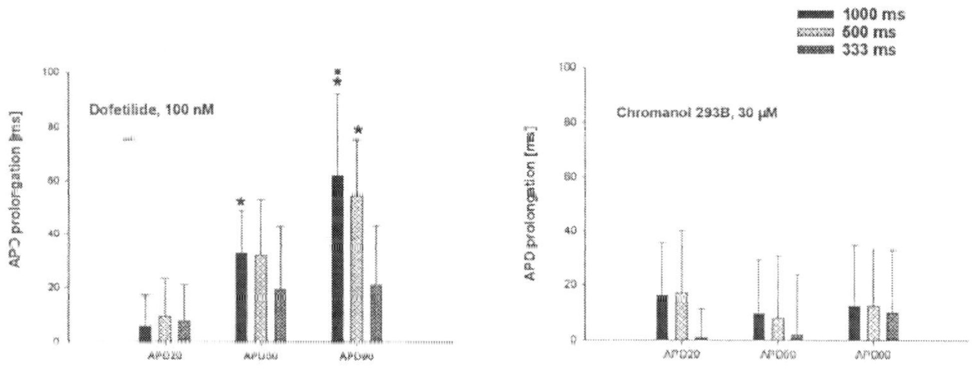

Figure 4. Rate-dependent prolongation of action potential durations (APD_{20}, APD_{50}, APD_{90}) after application of Dofetilide (100 nM) and Chromanol 293B (293B, 30 μM) at 1000, 500 and 333ms. Data are expressed as mean±SEM. *$p<0.05$ Dofetilide vs 293B, $p<0.05$ 333ms vs 1000ms.

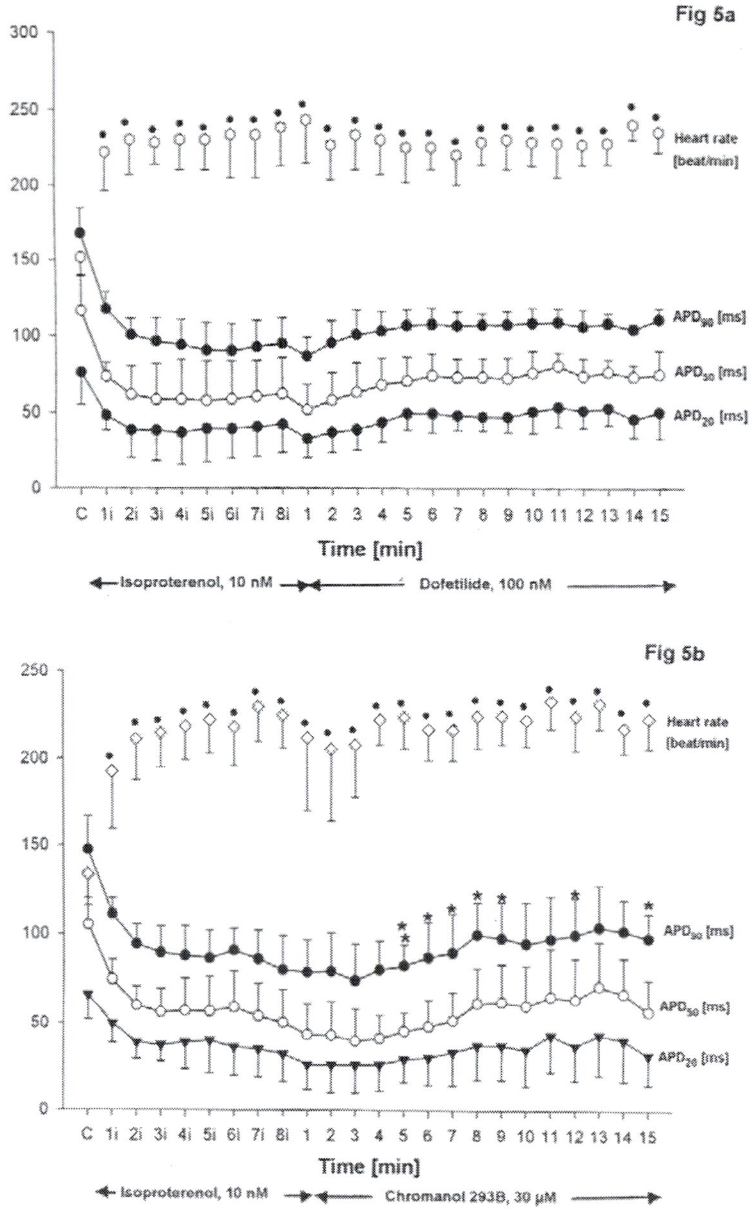

Figure 5. Effect of isoproterenol (10 nM, 8 min) and each of Dofetilide (100 nM, 15 min, Fig 5a) and Chromanol 293B (293B, 30 μM, 15 min, Fig 5b) on action potential durations (APD_{20}, APD_{50}, APD_{90}) and heart rate. Data are expressed as mean±SEM. •p<0.001 isoproterenol and isoproterenol+substance vs control, *p<0.05, **p<0.01 293B vs isoproterenol.

3. Effects of I_{Kr} and I_{Ks} Block under β-Adrenergic Stimulation

The increase in heart rate from 134 ± 17 to 225 ± 19 beats/min (p<0.001) induced by perfusing 10 nmol/l isoproterenol for 8 minutes was accompanied with a significant shortening of all measured APDs: For example, the APD_{90} was shortened from from 167.6 ±

17.2 ms to 95.0 ± 16.6 ms ($p<0.001$) in the dofetilide group (Figure 5a), and from 147.4 ± 19.0 to 80.4 ± 18.78 ms ($p<0.001$) in the 293B group (Figure 5b). Both APD_{50} and APD_{20} were also shortened to about half their control values. The 8-minute isoproterenol phase was followed by blocking either I_{Kr} or I_{Ks} for 15 minutes while perfusion was continued. Neither dofetilide nor 293B had an effect on heart rate (Figures 5a and 5b).

Blocking I_{Ks} with 293B was associated with a persistent lengthening of APD_{90}, (e.g. 29.7 ± 18.5 %, $p<0.05$ at the 8th min), whereas APD_{50} and APD_{20} where not affected (Figure 5a). I_{Kr} block did not induce any significant increase on any APD value (Figure 5b).

Discussion

The present study compared the concentration- and rate-dependent effect on the APD of two K channel targeting substances, dofetilide, blocking I_{Kr}, and 293B, blocking I_{Ks}. Both I_{Kr} and I_{Ks} are major repolarizing currents controlling action potential duration, but they differ markedly in their kinetiks (Jurkiewicz & Sanguinetti, 1993). At physiological rates, which are in the range of 140/min in the rabbits used in our experiments, I_{Kr} is able to activate rapidly and to reach a steady state, whereas I_{Ks} is incompletely deactivated (Capucci et al., 1998; Varró et al., 2000). As heart rate increases, i.e. when rising the pacing rate from 2 to 3Hz (which corresponds to cycle lengths of 500 and 333 ms respectively), I_{Ks} accumulates open and becomes the more important leading to the rate-dependent action potential abbreviation (Nattel & Singh, 1999). Thus, it was not surprizing to observe a significant shortening of APD as the hearts were paced at rates exceeding their physiological values.

1. Dose-Dependent Effects of I_{Kr} and I_{Ks} Block

In the isolated rabbit heart, dofetilide exhibited a dose-dependent lengthening of APD_{90} with an IC_{50} of 4.7 nM and, to a less extent of APD_{50}, while having no effect on APD_{20}. Such a potent effect was also described by Tande (Tande et al., 1990) in the guinea pig papillary muscle with a more pronounced effect on APD_{90} compared to APD_{50} and APD_{25}. On the other hand, it was recently reported by the group of Chen on a model of perfused rabbit ventricular wedge that dofetilide increased endo- and epicardial APD_{90} within clinically relevant concentration ranges (Chen et al., 2006). Moreover, a concentration-dependent increase of APD was published in the same year by So and coworkers. These authors calculated an IC_{50} of 15 nM for dofetilide (So et al., 2006), whereas a value of 10 nM was found by the group of Yang on AT-1 cells of the mice (Yang et al., 2001). Dofetilide is well-known as a selective and specific I_{Kr} blocker (Falk & Decara, 2000; Camm 2000; Lee et al., 2003; Gerlach, 2003). Therefore, it may act through a marked increase of APD (Jurkiewicz & Sanguinetti, 1993).

Compared to dofetilide, 293B resulted in no significant effect on both APD_{90} and APD_{50}. Concerning this point, the data already published exhibit many discripancies, which may be attributed to species differences, to the methodology applied, and to the problem of *in vitro* vs *in vivo* measurements. 293B seems to be more active on isolated cells (Busch et al., 1996). However, experiments on isolated dog ventricular myocytes (Varró et al., 2000) showed that 293B in a concentration of 10 μM resulted in an increase of APD which did not exceed 7%

over a wide range of pacing cycle lengths (300-5000 ms). In another study (Burashnikov & Anzelevitch, 2000) on transmural preparations from dog left ventricle and with the use of 293B in concentrations ranging from 1 to 30 μM, the only significant APD_{90} prolongation observed on each of epicardial and endocardial preparations needed 30 μM. These authors suggest – in reference to the data of Bosch et al. (1998) – that the concentration-response relationship of 293B could be shifted to higher concentrations in intact cardiac preparations versus isolated myocytes. It could be asked whether the same applies to our results.

Dofetilide induced no response at the level of APD_{20}, whereas 293B resulted in significant APD_{20} prolongation observed upon application of 100 nM 293B, concentration at which no effect was observed on both APD_{50} and APD_{90}. One explanation would be an eventual interaction with other channels, although patch-clamp measurements revealed no influence of 293B on either I_{Na} or L-type I_{Ca} at concentrations blocking I_{Ks} completely. The open channel block activity of 293B would also account for this effect (Fujisawa et al., 2000).

2. Rate-Dependent Effects of I_{Kr} and I_{Ks} Block

Reverse rate-dependence means that the effect of APD prolongation increases strongly at long diastolic intervals. Our results show clearly that I_{Kr} block is accompanied with reverse rate-dependence, while I_{Ks} is not. This phenomenon has been evidenced on various experimental models (Tande et al., 1990; Jurkiewicz & Sanguinetti, 1993; Bosch et al., 1998; Martin et al., 1996; Camm & Yap, 1999; Kalus & Mauro, 2000; Kovàcs et al., 2003) According to So and coworkers (2006), the reverse rate-dependence of I_{Kr} block could be caused by a compensatory increase in I_{Ks} during fast heart rates (which are favorable for its accumulation). Clinically, the phenomenen of reverse rate-dependence is a disadvantage: On the one hand, the substance is less effective in treating tachyarrhythmias, on the other hand, excessive APD prolongation at low frequencies constitutes a risk of Torsades de Pointes (Nattel & Singh, 1999; Kalus & Mauro, 2000; Singh & Wadhani, 2004). However, based on our results, one can remark that although the APD_{90} prolongation induced by dofetilide decreases significantly when pacing at 333 ms, a prolongation by 17% remains. This means that an effect persists at high rates (Lande et al., 1998). A parallel remark was made on humans in vivo: No rate-dependence of APD prolongation was observed between 75 and 120 beats/min (Sedgwick et al., 1992).

3. Effects of I_{Kr} and I_{Ks} Block under β-Adrenergic Stimulation

The acceleration of heart rate induced by 10 nM isoproterenol was accompanied with an immediate shortening of APD. Under these conditions, dofetilide failed to produce any significant prolongation of APD. Isoproterenol was found to antagonize the action of dofetilide on guinea pig papillary muscle (Schreieck et al., 1997) as well as on cells isolated from endocardial layers of the left ventricular myocardium of dogs (Marschang et al., 2000). Also, on isolated guinea pig atrium (Kovàcs et al., 2003) and on the right papillary muscle of rabbit (Kovàcs & Szenasi, 2006), isoproterenol (30 nM) abolished the effect of dofetilide in lengthening the effective refractory period. According to these experimental observations, it was suggested that the endogenous release of catecholamines and the concomitant β-adrenoceptor activation play an important role in the development of the reverse-phase dependence of dofetilide (Kovàcs et al., 2003).

The opposite was produced by 293B: The prolongation of APD under β-adrenergic stimulation started to be significant at the 5th minute continued up to the 15th minute. To our knowledge, such a kinetik study has not yet been performed on the isolated perfused rabbit heart. Our data are in accordance with those obtained on myocytes from guinea pig (Schreieck et al., 1997) or from human heart (Jost et al., 2005). Under β-adrenergic stimulation, I_{Ks} increases, while I_{Kr} remains unchanged (Sanguinetti et al., 1991). This explains that the 293B-induced APD_{90} prolongation (34%) exceeded by far that observed without β-adrenergic stimulation (7% at 333 ms cycle length). 293B does not affect normal ventricular muscle APD within a normal range of heart rates, however, it lengthens APD substantially by increased sympathetic tone. It has also been suggested that cAMP increases I_{Ks} and may alter its activation kinetics (Jost et al., 2005). One interesting observation concerning the weak effect of I_{Ks} blockade in the perfused heart is the sympathetic denervation (So et al., 2006). This could also explain some discrepancies between *in vivo* and *in vitro* experimental models.

4. Conclusion

In the present study, we investigated two substances susceptible to influence the repolarization but acting in different ways: The first one is the I_{Kr} blocker, dofetilide, acting as an antiarrhythmic agent through a marked prolongation of the repolarization which is the most accentuated at low frequencies. The second substance is the I_{Ks} blocker, 293B, which has practically no significant effect at resting heart rate, but plays a substantial role at high frequencies. It should be noted that even newer and potenter I_{Ks} blockers such as HMR 1556 (IC_{50}, 10.5 nM) (Thomas et al., 2003) also failed to increase APD at resting frequencies (So et al., 2006).

Dofetilide has proved a high efficiency in the treatment of atrial flutter and fibrillation (Lindeboom et al., 2000; Hohnloser et al., 2000; Falk & Decara, 2000; Elming et al., 2003), but its role in ventricular arrhythmias remains unclear (Khan et al., 2004). However, the potent effect of dofetilide is associated with two disadvantages: Firstly, the decrease of the effect at a higher heart rate, and, secondly, the excessive APD prolongation at long diastolic intervals, which can induce early after depolarizations, which in turn trigger Torsades de Pointes (Lengyel et al., 2001; Singh & Waldhani, 2004). Despite the incidence of Torsades de Pointes, which is estimated to be approximately 2% in patients with impaired ventricular function (Falke & Decara, 2000), dofetilide is considered to be effective and safe when an elaborate procedure for dosing is applied (Elming et al., 2003). Treatment with dofetilide was not associated with an increase in mortality rate in patients with reduced ejection fraction (Falke & Decara, 2000). Moreover, dofetilide is estimated to be the antiarrhythmic of choice for the treamtent of atrial fibrillation in patients with left ventricular dysfunction (Nacarelli et al., 2003).

I_{Ks} blockers, which show only a small effect at resting heart rates possess the big advantage to act increasingly at faster rates. Therefore, they are susceptible to provide a greater protection from tachyarrhythmias compared to I_{Kr} blockers. Additionally, they may be less proarrhythmic (Gerlach, 2003; Pajouh et al., 2005).

As new antiarrhythmic strategy, it has been suggested to combine I_{Ks}- with β-adrenoceptor blockers (Jost et al., 2005). Another proposal would be to increase rather than to block I_{Ks} (Jost et al., 2005). I_{Ks} constitutes a reserve current preventing the excessive prolongation of repolarization by I_{Kr} block particularly at slow heart rates (So et al., 2006). Therapeutic increase of I_{Ks} would reduce the risk of sudden cardiac death during progression of heart failure.

Acknowledgements

This investigation has been supported by a grant of *f*ortüne-program of the University of Tübingen (R.F.B., 480-0-0). The authors wish to thank Dr. Guiscard Seebohm (Institute of Physiology, Tübingen) for reading the manuscript and for his valuable comments.

References

Colatsky, TJ; Follmer, CH; Starmer CF. (1990) Channel specificity in antiarrhythmic drug action. Mechanism of potassium channel block and its role in suppressing and aggravating cardiac arrhythmias. *Circulation* **82**:2235-2242.

Sanguinetti, MC; Jurkiewicz, NK. (1990) Two components of cardiac delayed rectifier K^+ current: Differential sensitivity to block by class III antiarrhythmic agents. *J Gen Physiol* **96**: 194-214.

Jurkiewicz, NK; Sanguinetti, MC. (1993) Rate-dependent prolongation of cardiac action potentials by a methansulfonanilide class III antiarrhythmic agent. Specific block of rapidly activating delayed rectifier K^+ current by dofetilide. *Circ Res* **72**:75-83.

Nattel, S; Singh, BN. (1999) Evolution, mechanisms, and classification of antiarrhythmic drugs: Focus on class III actions. *Am J Cardiol* **84**:11R-19R.

Seebohm, G; Lerche, C; Busch, AE; Bachmann, A. (2001) Dependence of I_{Ks} biophysical properties on the expression system. *Pflügers Arch* **442**: 891-895.

Varró, A; Baláti, B; Iost, N; Takacs, J; Viràg, L; Lathrop, DA; Csaba, L; Talosi, L; Papp, JG. (2000) The role of the delayed rectifier component I_{Ks} in dog ventricular muscle and purkinje fibre repolarization. *J Physiol* **523**:67-81.

Lengyel, C; Iost, N; Viràg, L; Varró, A. (2001) Pharmacological block of the slow component of the outward delayed rectifier current (I(Ks)) fails to lengthen rabbit ventricular muscle QT(c) and action potential duration. *Br J Pharmacol* **132**: 101-110.

Kovàcs, A; Magyar, J; Bànyàsz, T; Nànàsi, P; Szénàsi, G. (2003) β-adrenoceptor activation plays a role in the reverse rate-dependency of effective refractory period lengthening by dofetilide in the guinea pig atrium, *in vitro*. *Br J Pharmacol* **139**: 1555-1563.

Kalus, JS; Mauro, VF. (2000) Dofetilide: A class III-specific antiarrhythmic agent. *Annal Pharmacother* **34**:44-56.

Bosch, RF; Gaspo, R; Busch, AE; Lang, HJ; Li, G-R;, Nattel, S. (1998) Effects of the chromanol 293B, a selective blocker of the slow component of the delayed rectifier K^+ current, on repolarisation in human and guinea pig ventricular myocytes. *Cardiovasc Res* **38**:441-450

Sanguinetti, MC; Jurkiewicz, NK; Scott, A; Siegl, PKS. (1991) Isoproterenol antagonizes prolongation of refractory period by the class III antiarrhythmic agent E-4031 in guinea pig myocytes. Mechanism of action. *Circ Res* **68**:77-84.

Fujisawa, S; Ono, K; Iijima, T. (2000) Time-dependent block of the slowly activating delayed rectifier K^+ current by chromanol 293B in guinea-pig ventricular cells. *Br J Pharmacol* **129**:1007-1013.

Jost, N; Viràg, L; Bitay, M; Takàcs, J; Lengyel, C; Biliczki, P; Nagy, Z; Bogàts, G; Lathrop, D: Rapp, J; Varró, A. (2005) Restricting excessive cardiac action potential and QT prolongation: A vital role for I_{Ks} in human ventricular muscle. *Circulation* **112**: 1392-1399.

Tande, PM; Bjørnstad, H; Yang, T; Refsum, H. (1990) Rate-dependent class III antiarrhythmic action, negative chronotropy, and positive inotropy of a novel I_K blocking drug, UK-68,798: Potent in guinea pig but no effect in rat myocardium. *J Cardiovasc Pharmacol* **16**:401-410.

Schreieck, J; Wang, Y; Gjini, V; Korth, M; Zrenner, B; Schömig, A; Schmitt, C. (1997) Differential effect of ß-adrenergic stimulation on the frequency-dependent electrophysiologic actions of the new class III antiarrhythmics dofetilide, ambasilide, and chromanol 293B. *J Cardiovasc Electrophysiol* **8**:1420-1430.

Gogelein, H; Bruggemann, A; Gerlach, U; Brendel, J; Busch, AE. (2000) Inhibition of I_{Ks} channels by HMR 1556. *Naunyn Schmiedebergs Arch Pharmacol* **362**: 480-488.

Chen, X; Cordes, JS; Bradley, JA; Sun, Z; Zhou, J. (2006) Use of arterially perfused rabbit ventricular wedge in predicting arrhythmogenic potentials of drugs. *J Pharmacol Toxicol Methods* **54**: 257-260.

Burashnikov, A; Antzelevitch, C. (2000) Block of I_{Ks} does not induce early afterdepolarization activity but promotes ß-adrenergic agonist-induced delayed afterdepolarization activity. *J Cardiovasc Electrophysiol* **11**:458-465.

Biliczki, P; Viràg, L; Iost, N; Papp, JG; Varró, A. (2002) Interaction of different potassium channels in cardiac repolarization in dog ventricular preparations: role of repolarization reserve. *Br J Pharmacol* **137**: 361-368.

Bauer, A; Becker, R; Karle, C; Schreiner, K; Senges, J; Voss, F; Kraft, P; Kuebler, W; Schoels, W. (2002) Effects of I_{Kr}-blocking agent dofetilide and of the I_{Ks}-blocking agent chromanol 293b on regional disparity of left ventricular repolarization in the intact canine heart. *J Cardiovasc Pharmacol* **39**: 460-467.

Valentin, JP; Hoffmann, P; De Clerck F; Hammond, TG; Hondeghem, L. (2004) Review of the predictive value of the Langendorff heart model (Screenit system) in assessing the proarrhythmic potential of drugs. *J Pharmacol Toxicol Methods* **49**: 171-181.

Lawrence, CL; Bridgland-Taylor, MH; Pollard, CE; Hammond, TG; Valentin, JP. (2006) A rabbit heart proarrhythmia model: predictive value for clinical identification of Torsades de Pointes. *Br J Pharmacol* **149**: 845-860.

Franz, MR;, Burkhoff, D; Spurgeon, H; Weisfeldt, ML; Lakatta, EG. (1986) *In vitro* validation of a new catheter technique for recording monophasic action potentials. *Eur Heart J* **7**:34-41.

Cappucci, A; Villani, GQ; Aschieri, D; Piepoli, M. (1998) Effects of class III drugs on atrial fibrillation. *J Cardiovasc Electrophysiol* **9**:S109-S120.

So, PP-S; Hu, X-D; Backx, PH; Puglisi, JL; Dorian, P. (2006) Blockade of I_{Ks} by HMR 1556 increases the reverse rate-dependence of refractoriness prolongation by dofetilide in isolated rabbit ventricle. *Br J Pharmacol* **148**: 255-263.

Yang, T; Snyders, D; Roden, D. (2001) Drug block of IKr: Model systems and relevance to human arrhythmias. *J Cardiovasc Pharmacol* **38**: 737-744.

Falk, RH; Decara, JM. (2000) Dofetlide: a new pure class III antiarrhythmic agent. *Am Heart J* **140**: 697-706.

Camm, AJ. (2000) Clinical differences between the newer antiarrhythmic agents. *Europace* **1** Suppl C: C16-C22.

Lee, K; Park, JY; Ryu, PD; Kwon, LS; Kim, HY. (2003) I_{Kr} channel blockers: novel antiarrhythmic agents. *Curr Med Chem Cardiovasc Hematol Agents* **1**: 203-223.

Gerlach, U. (2003). Blockers of the slowly delayed rectifier potassium I_{Ks} channel: potential antiarrhythmic agents. *Curr Med Chem Cardiovasc Hematol Agents* **1**: 243-252.

Busch, AE; Suessbrich, H; Waldegger, S; Sailer, E; Greger, R; Lang, H; Lang, F; Gibson, KJ; Maylie, JG. (1996) Inhibition of I_{Ks} in guinea pig cardiac myocytes and guinea pig I_{sK} channels by the chromanol 293B. *Pflüg Arch* **432**:1094-1096.

Martin, CL; Palomo, MA; McMahon, EG. (1996) Comparison of bidisomide, flecainide and dofetilide on action potential duration in isolated canine atria: Effect of isoproterenol. *J Pharmacol Exp Ther* **278**:154-162.

Camm, AJ; Yap, YG. (1999) What should we expect from the next generation of antiarrhythmic drugs? *J Cardiovasc Electrophysiol* **10**:307-317.

Lande, G; Maison-Blanche, P; Fayn, J; Ghandafar, M; Coumel, P; Funk-Brentano, C. (1998) Dynamic analysis of dofetilide-induced changes in ventricular repolarization. *Clin Pharmacol Ther* **64**:312-321.

Sedgwick, ML; Rasmussen, HS; Cobbe, SM. (1992) Effects of the class III antiarrhythmic drug dofetilide on ventricular monophasic action potential duration and QT interval dispersion in stable angina pectoris. *Am J Cardiol* **70**:1432-1437.

Marschang, H; Brachmann, J; Karolyi, L; Kübler, W; Schöls, W. (2000) Isoproterenol specifically modulates reverse rate-dependent effects of D,L- sotalol, D-sotalol, and dofetilide. *J Cardiovasc Pharmacol* **35**: 443-450.

Kovàcs, A; Szénàsi, G. (2006) Effects of dofetilide and EGIS-7229, an antiarrhythmic agent possessing class III, IV, and IB activities, on myocardial refractoriness in hyperkalemia, hypokalemia, and during beta-adrenergic activation in the rabbit papillary muscle *in vitro*. *J Pharmacol Sci* **100**: 303-309.

Lindeboom, J-E; Kingma, JH; Crijns, HJGM; Dunselman, PHJM. (2000) Efficacy and safety of intravenous *dofetilide* for rapid termination of atrial fibrillation and atrial flutter. *Am J Cardiol* **85**:1031-1033.

Hohnloser, SH; Li, Y-G; Bender, B; Grönefeld, G. (2000) Pharmacological management of atrial fibrillation: An update. *J Cardiovasc Pharmacol Therapeut* **5**:11-16.

Elming, H; Brendorp, B; Pedersen, OD; Kober, L; Torp-Petersen, C. (2003) Dofetilide: a new drug to control cardiac arrhythmias. *Expert Opin Pharmacother* **4**: 973-985.

Khan, MH. (2004) Oral class III antiarrhythmics: what is new? *Curr Opin Cardiol* **19**: 47-51.

Nacarelli, GV; Wolbrette, DI; Khan, M; Bhatta, L; Hynes, J; Samii, S; Luck, J. (2003) Old and new antiarrhythmic drugs for converting and maintaining sinus rhythm in atrial fibrillation: comparative efficacy and results of trials. *Am J Cardiol* **91**: 15D-26D.

Pajouh, M; Wilson, LD; Poelzing, S; Johnson, NJ, Rosenbaum, DS. (2005) I_{Ks} blockade reduces dispersion of repolarization in heart failure. *Heart Rhythm* **2**: 731-738.

In: Progress in Cardiac Arrhythmia Research
Editor: Ira R. Tarkowicz, pp. 183-205
ISBN: 1-60021-796-6

Chapter 8

Cardiac Arrhythmias in the Intensive Care Patient – A Review

Elisabeth Paramythiotou[1], Dimitrios Karakitsos[2], Evangelos Matsakas[3] and Andreas Karabinis[2]
[1] ICU Attikon University Hospital, Athens , Greece
[2] ICU George Gennimatas General Hospital, Athens, Greece.
[3]Cardiology department George Gennimatas General Hospital, Athens, Greece

Abstract

Cardiac arrhythmias are commonly observed in the intensive care unit (ICU) setting. These arrhythmias may result in life threatening events, hence requiring good knowledge of management strategies including urgent transcutaneous pacing. The types of arrhythmias which may be encountered in the ICU can be broadly divided into bradyarrhythmias and tachyarrhythmias. They could vary from "innocent" premature atrial contractions to ventricular tachycardia or complete atrio-ventricular block. It is of note that patients with an underlying disorder are more prone to develop life threatening arrhythmias than healthy subjects. However, there are certain subgroups of previously healthy critical care patients, such as patients with severe brain injury due to trauma, who exhibit a number of changes in heart rate and cardiovascular control. Furthermore, many factors may impair pacemaker automa-ticity or myocardial impulse conduction in critical care patients such as drugs, electrolyte and pH disturbances, myocardial ischaemia, anaesthesia, sepsis, shock, hypoxia, insertion of central venous catheters, trauma and head injury. Also, of great interest is the recent delineation of at least four different hereditary syndromes characterised by myocardial ion channel abnormalities. Clinically these syndromes manifest as a prolonged QT interval on surface electrocardiogram (ECG), associated with sudden death in some affected individuals. Other myocardial ion channel abnormalities such as the Brugada syndrome have been also reported in the ICU setting.

The purpose of this review is to provide a comprehensive update of the diagnosis, physiopathology and therapeutic strategies of cardiac arrhythmias in the ICU setting. In this review, we also discuss the occurrence of cardiac arrhythmias in unique subpopulations of critical care patients as well as management guidelines for potentially lethal arrhythmias.

Introduction

The critical care physician is often confronted with patients presenting with several cardiac problems especially arrhythmias and continuous electrocardiographic monitoring is an important tool for their diagnosis and treatment [1, 2]. Also, there are critical care patients who are extremely vulnerable to several types of arrhythmias while in the ICU, such as patients with a recent ischemic infarction, heart failure or finally those recovering from cardiac surgery. Nonetheless, patients previously healthy are also at risk of developing cardiac arrhythmias. Several inciting factors may contribute to the appearance of disturbances of cardiac rhythm. Among them, hypoxia, severe infection, acidosis or alkalosis, catecholamine excess (endogenous or exogenous), electrolyte abnormalities, severe brain injury, hypothermia, trauma and insertion of central venous lines are considered important in the ICU setting. Proper management of arrhythmias includes correction of underlying disorders as well as medical therapy directed at the arrhythmia itself.

The types of arrhythmias that physicians may encounter in the ICU can be broadly divided into tachyarrhythmias and bradyarrhythmias. The physiological impact of rhythm disorders depends on ventricular response rate, duration of arrhythmia and underlying cardiac function. Tachyarrhythmias may shorten diastolic filling time, reduce cardiac output significantly and result in a decline of arterial pressure, contributing therefore to morbidity and mortality of intensive care patients [3, 4]. Bradyarrhythmias may decrease cardiac output especially in patients who have relatively fixed stroke volume. If the arrhythmia has undesirable effects upon patients' cardiac status then an immediate intervention is necessary. Therefore, proper and early identification of disturbances of the normal cardiac rhythm and development of effective therapeutic strategies are of extreme clinical importance to all intensivists.

Tachyarrhythmias

The incidence of tachyarrhythmias in the ICU varies from 14.3% to 29.7% depending upon the population hospitalized and the inclusion criteria used in various studies [3, 5]. The therapeutic approach includes first an accurate interpretation of the arrhythmia itself. Determination of the cause of the arrhythmia and assessment of the patient's hemodynamic stability are the next important steps. If the hemodynamic status is compromised by the arrhythmia and all other causes are excluded, a pharmacological treatment or electrical conversion should be performed. However, one should always bear in mind that patients with arrhythmias and not arrhythmias themselves are treated and since treatment involves some risks, one must be sure that the risks of not treating the arrhythmias should outweigh the risks of therapy.

The mechanisms of tachycardias can be the result of increased automaticity in pacemaker cells (e.g. sinus tachycardias), triggered activity (e.g. ectopic impulses) or a process known as a re-entry [6]. Re - entry is the most common cause of clinically significant tachycardias. Premature beats can, in the presence of two electrophysiologically separate paths, initiate a re-entrant circuit that continually reactivates itself. Abnormal automaticity can lead to rapid rates and is responsible for multifocal atrial tachycardia, focal atrial tachycardia and torsades de pointes [7].

Tachycardias are divided into narrow complex tachycardias and wide complex tachycardias. Narrow complex tachycardias include sinus tachycardia, atrioventricular nodal reentry tachycardia (AVNRT), atrial flutter, atrial fibrillation, atrio-ventricular (AV) re-entry from the accessory pathway (Wolff - Parkinson White syndrome, WPW). Wide QRS tachycardias include monomorphic and polymorphic ventricular tachycardias, supraventricular tachycardias with pre-existing bundle branch block (SVTs), torsade de pointes tachycardia and AV re-entry from an antegrade accessory pathway (WPW).

Supraventricular tachycardias are recognized by a narrow QRS complex (< 0.12 sec). A 12 – lead ECG is necessary to establish the diagnosis of a tachycardia, since a rhythm strip from one monitor lead could lead to a wrong diagnosis given that the QRS width varies between one lead to another. Another clue to the diagnosis is a previous ECG helping, for example, to identify pre-existing bundle brunch block or QT interval prolongation.

Moreover, several manoeuvres are useful in the discrimination between supraventricular and ventricular tachycardias. Carotid sinus massage increase vagal tone, slow conduction time and increase refractoriness aiding in the diagnosis through demonstration of p waves or interruption of AVNRT or AV re-entrant tachycardia. Adenosine is another useful tool for the same purpose. It is given as a rapid intravenous bolus of 6 mg and a second dose of 12 mg can be given 1 to 2 minutes later. If the drug is given through a central venous line, the dosage is usually halved.

Adverse drug reactions of adenosine include facial flushing, bronchospasm, chest pain, dyspnea, bradycardia, arrhythmia (ventricular tachycardia or fibrillation) and a-trioventricular block [6, 8].

Narrow Complex Tachycardias

Tachycardias with a narrow QRS complex (< 0.12 sec) are divided into regular and irregular ones. Regular supraventricular tachycardias (SVTs) include sinus tachy-cardias, AV nodal reentrant tachycardia with rapid ventricular response, atrial flutter, atrial ectopic tachycardia, and preexcitation syndromes combined with atrial fibril-lation. Irregular narrow complex tachycardias include sinus tachycardia with frequent premature atrial complexes, multifocal atrial tachycardia, atrial flutter with variable block and atrial fibrillation.

Regular Rhythms

Sinus Tachycardia

Sinus tachycardia in adults is defined as a rate exceeding 100 beats / min. The discharge frequency varies between 100 and 180 beats/min. It occurs usually as a normal reaction to a variety of stresses such as fever, hypotension, hyperthyroidism, dehydration, hypovolemia, pain, hypoxia, thyrotoxicosis, hemopericardium etc. Other possible causes of sinus tachycardia in the ICU include various medications (e.g. vasopressors, inotropes) and reviewing them is necessary in order to exclude iatrogenic etiology of tachycardia. Identification and correction of the underlying di-sorder is the first step to be taken. In case of concomitant ischemia, b - blockers are considered the treatment of choice. Attention must be paid to the fact that sinus tachycardia is often an appropriate compensating hemodynamic response. In such a case the use of b-blockers could reduce cardiac output and lead to deleterious effects on the hemodynamic situation of the patient.

Atrioventricular Nodal Reentrant Tachycardia

Atrioventricular nodal reentrant tachycardia (AVNRT) is the most common type of paroxysmal supraventricular tachycardia and accounts for 50% to 60% of PSVT [9]. Usually, this is a tachycardia of supraventricular origin with sudden onset and termination, generally at rates of 150 to 250 beats/min (common rates between 180 to 200 beats/min). It is more prevalent in females and presents after the age of twenty while it is not usually associated with structural heart disease [10]. It involves dual AV nodal pathways and in most cases antegrade conduction proceeds via the posterior AV nodal approach and retrograde conduction via the anterior (fast) AV nodal pathway usually with slow conduction. Therefore, the key to treatment is to block AV conduction. Acute treatment includes vagal manoeuvres and IV adenosine (6 to 12 mg given rapidly) or verapamil (5 to 10 mg). Long-term preventive therapy includes either medications that suppress the initiating premature atrial contractions (b blockers) or slow AV conduction, or catheter ablation of one of the pathways.

Atrial Flutter

Atrial flutter is a regular tachycardia identified by the presence of recurring regular sawtooth flutter waves usually best seen in leads II, III, aV_f or V_1. The arrhythmia is now recognized as a macro – re-entrant rhythm. The atrial rate during typical atrial flutter is usually 250 to 350 beats/ min and in untreated patients the ventricular rate is half the atrial rate, i.e. 150 beats/ min. If the patient has not received any drugs, a significantly lower ventricular rate is suggesting abnormal AV conduction. If the ratio of conducted beats varies (usually as a result of Weckenbach AV block) the ventricular rhythm will be irregular. Synchronous direct-current (DC) cardioversion if the patient presents acute hemodynamic collapse or congestive heart failure is a treatment of choice since cardioversion effectively restores sinus rhythm with low energy (50J) and the success rate is considered high [11]. If the electrical shock results in atrial fibrillation, a second shock at a higher energy level is used to restore sinus rhythm. The reported frequency of atrial flutter in ICU patients is about 3.6% [5].

If cardioversion cannot be used, several antiarrhythmics are available. Intra-venous ibutilide is efficient in a percentage of 76% (with intravenous procainamide being efficient only in 14% of cases) but prolongs the QTc interval and can provoke sustained polymorphic VT in 1-2% of cases [12]. Ibutilide should not be used in patients with a prolonged QT interval or in those with underlying sinus node disease. Several trials showed efficacy rates of 38% to 76% for conversion of atrial flutter to sinus rhythm [12, 13]. Other antiarrhythmics such as procainamide, flecainide and propafenone were not as efficient as ibutilide for acute conversion [14 - 16]. Intravenous sotalol has a conversion rate varying from 20 to 40%, similar to placebo [17]. Verapamil and diltiazem can be also tried. Esmolol, a beta adrenergic blocker can be used to slow the ventricular rate. If a temporary or permanent pacemaker is in place, atrial overdrive pacing can sometimes restore rhythm. If the atrial flutter persists, diltiazem, verapamil, b- bloquers and digoxin can be used while flecainide can prevent atrial flutter but must be used in combination with atrio- ventricular blocking agents [11].

Irregular Rythms

Multifocal (chaotic) Atrial Tachycardia

Multifocal (chaotic) atrial tachycardia (MAT) is characterized by atrial rates between 100 and 130 beats / min with marked variation in P wave morphology and irregular P – P waves. P waves are nonsinus and at least three P wave contours are noted. The arrhythmia is easily confused with atrial fibrillation. MAT is more common in older patients suffering from chronic obstructive pulmonary disease [18] and congestive heart failure. It is also caused by digitalis and theophylline toxicity. Other possible causes include use of b-agonists and electrolyte abnormalities (hypomagnesemia and hypokalemia) [19]. Correction of the underlying cause is the first goal of therapy. Drugs used for rate control are beta - adrenoreceptor blockers (if bronchospastic pulmonary disease is absent) or verapamil. Potassium and magnesium supplements may help control the tachycardia [20]. Amiodarone has been also used to suppress the tachycardia.

Atrial Fibrillation

Atrial fibrillation is the most common narrow complex tachyarrhythmia encountered in hospitalized patients. A percentage of 47.4% is reported in a medical – cardiological ICU by Reinelt P and colleagues [5]. Knotzer H et al report that AF was observed in 60.7% of cases in a surgical ICU in one year time period [21] while Seguin et al report a percentage of 5. 3% in a six month study [22].

The prevalence of AF in the general population increases with age, from 0.9% at age 40 to 5.9% in those over 65 years [23]. Common risk factors for the development of AF in the general population are structural heart disease, arterial hypertension, valvular heart disease, left atrial enlargement and left ventricular hypertrophy while sepsis, SIRS and blunt thoracic trauma are among the most significant risk factors for the development of AF in ICU patients [22, 24].

The first step in the approach of a patient with AF in ICU includes i-dentification of a possible cause (for example fluid or electrolyte disturbances, hypoxia, sepsis etc) and its correction if possible. Patients with increased circulating catecholamines (exogenous or endogenous) and multi organ failure might not respond to attempts of restoration of sinus rythm.

In hemodynamically unstable patients presenting with significantly low arterial pressure or signs of congestive heart failure, cardioversion should be applied in a synchronized mode after the administration of an anesthetic agent. Anticoagulation with intravenous heparin for the prevention of embolic phenomena during DC cardioversion of AF that has persisted for more than 48 hours is necessary [25]. The risk of stroke in patients between the ages of 60 and 75 years with lone atrial fibrillation is low (~ 2% per year) and they can be protected by aspirin therapy. Patients with other risk factors for stroke (prior stroke or transient ischemic attack, significant valvular heart disease, hypertension, diabetes, age older than 65 y, coronary artery disease, and congestive heart failure) should be treated with warfarin anticoagulation [26].

In patients with hemodynamically stable situation and recent onset of AF, DC cardioversion should be also considered but pharmacologic conversion to sinus rythm with antiarrhythmic drugs is used more commonly. One of the most frequently used medications is amiodarone with reported conversion rates in AF of up to 80% [27]. However only a single retrospective study including ICU patients with left ventricular failure has been published [28] and no prospective randomized studies have been reported. Amiodarone is widely used in ICUs for the conversion of AF to a regular rhythm and although it is generally considered as a safe drug, an increasing number of reports are calling attention to its use because of reported serious acute pulmonary toxicity in ICU patients [29, 30, 31]. Patients receiving high concentrations of oxygen are at increased risk of presenting this syndrome and early discontinuation of the drug is suggested in such cases [30]. Other side effects of the drug include hypotension, phlebitis, bradycardia and elevated liver enzymes. Ibutilide is a relatively new class III antiarrhythmic agent that has been reported to have high conversion rates but with proarrhythmic effects of a relatively high rate (5 to 7%) and therefore requiring careful monitoring. Despite that, Hennesdorf et al studied 26 patients who developed atrial fibrillation or flutter in the ICU and initially received amiodarone. Because of persistent arrhythmia, ibutilide was administered with a conversion rate of 81.5% while a relatively low rate of proarrhythmic effect due to the drug was noticed [32].

Apart from rhythm control, hemodynamically stable patients can also benefit from rate control. Besides, a rapid ventricular response may be poorly tolerated along with the loss of atrial synchrony in hemodynamically compromised patients. Pharmacological agents for acute rate control include b-bloquers, diltiazem, verapamil, and digoxin. Beta bloquers are more effective at rest and during exercise. Metoprolol can be given intravenously at a dose of 2.5 to 5.0 mg over 1 to 2 min every 5 to 10 min for a total of 15 mg. Esmolol is started with a bolus of 0.5 mg/kg, followed by an infusion of 0.05 mg/kg/min. Given the more rapid onset and offset of its action, esmolol is probably a better choice for unstable patients, a usual category in ICU. Diltiazem and verapamil are effective nodal bloquers. Verapamil may induce hypotension in patients with left ventricular dysfunction and borderline arterial pressure. In these patients it is preferable to use diltiazem which can be used as a continuous infusion at a rate of 5 to 15 mg per hour. Digoxin acts directly on the AV node. Digoxin is given in an initial dose of 0.5 mg and after 30 min 0.25 mg will be administered again.

It is of note that two important studies have compared the results of the rhythm and rate control in patients with AF [33, 34]. Although these studies were not performed in critically ill patients, they have many implications in the management of patients with atrial fibrillation arriving in an ICU [27]. According to the results of these studies rhythm control is not superior to rate control for the prevention of death and morbidity.

Atrial fibrillation after cardiac or thoracic surgery occurs in 25 to 40% of patients, with peak incidence on day 2 while it increases the risk for stroke, prolongs ICU stay and increases hospital costs [35]. In patients with a recent onset of AF and hemodynamically unstable situation resulting in angina, myocardial ischemia, shock or pulmonary edema, immediate cardioversion should be performed. Otherwise drugs which establish rate control (diltiazem, esmolol, metoprolol, propranolol, verapamil, digoxin) can be used initially IV and then per os. Preoperative use of b blockers, sota-lol and amiodarone has been also tried with satisfactory results [36]. This arrhythmia is usually self – limited and more than 90% of patients will convert to sinus rhythm within 6 to 8 weeks [37].

Wide Complex Tachycardia

Wide QRS complex tachycardia may be defined as a tachycardia with QRS duration greater than 120 ms (0.12 sec). The intensivists first step in the evaluation of a patient with a wide complex tachycardia should be to discriminate between a ventricular tachycardia and a supraventricular with aberrancy (with permanent or rate – dependent right or left bundle branch block).

Ventricular tachycardia (VT) arises in the specialized conduction system, in ventricular muscle, or in combination of both tissue types. VT is defined as three or more consecutive ventricular beats. In *monomorphic VT*, QRS complexes are uniform in size and shape while in *polymorphic VT*, the QRS morphology changes con-tinuously [6]. Sustained ventricular tachycardia is defined arbitrarily as lasting more than 30 seconds of ventricular beats at a rate of more than 100 bpm or nonsustained when it stops spontaneously in less than 30 sec. The establishment of diagnosis is essential because VT is more ominous than supraventricular tachycardia with aberration. Initially a 12 - lead ECG should be obtained and any electrolyte abnormalities (potassium, calcium, magnesium) corrected. Distinction between VT and SVT with aberration can be difficult at times and a SVT can mimic the criteria established for VT. It is important to emphasize that ventricular tachycardia is the most common cause of a wide QRS complex tachycardia [38]. Moreover the following points must be taken into account. A past history of *myocardial infarction* or the presence of Q waves makes the diagnosis of VT more likely [5, 39, 40]. *Circulatory collapse* is more common with SVT with aberration, but patients with VT may maintain normal blood pressure. The presence of *fusion beats and capture beats* provides maximum support for the diagnosis of VT. Fusion beats indicate activation of the ventricle from two different foci. Capture beats are occasional beats conducted with a narrow complex, ruling out a fixed bundle branch block. *QRS contours* can also be helpful, for example QRS contours suggesting a ventricular tachycardia include a QRS width exceeding 140 m/sec with right bundle branch block or 160 msec during left bundle branch block. *Triggering vagal reflexes* would terminate the supraventricular tachycardia but uncommonly a ventricular tachycardia would be stopped in a similar manner. If patient is hemodynamically stable intravenous *adenosine* can help to unmask a paroxysmal supraventricular tachycardia. Adenosine will not terminate VT but it will abruptly terminate most cases of paroxysmal SVT.

In general if one is not certain about the diagnosis, it is better to treat a wide QRS complex tachycardia as a ventricular tachycardia because several adverse events are associated with the misdiagnosis of a VT as SVT and treatment of VT with calcium channel blockers [41].

Nonsustained Ventricular Tachycardia

Nonsustained ventricular tachycardia (NSVT) is one of the common clinical problems in modern cardiology, encountered equally in men and women. It is defined as 3 or more consecutive beats arising below the atrioventricular node with a rate > 120 beats/min and lasting less than 30 msec [42, 43]. It is encountered with an incidence of 0 to 4% in the general population [44] and it can be associated with a wide range of clinical conditions, from patients with significant heart disease and annual mortality rates exceeding 50% to asymptomatic, apparently healthy, young individuals.

The physician attending a patient with an episode of NSVT has to establish whether a structural heart disease exists and in such a case to risk – stratify the patient for appropriate management. A thorough history and physical examination, echocar-diography and stress testing are usually sufficient to exclude significant heart disease.

Generally, it seems that if occult ischemia or structural heart disease are excluded, prognosis is not affected adversely [45]. In ischemic heart disease the occurrence of NVST though not very rare (40% to 70% of patients) during the first day of acute myocardial infarction, it is not associated with increased risk for subsequent mortality. Following the first 24 h postinfarction, NSVT is detected in 5 -10% of patients, particularly during the first months and has been considered to have adverse prognostic significance [46 - 48]. On the other hand, NVST occurring more than a week after MI doubles the risk of sudden cardiac death in patients with preserved left ventricular function [49]. In dilated cardiomyopathy up to 80% of patients' present ventricular arrhythmia [50] but the prognostic significance of these arrhythmias is difficult [45]. Furthermore, neither the use of amiodarone nor the implantation of an internal cardiac defibrillator (ICD) has shown satisfactory results in decreasing the mortality in these patients [51, 52].

In hypertrophic cardiomyopathy 20 -30% of patients may have NSVT and it is suggested that NSVT has prognostic importance when it is repetitive, prolonged or symptomatic [11, 45]. It seems that NSVT is associated with a substantial increase in risk for sudden death and the implantation of a defibrillator seems justified [53].

Patients with valvular disease present a considerable incidence of NSVT (20% of patients with mitral valve prolapse and mitral regurgitation and 5% with aortic stenosis) but the arrhythmia does not appear to be associated with sudden cardiac death [54]. Other possible causes of NSVT include arterial hypertension, with or without ventricular hypertrophy and repaired congenital abnormalities.

Monomorphic Ventricular Tachycardia

In monomorphic ventricular tachycardia all ventricular complexes have a uniform QRS morphology. The rate ranges between 100 and 150 beats /min and occasionally becomes as rapid as 250 beats / min. If the tachycardia becomes sustained (defined arbitrarily as lasting more than 30 msec) its importance and symptoms depend on the duration of tachycardia, ventricular rate and the underlying heart disease. Sustained ventricular tachycardia (SVT) is usually associated with ischemic heart disease and in such cases re-entry has been suggested as the possible underlying mechanism [55]. Other causes of SVT include dilated and hypertrophic cardiomyopathies, valvular heart disease, mitral valve prolapse and miscellaneous causes.

Treatment of SVT depends on the presence of hemodynamic instability, pulmonary congestion and decreased level of consciousness or myocardial ischemia. If such symptoms are present, synchronized cardioversion is indicated. Cardioversion should begin with an initial shock of 100J, followed by repetitive shocks of 200, 300 and 360J. Stable patients can be medically treated with lidocaine, procainamide, sotalol or amiodarone [56]. The choice of the drug depends on the left ventricular function. In case the latter is impaired, sotalol and procainamide should not be used. Amiodarone has replaced lidocaine as the antiarrhythmic of choice for terminating a ventricular tachycardia according to the most recent guidelines [57]. Amiodarone can be given at initial doses of 5 to 10 mg /kg over 20 to 30 minutes followed by an infusion of 1mg/min for 6 hours, then 0.5 mg/min infusion for 18 hours. Additional doses of 150 mg IV can be given every 10 min as needed. Maximum daily dose is 2.2 gr. Lidocaine is administered at an initial dose of 1 to 1, 5 mg /kg by bolus injection. After 5 minutes a second dose of 0.05 to 0.75 mg/kg can be given if needed followed by continuous infusion of 2 to 4 mg/min. Procainamide is considered a second – line drug because it cannot be administered rapidly. It is infused at a rate of 20 mg/min IV for a loading dose of 17mg/kg, then continued as an infusion at 1 to 4mg /min. Procainamide may cause hypotension and proarrhythmic effects. It is contraindicated in patients who are elderly, present renal dysfunction or with a prolonged QT interval. For special cases of monomorphic ventricular tachycardia rhythms (bundle branch reentrant VT, right ventricular outflow tract VT and idiopathic left ventricular tachycardia) treatment with radiofrequency ablation can be performed [58].

The incidence of ventricular tachycardia in general ICUs varies widely between 9.4% according to a study by Artucio H et al in a population of 2820 consecutive patients hospitalized in a 12 - year period [3] and 40.6% in 133 patients in a 3 year period [5].

Polymorphic Ventricular Tachycardia

Polymorphic ventricular tachycardia (PMVT) is defined as a ventricular rhythm faster than 100 beats/min characterized by clearly defined QRS complexes with a random variation of QRS contour. PMVT may range from a brief, asymptomatic, self- terminating episode, to recurrent episodes leading to syncope or sudden cardiac death [59].

Polymorphic ventricular tachycardia is divided into PMVT with a normal Q – T interval and PMVT with a long Q – T interval. The Q – T interval depends upon the heart rate, age and gender and it also exhibits diurnal variation [60 – 63]. The Q – T interval measures the time between the initiation of the QRS complex and the termination of the T wave. The rate - corrected Q- T interval (Q – Tc) may be calculated from the observed QT interval using several formulas, usually the formula of Bazett, $QTc = QT/\sqrt{RR}$ [64]. A prolonged Q- Tc interval is defined as longer than 0.44 seconds [65]. PMVT with a normal Q - T interval is considered to be an ischemic rhythm that typically degenerates into ventricular fibrillation. This form of tachycardia is almost never asymptomatic and DC cardioversion is the initial recommended treatment if there is evidence of hemodynamic compromise. Patients with myocardial ischemia presenting with polymorphic VT are in a greater danger than patients with monomorphic VT. Patients in ICU may be taking medications that might predispose to ischemia, such as inotropes or vasopressors. These drugs should be stopped or tapered if possible. If withdrawal of such medications is contraindicated, IV infusion of lidocaine or amiodarone should be initiated. Other causes of PMVT with a normal Q – T include myocardial reperfusion, organic heart disease, catecholaminergic PMVT, idiopathic PMVT, and Brugada syndrome.

PMVT with a prolonged Q – T interval is commonly known as torsades de pointes and may be congenital or acquired.

Brugada Syndrome

In 1992 Brugada and Brugada described a new syndrome consisting of syncopal episodes and / or sudden cardiac death in patients with a structurally normal heart and an ECG characterized by ST segment elevation in the right precordial leads (V1 to V3) and right bundle branch block [66]. The syndrome which is inherited in the autosomal dominant character is associated with a poor prognosis and it appears to be a congenital ion channel disorder since mutations in the cardiac sodium channel gene SCN5A have been reported. The diagnosis is based on the history of aborted sudden death with the typical electrocardiographic pattern. The syndrome seems to be more prevalent in Japan and Southeast Asia. The age at onset of clinical manifestations is the third to fourth decade of life and cardiac events typically occur during sleep or at rest. Symptoms include syncope, cardiac arrest or sudden death due to ventricular fibrillation.

The diagnosis of the syndrome is complicated by the intermittent nature of the ECG pattern. The complete syndrome is characterized by episodes of rapid polymorphic VT in patients with an EEG pattern of right bundle branch block and ST segment elevation in V1 to V3. In other individuals the atypical ECG is detected during routine examination [67]. Concealed forms may be unmasked by provocative drug testing with selected Class IC drugs (ajmaline, flecainide, procainamide) [66]. Therefore critical care patients with Brugada syndrome may present with a normal baseline ECG. In such cases the characteristic features of the syndrome may be revealed after a febrile episode [68, 69], following a tricyclic antidepressant overdose [70, 71] or a septic shock [72]. Additionally the ECG pattern of the critical care patient with Brugada syndrome may occasionally imitate acute myocardial infarction [73].

Long Q – T Syndrome (LQTS) and Torsades de Pointes

The congenital long QT syndrome is an inherited arrhythmogenic disease characterized by susceptibility to life – threatening ventricular arrhythmias. Two major forms of LQTS have been identified; one transmitted as an autosomal dominant trait (Romano – Ward syndrome) [74] and the second transmitted as an autosomal recessive disease (Jervell – Lange – Nielsen syndrome) [61]. In these patients chromosome abnormalities have been identified that affect sodium and potassium channels. Beta blockade prevents new syncope in 75% of patients while permanent pacemakers and left cervicothoracic sympathetic gangliectomy consist other treatment options. Implantation of a cardioverter defibrillator is also increasingly used in this group of patients [58].

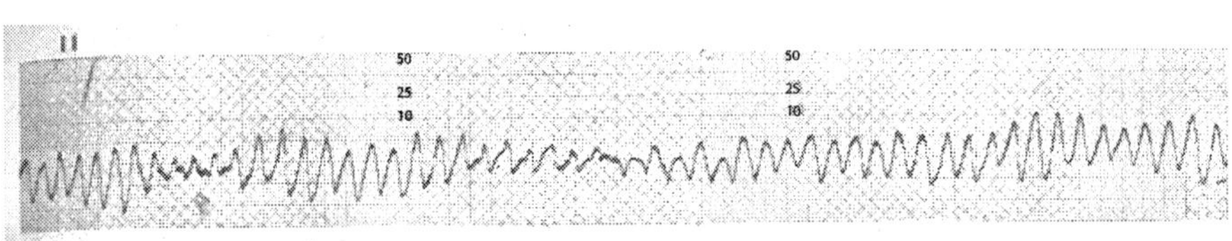

Figure 1. Torsades de pointes in a patient with ischemic heart disease who was given amiodarone for recurrent ventricular tachycardia.

The acquired syndrome may be due to various medications causing a long Q – T interval such as quinidine, procainamide, sotalol, ibutilide, amiodarone, phenothiazines, antibiotics (makrolides and fluoroquinolones, pentamidin, ketokona-zole, metronidazole, TMP- SMX) [75,76], [figure 1] antihistamines (terfenadine, astemizole) and tricyclic antidepressants [77]. Other etiologies include electrolyte disturbances (hypokalemia, hypocalcemia, hypomagnesemia), cerebrovascular abnormalities (subarachnoid hemorrhage, stroke, intracranial trauma) and insecticide poisoning.

The patient with LQTS (congenital or acquired) is at risk for torsades de pointes. The term “torsades de pointes” is a French term translated as “twisting of the points”. It is a ventricular tachycardia first described in 1966 [78], characterized by QRS complexes of changing amplitude that appear to twist around the isoelectric line and occur at rates of 200 to 250/min. The term “torsades de pointes” connotes generally a syndrome not simply an ECG description. Prolonged ventricular repolarization with Q-T interval usually exceeding 500msec occurs as part of the syndrome. The arrhythmia is more common in women and it is usually self – terminated but may degenerate into ventricular fibrillation or more rarely sustained monomorphic ventricular tachycardia. Correction of any underlying factors and normalization of electrolyte abnormalities is the base of the treatment. Intravenous magnesium has been successful and it should be given in doses of 1 to 2 gr over 30 to 60 minutes followed by a continuous infusion of 1 gram/hour for the next 6 hours. Magnesium should be given with caution in patients with renal failure. Other potential treatment may include lidocaine, overdrive pacing or isoproterenol to increase heart rate and thus shorten QTc. Although amiodarone may increase the Q – T interval and has been implicated in the initiation of torsades de pointes, successful suppression of drug – induced torsades de pointes with this drug has been also reported [59].

Preexcitation Syndrome and Wolff–Parkinson White

Preexcitation syndrome occurs when the atrial impulse activates the whole or some part of the ventricle or the ventricular impulse activates the whole or some part of the atrium, earlier than would be expected if the impulse travelled by way of the normal specialized conduction system only. Myocardial fibers connect atrium and ventricle and they are named *accessory atrioventricular pathways* or Kent bundles [79]. The term Wolff – Parkinson – White (WPW) syndrome is applied when the patient is symptomatic due to tachyarrhythmias. In patients with WPW syndrome there is a P- R interval less than 120 msec during sinus rythm, QRS complex duration > 120 msec with a slurred onset of the QRS in some leads, (delta wave) and secondary ST – T wave changes.

The most common tachycardia is atrioventricular reciprocating tachycardia (AVRT) involving a concealed bypass tract. Patients with WPW syndrome present atrial fibrillation in 20 – 30% of cases [80]. Atrial fibrillation may generate a rapid ventricular response and degenerate into ventricular fibrillation and consequently to syncope or sudden cardiac death. Agents preferred for treatment of the syndrome are procainamide, ibutilide and flecainide because they prolong the refractory period in the accessory pathway. On the contrary, drugs like digitalis that prolong the refractoriness in the AV node but may shorten the refractoriness in the accessory pathway should not be used. Calcium channel blockers are also contraindicated. Adenosine is useful for orthodromic AVRT with a narrow QRS complex but it might precipitate AF with a rapid ventricular response [81, 82]. If a rapid ventricular response is present, electrical cardioversion is the initial treatment. For long term therapy class IC drugs and amiodarone can be effective. Patients with frequent symptomatic arrhythmias that cannot be fully controlled by drugs must be submitted to ablation of the accessory pathway.

Ventricular Flutter and Fibrillation

Ventricular flutter is manifested as regular large oscillations occurring at a rate of 150 to 300 /min. Ventricular fibrillation is recognized by the presence of irregular undu-lations of varying contour and amplitude. Distinct QRS complexes, ST segments, and T waves are absent. The distinction between rapid VT and ventricular flutter is of no significance since hemodynamic collapse is present in both. Therapy includes immediate nonsynchronized DC electrical shock 200 to 400 J.

Incidence of ventricular flutter and fibrillation in general ICUs varies between 9.4% [3] and 4.5% [5].

Unusual Causes of Wide - Complex Tachycardia in the ICU

The critical care physician may encounter several causes of wide complex tachycardia (WCT) apart from SVT and PSVT with aberrancy [83]. These tachycardias require a specific therapy and therefore clinicians must be able to recognize them early on and be prepared for their acute management.

Hyperkalemia is a common electrolyte disorder that can lead to lethal cardiac arrhythmias. Potassium levels of 6.5 to 7.7 meq / lt will present with tall peaked T waves, short QT interval and prolonged PR interval [figure 2]. If serum potassium levels exceed 7.5 and 8.0 meq/lt a wide QRS complex will follow with loss of P wave, second or third degree of AV block, ventricular fibrillation and asystole. Arrhythmias will appear sooner if the rise in the serum potassium is rapid while there is a variable relationship between the degree of hyperkalemia and the ECG changes. In rare cases the ECG may be normal despite high potassium levels. A major cause of hyperkalemia is impaired potassium excretion due to renal insufficiency. Other possible causes in the ICU setting include rhabdomyolysis (table 1) and several causes of iatrogenic hyperkalemia including massive blood transfusions or drugs (table 2). Management depends on patients' clinical situation and ECG findings. Intravenous calcium in the form of calcium chloride or calcium gluconate should be administered as a first measure in order to restore an appropriate electrical gradient across the cell membrane. Medications that are capable of moving the potassium into the cell and transiently lower its levels in the serum include glucose, insulin, b - adrenergic agonists, magnesium, sodium bicarbonate and intravenous saline. Of note that repeated administration of these agents may be necessary until removal of the electrolyte is achieved via urine excretion with the aid of loop diuretics or the initiation of some form of hemodialysis.

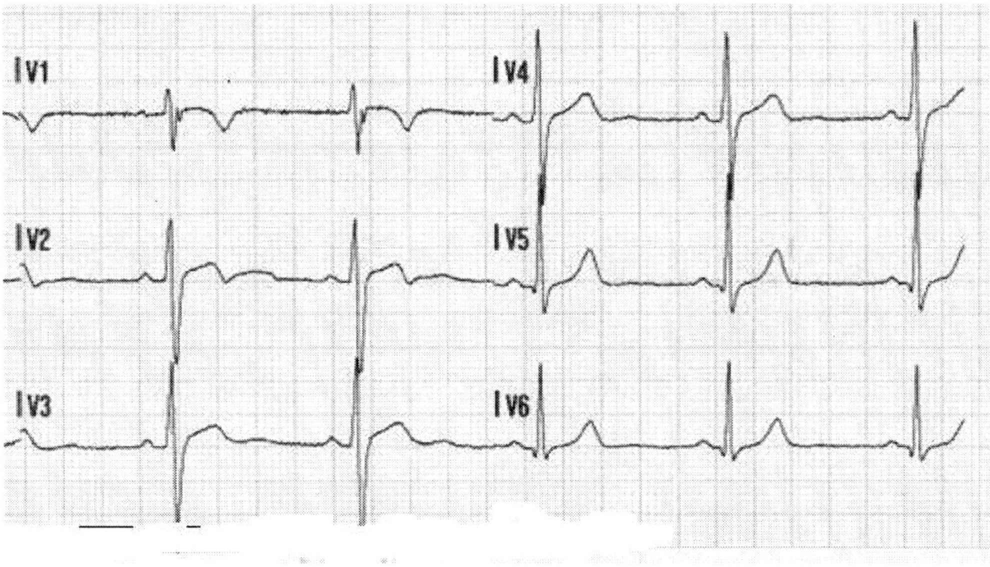

Figure 2. Presence of wide and tall T waves in a patient with hyperkalemia.

Several medications produce myocardial sodium channel blocking and influence other myocardial ion channels such as the calcium influx and potassium efflux channels. As a result, a prolongation of the QRS complex ensues which may result in a sine - wave pattern and eventual asystole. A diverse group of pharmaceu-tical agents are comprised in these myocardial sodium blocking agents. Examples include tricyclic antidepressants (amitriptyline, imipramine e.t.c) carbamazepine, chloroquine, class IA antiarrhythmics, and antihistamines like diphenhydramine, orphenadrine and cocaine. Consequently, poisoning with these agents can result in several kinds of toxicity including central nervous system toxicity and cardiac toxic effects. As a matter of fact, up to 50% of the poisoning admitted in the ICU is associated with acute antidepressant overdose [84]. Management of intoxication with these agents include the administration of sodium and the induction of metabolic or respiratory alkalosis. Infusion of sodium bicarbonate in the form of intermittent bolus or continuous infusion should be considered if the QRS complex lasts more than 100 ms, dysrhythmias are present or the hypotension is not corrected after adequate hydration. Alkalosis with a pH between 7.5 and 7.6 must be achieved while a close monitoring of electrolyte, pH and fluid balance is performed. Iatrogenic respiratory alkalosis achieved through hyperventilation has also shown to be effective.

Table 1. Usual causes of rhabdomyolysis

mechanical	Crush injury, excessive exertion, intractable convulsions, surgery, compression by a tourniquet, local muscle compression due to comatose states, compartment syndrome, malignant neuroleptic syndrome
physical	High fever or hyperthermia, electric current
chemical	Metabolic disorders, anoxia of the muscle due to toxins, special kind of mushrooms, alcohol ingestion

Table 2. Drugs causing hyperkalemia.

ACE inhibitors	Heparin
Angiotensin inhibitors	Non steroidal anti-inflammatory drugs
B - blockers	Potassium penicillin
cyclosporine	Trimethoprim - pentamidine
digitalis	Succinylcholine
K sparing diuretics	Barbiturates

Cardiac arrest is a major public health problem in the Western societies. It is reported that approximately 1000 people in the United States experience cardiac arrest each day [37] which in most cases is the result of acute myocardial infarction and accompanying ventricular fibrillation or unstable ventricular tachycardia. Initial resuscitation is achieved in 20 – 40% of cases while fewer patients survive to hospital discharge. Several dysrhythmias follow the resuscitation of patients including wide complex tachycardia, narrow complex tachycardia and bradycardia. The morphology of the wide QRS complex is supposed to be due to an acute bundle dysfunction which is related to the cardiac arrest and the defribillatory shocks delivered across the heart [83].

Bradyarrhythmias

Bradyarrythmias in the ICU are much less common than tachyarrhythmias. Reinelt et al report only 32 bradycardic events versus 278 tachycardic [5]. Bradycardias include sinus bradycardia, second and third degree atrioventricular block, asystole, atrial fibrillation, and ventricular escape rhythm. Sinus bradycardia (SB) exists in an adult when the sinus discharges at a rate less than 60 beats/min. It is the result of excessive vagal tone or decreased sympathetic tone, as an effect of medications or from anatomical changes in the sinus node. Acute myocardial infarction, intracranial tumors, raised intracranial pressure, meningitis , prolonged and excessive hypothermia, gram negative sepsis, and sleep apnea during apneic periods are common causes of sinus bradycardia in ICU patients. Several drugs usually administered in ICU can also produce SB. Propofol, remifentanil, b - bloquers, amiodarone, calcium channel blockers and clonidine are typical examples. Sinus bradycardia in such cases is usually terminated if the underlying cause is corrected and treatment is seldom necessary. If cardiac output is not adequate or if escape ventricular arrhythmias are associated with this low rate, low doses of atropine IV at a dose of 0.6 mg - 3mg or IV isoprenaline at an infusion of 0.5 – 10 mcg/min may be useful (the drug must be given with caution in ischemic heart disease). If the patient presents heart failure, syncope or other symptoms accompanying bradycardia, electric pacing is necessary.

Other causes of bradyarrhythmia in ICU patients include several degrees of atrioventricular (AV) block. Possible causes of complete AV block (CHB) in the ICU include electrolyte abnormalities (e.g. severe hyperkalemia) cardiac surgery, various medications (b-blockers, calcium channel bloquers, amiodarone) or insertion of central venous catheters especially pulmonary artery catheters (PAC). Patients with pre-existing left bundle branch block are at greater risk to present a complete block in the last case [85, 86], but CHB has been also described during the insertion of a central venous line in a previously healthy adult

[87] [figure 3]. The use of a temporal pacemaker is seldom necessary and arrhythmias usually resolve with catheter movement. Indications of permanent pacing in AV block according to American Heart Association and the American college of cardiology include three categories: "generally indicated", "may be indicated" and "not indicated." Insertion of pacemaker is considered necessary (class I indications) in complete AV block congenital or acquired, atrial fibrillation with CHB, neuromuscular diseases with AV block, symptomatic AV second degree AV block and asymptomatic advanced second degree block with asystole > 3.0 sec or escape rate < 40 beats/min [88].

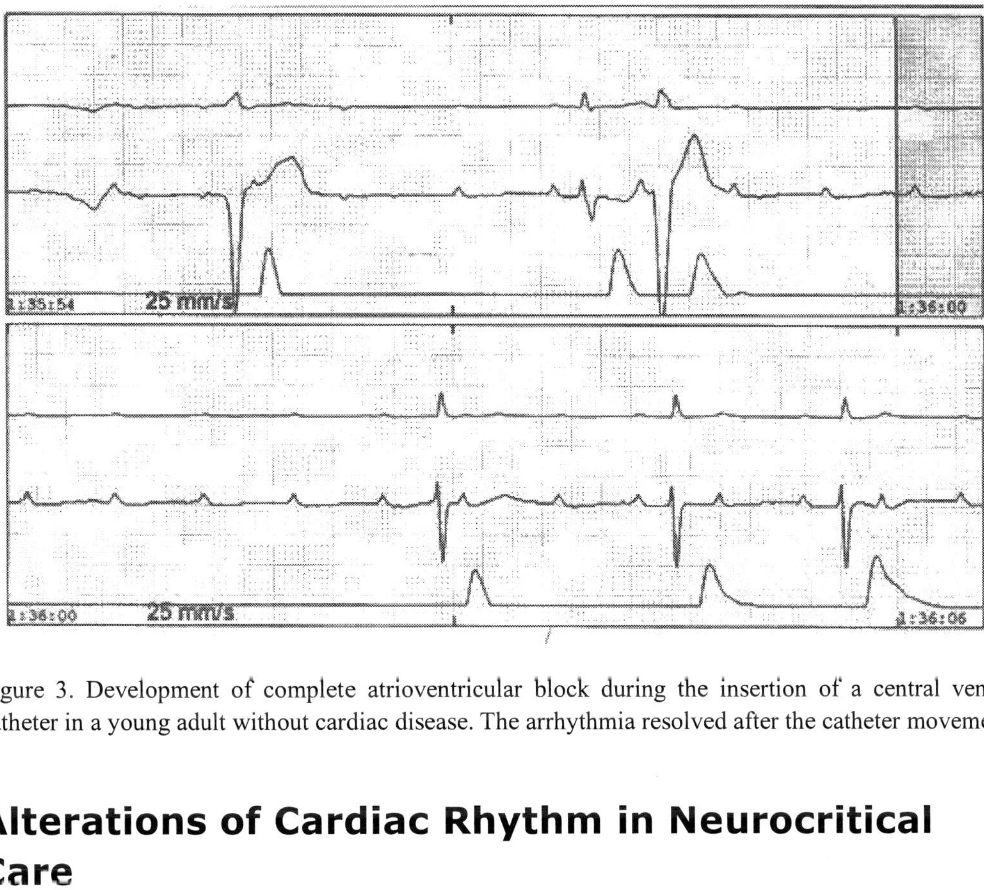

Figure 3. Development of complete atrioventricular block during the insertion of a central venous catheter in a young adult without cardiac disease. The arrhythmia resolved after the catheter movement.

Alterations of Cardiac Rhythm in Neurocritical Care

CNS Disease

Electrocardiographic abnormalities after cerebrovascular accidents especially subarachnoid haemorrhage (SAH) have been recognized since several decades when Burch et al [89] described an ECG pattern of Q-T prolongation and T wave inversion in 17 patients with SAH while identical changes were described previously in case reports [90,91]. Subsequent investigations have determined that ECG abnormalities occur in 25 to 75% of patients with SAH [92] while a wide variety of ECG changes has been reported, including atrioventricular conduction block, abnormal T waves, QT prolongation, prominent U waves, ST segment changes, and ventricular tachycardia [93,94]. Other studies [95-97] have also described paroxysmal atrial fibrillation and SVT, sinus brady – tachycardia, several degrees of A – V block, torsades de pointes, ventricular flutter and ventricular fibrillation. Therefore continuous electrocardiographic monitoring should be available in the acute phase since life threatening arrhythmias may occur during the first 48 hours [98].

The variety of arrhythmias observed, reflect perhaps the autonomic imbalance and the secretion of catecholamines that often accompanies SAH [94, 97-99] while hypokalemia has been observed in patients with SAH and ventricular arrhythmias [97]. Some studies reported that there was no correlation between the concentrations of plasma catecholamines and ECG abnormalities [98,101] while other suggest that not only sympathetic activity but also vagal activity is enhanced during the acute phase of SAH [102]. Additionally, an increased QT dispersion which has been documented in patients with SAH may predispose to cardiac arrhythmias [103,104]. The abnormalities observed in the ECG are attributed, according to existing evidence, to myocardial damage due to excessive sympathetic tone and catecholamine produ-ction.

Other cerebrovascular disorders associated with arrhythmias (mostly atrial fibrillation, ventricular premature beats and paroxysmal atrial tachycardia) include intracranial hemorrhage, head trauma, neurosurgical procedures, acute meningitis, intracranial hypertension, epilepsy and intracranial tumors [105].

Myocardial Contusion Injury

Myocardial contusion injury (MCI) is usually a complication of blunt thoracic trauma caused by motor vehicle accidents or work related injuries. A direct blow to the chest from a steering wheel, rapid deceleration of the car or deceleration caused by a fall, may result in blunt cardiac injury.

The incidence of MCI in patients with blunt chest trauma varies greatly depending on the diagnostic criteria used. Percentages reported range from 0% to 76% [106], 8.2 % to 75% [107] while in a recent study Boeken et al [108] report a percentage of 16.9%. Mechanism of contusion involves the compression of the heart between the sternum and the spine because of a blow to the precordium or the force exerted on the thoracic wall. The right ventricle and the mitral and aortic valves are more vulnerable because of their location. Arrhythmias and cardiac failure are possible complications of cardiac injury. Arrhythmias constitute the most common abnormality observed in the electrocardiogram and they usually occur in the first 24 – 48 hours [109]. The severity of arrhythmia varies. Sinus tachycardia, atrial and ventricular extrasystoles are most frequently observed while more serious arrhythmias such as atrial fibrillation, ventricular fibrillation, right bundle branch block, various degrees of atrioventricular block [106] might also occur and result in sudden death [110]. Notably, paucity of symptoms does not exclude cardiac contusion and life threatening arrhythmias can occur even without any symptoms [111]. Moreover, it seems that no correlation exists between ECG alterations and cardiac complications [112] while other possible sources of ECG abnormality must be always taken into account such as previous heart disease, electrolyte abnormalities, craniocerebral injury, haemorrhage, hypoxia etc.

Conclusion

Though serious or life - threatening arrhythmias are uncommon events in critical care patients, they demand rapid diagnosis and intervention. Consequently the critical care physician must have an understanding of basic arrhythmia mechanism and therefore be able to identify the exact type of each abnormal cardiac rhythm. Furthermore, adequate knowledge of antiarrhythmic medications as well as their adverse effects is also of paramount importance for the proper management of rhythm disturbances in the critically ill, while the development of management strategies for the medical or invasive treatment of potentially lethal arrhythmias is a critical training element in the continuous medical education of all intensivists.

References

[1] Van Mieghem, C; Sabbe, M & Knockaert, D. The clinical value of the ECG in noncardiac conditions. *Chest*, 2004; 125: 1561- 1576.

[2] Balaji, S ; Ellenby, M; McNames, J & Goldstein B. Update on Intensive Care ECG and Cardiac Event Monitoring. *Cardiac Electrophysiology Review*, 2002; 6: 190 -195.

[3] Artucio, H & Pereira, M. Cardiac arrhythmias in critically ill patients: Epidemiologic study. *Crit Care Med*, 1990; 18:1383-1388.

[4] Brathwaite, D & Weissman, C. The new onset of atrial arrhythmias following major cardiothoracic surgery is associated with increased mortality. *Chest*, 1998 ; 114: 462- 468.

[5] Reinelt, P; Karth, GD; Geppert, A; Heinz, G. Incidence and type of cardiac arrhythmias in critically ill paients: a single center experience in a medical – cardiological ICU. *Intens Care Med,* 2001 ; 27: 1466- 1473.

[6] Marino P. The ICU book. Third edition. Tachyarrhythmias chapter 18. Pages 343- 363. Lippincott Williams and Wilkins, Philadelphia, PA 19106 2007.

[7] Reising S, Kusumoto F, Goldschlager N. Life – threatening arrhythmias in the Intensive Care Unit. *J Intens Care Med*, 2007 ; 22 (1). P. 3 – 13.

[8] Zipes: Braunwald's Heart Disease: A Textbook of Cardiovascular Medicine. Chapter 30. WB Saunders, an imprint of Elsevier. 7th edition. Copyright 2005.

[9] Trohman, RG. Supraventricular tachycardia: implications for the intensivist *Critical Care Medicine* 2000; 28 (10) suppl. N129 – N135.

[10] Blomstrom - Lunqvist, C; Scheinmann, MM; Haliot, EM et al. ACC/AHA/ ESC guidelines for the management of patients with supraventricular arrhythmias: a report of the American College of Cardiology / American Heart Association. Task force on practice guidelines and the European society of cardiology committee on practice guidelines 2003. American college of cardiology website. http:// www.acc.org /clinical /guidelines /arrhythmias /sva_ index.pdf.

[11] Tarditi,DJ. & Hollenberg, SM. Cardiac arrhythmias in the Intensive Care Unit. *Semin Respir Crit Care Med*, 2006; 27: 221 -229.

[12] Ellenbogen, KA; Stambler, BS; Wood, MA et al. Efficacy of intravenous ibutilide for rapid termination of atrial fibrillation and atrial flutter: a dose – response study. *J Am Coll Cardiol*, 1996; 28: 130- 136.

[13] Stambler, BS; Wood, MA; Ellenbogen, KA et al. Efficacy and safety of repeated doses of ibutilide for rapid conversion of atrial flutter or fibrillation. Ibutilide repeat dose study Investigators. *Circulation*, 1996; 94: 1613-1621.

[14] Sung, RJ; Tan, HL; Karagounis, I et al. Intravenous sotalol for the termination of supraventricular tachycardia and atrial fibrillation and flutter: a multicenter, randomized, double-blind, placebo – controlled study. Sotalol Multicenter Study Group. *Am Heart J*, 1995; 129: 739-748.

[15] Kingma, J & Suttorp, MJ. Acute pharmacologic conversion of atrial fibrillation and flutter: the role of flecainide, propafenone and verapamil. *Am J Cardiol*, 1992 ;70: 56A-60 A.

[16] Suttorp, MJ; Kingma, JII; Jessuron, ER et al. The value of class IC antiarrhythmic drugs for acute conversion of paroxysmal atrial fibrillation or flutter to sinus rhythm. *J Am Coll Cardiol*, 1990;16: 1722 – 1727.

[17] Vos, MA; Golitsyn, SR & Stangl, K. Superiority of ibutilide (a new class III agent) over DL sotalol in converting atrial flutter and atrial fibrillation. The ibutilide /sotalol comparator study group. *Heart*, 1998; 79: 568-575.

[18] Kastor, J. Multifocal atrial tachycardia. *N Engl J Med*, 1990 ; 322 : 1713 – 1720.

[19] Cord, J.M & Borzac S. Multifocal atrial tachycardia. *Chest*, 1988 ; 113: 203-9.

[20] Iseri, LT; Fairshter, RD; Hardeman, JL et al. Magnesium and potassium therapy in multifocal atrial tachycardia. *Am Heart* J, 1985; 312: 21- 26.

[21] Knotzer, H; Mayr, A; Ulmer, H et al. Tachyarrhythmias in a surgical intensive care unit: a case – controlled epidemiologic study. *Intens Care Med*, 2000; 26: 908-914.

[22] Seguin, KI; Signouret, T; Laviolle, B et al. Incidence and risk factors of atrial fibrillation in a surgical intensive care unit. *Crit Care Med*, 2004;32: 722 – 726.

[23] Feinberg, WM; Blackshear, JL; Laupacis, A; Kronmal, R; Hart, RG. Prevalence, age distribution, and gender of patients with atrial fibrillation : analysis and implications. *Arch Intern Med*, 1995 ; 155: 469 – 473.

[24] Bruins, P; Te Velthuis, H; Yazdanbakhsh, AP et al. Activation of the complement system during and after cardiopulmonary bypass surgery – postsurgery activation involves C reactive protein and is associated with postoperative arrhythmia. *Circulation*, 1997; 96: 3542-3548.

[25] Arnold, AZ; Mick, MJ; Mazurek, RP et al. Role of prophylactic anticoagulation for direct current cardioversion for refractory atrial fibrillation. *J Am Coll Cardiol*, 1999; 34: 2031- 2034.

[26] Cage, BF; Waterman, AD; Shannon, W et al. Validation of clinical association schemes for predicting stroke: results from the National Registry of Atrial Fibrillation. *JAMA*, 2001; 285 : 2864 – 2870.

[27] Trappe, HJ; Brandts, B & Weismueller, P. Arrhythmias in the intensive care patient. *Curr Opin Crit Care,* 2003; 9: 345 – 355.

[28] Clemo, HF; Wood, MA; Gilligan, DM & Ellenbogen, KA. Intravenous amiodarone for acute heart rate control in the critically ill patients with atrial tachyarrhythmias 1998, *Am J Cardiol* **81**: 594-598.

[29] Skroubis, T; Galiatsou, E; Metafratzi, Z et al. Amiodarone-induced acute lung toxicity in an ICU setting. *Acta Anesthesiol Scand* 2005; 49: 569-571.

[30] Donaldson, L; Grant, IS; Naysmith, M.R & Thomas, J.S.J. Acute amiodarone – induced lung toxicity. *Intensive Care Med* 1998; 24: 626-630.

[31] Ashrafian, H & Davey, P. Is amiodarone an underrecognized cause of acute respiratory failure in the ICU? *Chest*, 2001; 120: 275-82.

[32] Hennersdorf, M; Perings, S; Zuhlke, C; Heidland, U; Perings, C; Henitzen, M; & Strauer, B. Conversion of recent – onset atrial fibrillation or flutter with ibutilide after amiodarone has failed. *Intens Care Med*, 2000; 28: 925 – 929.

[33] The atrial fibrillation follow – up investigation of Rhythm Management (AFFIRM) Investigators. A comparison of rate control and rhythm control in patients with atrial fibrillation. *N Engl J Med*, 2002; 347: 1825-1833.

[34] Van Gelder, IC; Hagens, VE; Bosker, HA et al. Crihns HJGM for the Rate Control versus Electrical Cardioversion for Persistent Atrial Fibrillation Study Group. A comparison of rate control and rhythm control in patients with recurrent persistent atrial fibrillation. *N Engl J Med*, 2002; 347: 1834 -1840.

[35] Ommen, SR; Odell, JA &. Stanton, MS. Atrial tachyarrhthmias after cardiothoracic surgery. *N Engl J Med*, 1997 ; 336: 1429 -1434.

[36] Crystal, E; Connolly, SJ; Sleik, K; Ginger, TJ &Yusuf S. Interventions on prevention of postoperative atrial fibrillation in patients undergoing heart surgery: a meta – analysis. *Circulation*, 2002 ; 106:75 - 80.

[37] Fuster V, Ryden LE, Ansinger RW, et al. ACC/AHA/ESC guidelines for the management of patients with atrial fibrillation: a report of the American College of cardiology/ American Heart Association task force on practice guidelines and the European society of cardiology committee on practice guidelines and policy conferences. J Am Coll Cardiol 2001; 38: 1266i-1xx. http:// www.acc.org/clinical guidelines /atrial fib/as_ index.htm).

[38] Akhtar, M. Electrophysiological basis for wide QRS complex tachycardia. *Pacing Clin Electrophysiol*, 1983; 6: 81 – 98.

[39] Wellens, HJ & Brugada, P. Diagnosis of ventricular tachycardia from the 12 – lead electrocardiogram. *Cardiol Clin,* 1987; 64: 27 – 33.

[40] Tchou,P; Young, P; Mahmud, R; Denker, S; Jayazeri, M & Akhtar, M. Useful diagnostic criteria for the diagnosis of ventricular tachycardia. *Am J Med*, 1988; 84: 53 - 56.

[41] Buxton, AE; Marchlinsky, FE; Doherty, JU et al. Hazards of intravenous verapamil for sustained ventricular tachycardia. *Am J Cardiol*, 1987; 59: 1107 – 1110.

[42] Buxton, AE; Duc, J; Berger, EE et al. Nonsustained ventricular tachycardia. *Cardiol.Clin*, 2000; 18: 327-36.

[43] Kinder, C; Tamburro, P; Kopp, D et al. The clinical significance of nonsustained ventricular tachycardia: current perspectives. *PACE* 1994 ;17:637 64.

[44] Kostis, JB; Mc Cronne, K; Moreyra, AE et al. Premature ventricular complexes in the absence of identifiable heart disease. *Circulation*, 1981; 63: 1351- 1356.

[45] Katritsis, D & Camm, J. Nonsustained tachycardia: where do we stand? Europ.Heart *Journal*, 2004 ; 25: 1093 –1099.

[46] Cheema, AN; Sheu, K; Parker, M et al. Nonsustained ventricular tachycardia in the setting of acute myocardial infarction: tachycardia characteristics and their prognostic implications. *Circulation*, 1995; 98: 2030-6.

[47] Bigger, JT; Fleiss, JL; Rolnitzky, LM. Prevalence, characteristics and significance of ventricular tachycardia detected by 24 – hour continuous electrocardiographic recordings in the late hospital phase of acute myocardial infarction. *Am J Cardiol*, 1986; 58 :1151- 60.

[48] Maggioni, AR; Zuanetti, G; Franzosi, MG et al. On behalf of GISSI - 2 Investigators. Prevalence and prognostic significance of ventricular arrhythmias after acute myocardial infarction in the fibrinolytic era: GISSI results. *Circulation*, 1993; 87: 312-322.

[49] Anderson, KP; De Camilla, J & Moss, AJ. Clinical significance of ventricular tachycardia detected during ambulatory monitoring after myocardial infarction. *Circulation*, 1978 ; 57:890-897.

[50] Singh, SN; Fletcher, RD; Fisher, SG et al. Amiodarone in patients with congestive heart failure and asymptomatic ventricular arrhythmia. Survival trial of Antiarrhythmic Therapy in congestive heart failure. *N Engl J Med*, 1995 ; 333:77 - 82.

[51] Doval, HC; Nul, DR; Grancelli, HO et al. Nonsustained ventricular tachycardia in severe heart failure. Independent marker of increased mortality due to sudden death.GESICA – GEMA Investigators. *Circulation*, 1996 ; 94: 3198 – 3203.

[52] Bansch, D; Antz, M; Bach, J et al. Primary prevention of sudden cardiac death in idiopathic dilated cardiomyopathy: the Cardiomyopathy Trial (CAT). *Circulation*, 2002; 105: 1453 -8.

[53] Maron, BJ; Shen, WK; Link, MS et al. Efficacy of implantable cardioverter-defribrillators for the prevention of sudden death in patients with hypertrophic cardiomyopathy. *N Engl J Med*, 2000; 342:365 – 73.

[54] Wolfe, RR; Driscoll, DJ ; Gersony, WM et al. Arrhythmias in patients with valvar aortic stenosis, valvar pulmonary stenosis and ventricular septal defect: results of 24-hour ECG monitoring. *Circulation*, 1993 ; 87:189- 101.

[55] Gupta, AK & Thakur, RK. Wide QRS complex tachycardias. *Med Clin North Amer,* 2001; 85: 245 – 266.

[56] Caron, MF; Kluger, J & White, CM. Amiodarone in the new AHA guidelines for ventricular tachyarrhythmias. *Ann Pharmacother*, 2001 Oct; 35 (10) : 1248 – 54.

[57] 2005 American Heart Association Guidelines for cardiopulmonary Resuscitation and Emergency cardiovascular care. Part 7.3 management of symptomatic bradycardia and tachycardia. Circulation 2005; 112 (sup II) IV 67 – IV 77. (http//circ.ahajournals.org/ content /vol 112/24 – suppl.

[58] Hammill, SC & Hubmayr, RD. The rapidly changing management of cardiac arrhythmias. *Am J Respir Crit Care Med*, 2000; 161: 1070 – 1073.

[59] Passman, R & Kadish, A. Polymorphic ventricular tachycardia, long Q – T syndrome , and torsades de pointes. *Med.Clin.North.Am.* 2001 March; 85 (2). 321- 41.

[60] Burke, JH; Ehlert, FA; Kruse, JT et al. Gender –specific differences in the QT interval and the effect of autonomic tone and menstrual cycle in healthy adults. *Am J Cardiol,* 1997; 79: 178 – 181.

[61] Jervell, A & Lange – Nielsen, F. Congenital deaf mutism, functional heart disease with prolongation of the QT interval and sudden death. *Am Heart J,* 1957; 54: 59.

[62] Larsen, JA & Kadish, AH. Effects of gender on cardiac arrhythmias. *J Cardiovasc Electrophysiol*, 1998 ; 9: 655 – 664.

[63] Molnar, J ; Zhang, F; Weiss, J et al: Diurnal pattern of QTc interval: How long is prolonged? Possible relation to circadian triggers of cardiovascular events. *J. Am Coll* Car*d*iol, 1996; 27: 76 – 83.

[64] Bazett, HC. An analysis of the time relations of electrocardiograms. *Heart*, 1918; 7: 353 – 370.

[65] Garson, AJr. How to measure the QT interval: what is normal? *Am J Cardiol* 1993; 26 : 14B – 16B.

[66] Brugada P, Brugada J. Right bundle branch block, persistent ST segment elevation and sudden cardiac death. A distinct clinical and electrocardiographic syndrome. *J Am Coll Cardiol*, 1992; 20: 1391- 1396.

[67] Brugada, J; Brugada, P & Brugada, R. Brugada syndrome: the syndrome of right bundle branch block, ST segment elevation in V1 to V3 and sudden death. *Indian pacing electrophysiol J,* 2001; 1: 6 -11.

[68] Karakitsos, D; Patrianakos, A; Poularas, J & Karabinis, A. Brugada – like electrocardiographic pattern unmasked by fever in a critical care patient. *Acta Anaesth Scand*, 2006; 50 : 1038 – 9.

[69] Porres, JM ; Brugada, J; Urbistondo, V et al. Fever unmasking the Brugada syndrome. *Pacing and clinical electrophysiology*, 2002; 25: p.1646.

[70] Bigwood, B; Galler, D; Amir, N & Smith, W. Brugada syndrome following tricyclic antidepressant overdose. *Anesthesia and intensive care*, 2005 ; 33 : 266 – 270.

[71] Monteban – Kooistra, W; van den Berg, M; Tulleken, J et al. Brugada electrocardiographic pattern elicited by cyclic antidepressants overdose. *Intensive Care Medicine*, 2006; 32 : 281 – 285.

[72] Terajima, K; Yamamoto, T; Onodera, H et al. Unmasking of Brugada syndrome by an antiarrhythmic drug in a patient with septic shock. *Anesth Analg,* 2006 ; 102 : 233 - 6.

[73] Glatter, K & Chiamvimonvat, N. Evaluation of the critical care patient with Brugada syndrome. *Crit Care Med*, 2005 ; 33 : 1666 – 1667.

[74] Romano, C; Gemme, G & Pongiglione R. Aritmie cardiache rare in eta pediatrica. *Clin Pediatr* , 45: 656, 1963.

[75] Justo, D & Zeltser, D. Torsades de pointes induced by antibiotics. *Europ Journ Intern Med*, 2006; 17 : 254- 259.

[76] Frothingham, R. Rates of torsades de pointes associated with ciprofloxacin, ofloxacin, levofloxacin, gatifloxacin, and moxifloxacin. Pharmacotherapy, 2001; 21: 1468 – 1472.

[77] Roden, DM. Drug – induced prolongation of the QT interval. *N Engl J Med,* 2004; 350: 1013- 1022.

[78] Dessertenne T. La tachycardie ventriculaire a deux foyers variables. *Arch Mal Coeur,* 1966 ; 59: 263-272.

[79] Braunwald E (Editor), Heart Disease. A Textbook of cardiovascular medicine, Fourth edition, p.693, Philadelphia, WB Saunders Co, 1992, ISBN 0-7216-4407-4.

[80] Conti, CR. Editors note: what happened to the Wolff – Parkinson – White syndrome? *Clin Cardiol*, 2001 ; 24 : 531- 2.

[81] Gupta, AK; Shah, CP; Maheshwari, A; Thakur, RK; Hayes, OW & Lockhandwala YY. Adenosine induced ventricular fibrillation in Wolff- Parkinson – White syndrome. *Pacing Clin Electrophysiol*, 2002 ; 25 : 477 – 80.

[82] Exner, D; Muzyka, T & Mc Gillis A. Proarrhythmia in patients with the Wolff – Parkinson – White syndrome after standard doses of intravenous adenosine. *Ann Intern Med*, 1995 ; 122 : 351 – 352.

[83] Hollowell, H; Mattu, A; Perron, A et al. Wide – complex tachycardia: beyond the traditional differential diagnosis of ventricular tachycardia vs supraventricular tachycardia with aberrant conduction. *Am J Emerg Med*, 2005; 23: 876- 889.

[84] Arranto, CA; Mueller, C; Hunziker, PR; Marsch, SC & Erikson, U. Adverse cardiac events in ICU patients with presumptive antidepressant overdose. Swiss Med Wkly 2003; 133: 479 - 483.

[85] Unnikrishnan, D; Idris, N & Varshneya N. Complete heart block during central venous catheter placement in a patient with pre-existing left bundle branch block. *Br J Anesth*, 2003; 91:747 – 9.

[86] Morris, D; Mulvihill, D & Lew WY. Risk of developing complete heart block during bedside pulmonary artery catheterization in patients with left bundle-branch block. *Arch Intern Med*, 1987 ; 147 : 2005 – 10.

[87] Paramythiotou, E; Poularas, I; Kalogeromitros A et al. Images in cardiology. An unexpected complication during right jugular vein cannulation in a young adult. *Heart*, 2006; 92 (1): 10.

[88] Gregoratos, G; Abrams, J; Epstein, AE et al. ACC/AHA /NASPE 2002 guideline update for implantation of cardiac pacemakers and antiarrhythmia devices : summary article. A report of the American College of Cardiology / American Heart Association Task force on Practice Guidelines. *J Cardiovasc Electrophysiol*, 2002 ;13: 1183 – 99.

[89] Burch, GE; Meyers, R & Abildskov. JA: A new electrocardiographic pattern observed in cerebrovascular accidents. *Circulation*, 1954; 9:719-723.

[90] Byer, E; Ashman, R & Toth LA. Electrocardiogram with large upright T waves and long Q – T intervals. *Am Heart J,* 1947 ; 33: 796 – 799.

[91] Levine H. Non – specificity of the electrocardiogram associated with coronary artery disease. *Am J Med*, 1953; 15: 344 – 354.

[92] Zaroff, JG; Rordorf, GA; Newell, JB et al. Cardiac outcome in patients with subarachnoid hemorrhage and electrocardiographic abnormalities. *Neurosurgery*, 1999; 44 : 34-39.

[93] Marion, DW; Segal, R & Thompson, ME: Subarachnoid hemorrhage and the heart. *Neurosurgery*, 1986;18: 101 – 106.

[94] Stober, T; Anstatt, T & Sen, S et al. Cardiac arrhythmias in subarachnoid haemorrhage. *Acta Neurochir (Wien),* 1988; 93: 37 – 44.

[95] Svigelj, V; Grad, A & Kiauta, T. Heart rate variability, norepinephrine and ECG changes in subarachnoid hemorrhage patients. *Acta Neurol Scand*, 1996; 94: 120 -6.

[96] Lanzino, G; Kongable, GL & Kassell, NF. Electrocardiographic abnormalities after nontraumatic subarachnoid hemorrhage. *J Neurosurg Anesthesiol*, 1994; 6: 156 -62.

[97] Andreoli, A; di Pasquale, G; Pinelli, G et al. Subarachnoid hemorrhage: frequency and severity of cardiac arrhythmias. A survey of 70 cases studied in the acute phase. *Stroke*, 1987; 18: 558 – 64.

[98] DiPasquale, G; Pinelli, G ; Andreoli, A et al. Holter detection of cardiac arrhythmias in intracranial subarachnoid hemorrrhage. *Am J Cardiol*, 1987;59:596 -600.

[99] Brouwers, PJAM; Wijdicks, EFM ; Hasan, D et al. Serial electrocardiographic recording in aneurysmal subarachnoid hemorrhage.*Stroke*, 1989; 20: 1162 – 1167.

[100] Cruickshank, JM & Dwyer GN. Electrocardiographic changes in subarachnoid hemorrhage: role of catecholamines and effect of beta blockade. *Br Heart J*, 1974;36: 697 – 706.

[101] Grad, A; Kiauta, T & Osredkar J. Effect of elevated plasma norepinephrine on electrocardiographic changes in subarachnoid hemorrhage: frequency and severity of cardiac arrhythmias. *Stroke*, 1987;18: 558-564.

[102] Kawahara, E; Ikeda, S; Miyahara, Y & Kohno S. Role of autonomic nervous dysfunction in electrocardiographic abnormalities and cardiac injury in patients with acute subarachnoid hemorrhage. *Circ J,* 2003; 67: 753- 756.

[103] Randell, T; Tansknanen, P; Scheinin, M et al. QT dispersion after subarachnoid hemorrhage. *J Neurosurg Anesthesiol*, 1999 ; 11 : 163- 166.

[104] Perkiomaki, JS ; Huikuri, HV; Koistinen, JM et al. Heart rate variability and dispersion of QT interval in patients with vulnerability to ventricular tachycardia and ventricular fibrillation after previous myocardial infarction. *J Am Coll Cardiol*, 1997; 30: 1331 - 8.

[105] Oppenheimer, SM; Cechetto, DF & Hachinski, VC. Cerebrogenic cardiac arrhythmias: cerebral electrocardiographic influences and their role in sudden death. *Arch Neurol*, 1990; 47: 513 – 519.

[106] Bansal, MK; Maraj, S; Chewaproung, D & Amanullah A. Myocardial contusion injury: redefining the diagnostic algorithm. *Emerg Med J,* 2005; 22 : 465 – 469.

[107] Mc Donald, RC; O Neill, D; Hanning, CD et al. Myocardial contusion in blunt chest trauma: a ten – year review. *Intens Care Med* ,1981; 7:265 -8.

[108] Boeken, U; Feindt, P; Gramsch – Zabel, H et al. The incidence of myocardial contusion in 160 patients with blunt chest trauma. Diagnostic criteria and outcome. *European Journal of Trauma*, 2000 ; 26: 111 -5.

[109] Kaye, P & O 'Sullivan, I. Myocardial contusion: emergency investigation and diagnosis. *Emerg Med J,* 2002; 19: 8 -10.

[110] Illig, KA; Swierzeski, MJ ; Feliciano, DV et al. A rational screening and treatment strategy based on the electrocardiogram alone for suspected cardiac contusion. *Am J Surg*, 1991; 162: 537 - 44.

[111] Sybrandy, KC; Cramer, MJ & Burgersdijk C. Diagnosing cardiac contusion : old wisdom and new insights. *Heart*, 2003; 89: 485 – 489.

[112] Fegheli, NT & Prisant, LM. Blunt myocardial injury. *Chest*, 1995; 108:1673 – 77.

In: Progress in Cardiac Arrhythmia Research
Editor: Ira R. Tarkowicz, pp. 207-234
ISBN: 1-60021-796-6

Chapter 9

Sudden Cardiac Death Syndrome- Arrhythmogenic Right Ventricular Dysplasia/Cardiomyopathy as most Frequent Cause of Fatal Arrhythmias

Ivana I. Vranic [*] ***and Tijana Simic***
University Clinical Center of Serbia, Institute for Cardiovascular Diseases,
Clinic for cardiosurgery
Belgrade, Serbia

Abstract

In the United States 350 000 people die annually of SCD which does not spare any age, gender, or socioeconomic group. The major cause of SCD is CAD, but a small percentage is due to cardiac diseases other then CAD. The main substrate of the latter are cardiac arrhythmias, mainly caused by ARVD/C, Long QT sy and WPW sy in this otherwise healthy population. A special problem exists in professional sports and dicing during sport activities, in spite of regular thorough examinations.

The most mysterious among aforementioned is arrhythogenic right ventricular dysplasia and/or cardiomyopathy (21 clinical genotype types) which unfortunately, apparently, has no clinical warning sign at the early stage, sometimes having SCD for the first and only presenting dramatic event. The arrhythmias leading to SCD may be identified by electrophysiological testing, and significant percentage of patients can have polymorphic VT or VF as the only inducible arrhythmia, which seems to be the exact scenario for the fatal outcome in the whole group of patients. So what might be the underlying cause and could it be prevented?

ARVD/C is a genetically inherited condition with autosomal-dominant pattern of inheritance (as most common), as consequence of single gene mutations which lead to complex patterns of

[*] E-mail address: ivvra@beotel.yu. Correspondence concerning this article should be addressed to: Ivana I Vranic, Koste Todorovica 8, 11 000 Belgrade, Serbia, Europe.

altered localization of desmosomal proteins. These mutations may change cytosolic pools of cell-cell junction proteins which lead to desmosome disorganization and gap junction distortion. Latter is explanation for loss of contact between cardiomyocytes and earlier start of apoptosis. Pathological hallmark of ARVD/C is the atrophy of myocytes with fatty or fibro-fatty infiltration of the right ventricle. Typical clinical picture encompasses arrhythmias with left bundle branch block morphology and ventricular tachyarrhythmias, while less frequent presentation are signs of right heart failure (fatigue and shortness of breath). The disease may be localized or widespread, with biventricular involvement in some cases.
Valid WHO criteria during last 12 years failed to detect disease at its early stage and recommended diagnostic methods were shown to have low sensitivity for the majority of patients even in its overt phase (because of lack of scoring system). Investigation of this population is further complicated by disease rarity and lack of large databases. New research published data give priority to vectorcardiography and ultrasound.
The possible explanation for this lies in the existence of specific place in the heart exposed to most physical forces during cardiac cycle. Nevertheless, this place is *locus minoris rezistentiae* during contraction and relaxation of the heart. It is presently the focus of an ongoing clinical study regarding two aforementioned methods in detecting early stage of ARVD/C. It is also registered by WIPO as SOPHIE methodology (suggesting wisdom to detect). Soon enough we can expect this technique to be incorporated in newly medical equipment (for stratification of risk for SCD).

Background

Sudden cardiac death does not respect geographic boundaries and it continues to represent an important challenge because of major difficulties in identifying those individuals at risk and in responding by timely prevention of a catastrophic event.

The mode and time of SCD are unexpected, which is a generally accepted definition for death heralded by abrupt loss of consciousness within an hour of the onset of acute symptoms. Clinical, scientific, medico-legal and social issues must be considered to give a full definition for SCD: prodromes, onset, cardiac arrest, and progression to biological death [1].

Incidence

The incidence of SCD is approximately 300 000- 350 000 annually which accounts for an incidence 0,1-0,2% per year among the population >35years of age. The overall incidence is 1 to 2 / 1000. Various estimates suggest that at least two-thirds of all SCDs occur due to coronary heart disease as a first clinical event or among subgroups of pts thought to be at a relatively low risk for SCD [2,3].

Circadyal Rhythm

Circadyal rhythm analysis produces definite diurnal, weekly and seasonal pattern. Throughout the day, peak incidence occurs during the early morning hours, and at night, soon after midnight [4]. This phenomena can be explained by hormonal disbalance in their prevalence: adrenalin/noradrenalin steep rise in the morning and prolactin peak during the night. Nevertheless, it might point to susceptibility of electrical conduction delay to hormone stimulation and activity of sympatico-parasympatetic ascendancy. In 7 days of the week, it is stress activated Monday syndrome obviously initiated by sympathetic activity, and weekends of stress nivelation by natural antioxydative substances like prostacyclin and adenosine (endothelial derived preservation parahormones). Seasonal pattern is preponderant to winter months because of usual low temperatures in the northern hemisphere, and also of the Moon and Sun influence during the year.

Age

There are two ages of clusterring registered for SCD: between birth and 6 months of age (the sudden infant death syndrome) due to concealed congenital heart disease like Uhl's anomaly, and between 45 and 75 years of age, due to CAD and ARVD. The incidence of SCD is 100-fold less in adolescents and adults below 30 years of age, than in adults above 35 [5]

Etiology: Genetics, Mutations, Desmosomal Cytosolic Changes

ARVD/C is a genetically inherited condition with autosomal-dominant pattern of inheritance (as most common), as consequence of single gene mutations witch lead to complex patterns of altered localization of desmosomal proteins.The linkage analysis in the ARVD affected families focused on chromosome 14 and located the ARVD gene in the proximity of D14S42 locus 14q23-q24 [6]. That region includes genes for beta-spectrin and for alpha-actinin.The existing hypothesis confirmed the possibility of mutation in that region to be involved in pathogenesis of ARVD, by assumption that functionally related genes are often located on the same chromosome.

The degeneration of skeletal muscle seen in Duchenne/Becker muscular dystrophy, similar to process in cardiomyocytes in ARVD, and structural similarities between alpha-actinin and N-terminal domain of dystrophin, postulated another possibility, the involvement of alpha–actinin gene mutation in ARVD patients [6,8]. However, published research data found alpha -actinin molecule in different isoforms, which led to conclusion that the mutation on the specific gene does not cause functional alteration in all isoforms.

Recently, more attention was paid to the well known clinical fact of right ventricular early involvement in Becker's dystrophy. Precisely, the right ventricle undergoes maximal streching of myocardial tissue during cardiac cycle and published data confirmed that dystrophin complex was related to stretch/modulated calcium channel in sarcolaema [6,8]. A possible explanation implied is intense stretching of myocardial fibers affecting stretch/modulated calcium channels in membrane and affecting dystrophin complex intracellulary. By analogy with right ventricular involvement in Becker's dystrophy, ARVD was found to be with similar scenario of having a product of ARVD gene as a component of dystrophin complex.

Synchronous propagation of electrical current in cardiomyocytes is highly dependent on number and spatial distribution of gap junction channels, the only place in membrane where transfer of depolarizing current can occur. These membrane areas with maximal possible amount of proteins in lipid bilayer are thus rigid and susceptible to fragmentation in response to shear stress of contracting ventricular myocardium.Concerning physiology, it is of utmost importance to secure areas of gap junctions by developing cell to cell adhesion junctions that stabilize sarcolemma. Gap junctions are dependent on structure and function of adhesion junctions specially in the cardiomyocytes.

It was postulated that the extent of electrical coupling at gap junctions is determined by the extent of mechanical coupling i.e.cell to cell adhesion junctions in cardiac myocytes [7].

Both mechanical junctions responsible for intercellular adhesion of cardiomyocytes (fascia adherens junctions and desmosomes) consist of three components: adhesion molecules, linker proteins and citoscletal proteins.

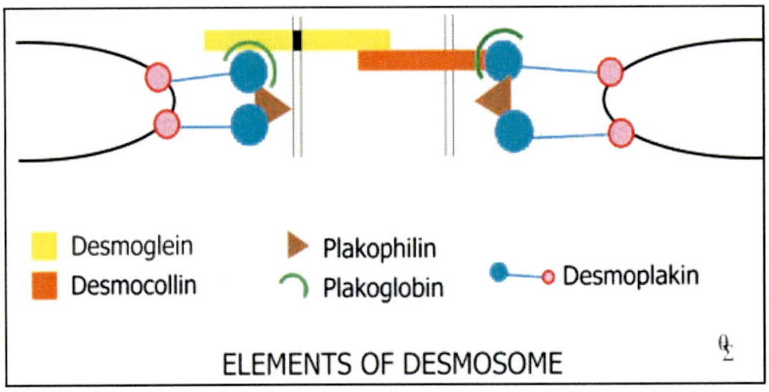

Figure 1. Schematic view of desmosome components.

A genetic defect in expression of one of these components cause an abnormal linkage between mechanical junctions and cytoskeleton progressively remodeling the myocite gap junctions at intercalated discs , thus compromising normal conduction and creating a highly arrhythmogenic substrate. Good example is Naxos disease [9] where mutation of the gene responsible for encoding plakoglobin, intercellular linkage protein and component of desmosome, leads to remodeling of cardiomyocite gap junctions and disruption of membrane leads to mechanical and electrical mismatch in like manner leading to arrhytmogenesis and enhancing the risk for SCD.

There are two distinctive disease mechanisms in the cell-cell junction cardiomyopathies that could be descriebed with certainity: first, mechanical, that explains discontinuities between cytoskeleton because of the abnormal adhesion of desmosomal proteins; and second nuclear signaling hypothesis that finds deficit of γ-catenin (plakoglobin) and β-catenin that contribute to disease pathogenesis. The above mentioned mutations may change cytosolic pools of cell-cell junction proteins which may lead to desmosome disorganization and gap junction distortion [Fig 1]. The latter may be the explanation for loss of contact between cardiomyocytes and earlier start of apoptosis. If the desmosomes are disorganized, the gap junctions should be distorted. Gap junctions play a key role in electrical coupling of cardiomyopathies which may explain slow conduction. Specific patterns of altered localization of cell-cell junction proteins correlate with disease phenotypes and 21 clinical forms of ARVD/C [7].

Apoptosis in the Heart

Morphogenesis and remodeling during heart development involve coordinated regulation of cell proliferation and apoptosis. Apoptosis, or programmed cell death, undergoes a characteristic cascade of biochemical events in which specific membrane phospholipids are exposed to cleavage of specific caspase enzymes. In the heart, clear evidence points toward focal apoptosis as a contributor to development of the embryonic outflow tract, cardiac valves, conducting system, and the developing coronary vasculature [10]. Much has been discovered about the molecular control of apoptosis since its initial description as a series of morphological events, that play a critical role in heart formation, such as formation of septa between cardiac chambers and valves [11].

The adult cardiomyocite has limited (if any) ability to proliferate. Correspondingly, apoptosis is observed infrequently in adult hearts. The finding that cardiomyocyte apoptosis occurs in the end stage human heart indicates that mechanical stretch with volume overload and raised ventricular end diastolic pressure as well as catecholamine stimulation are trigger factors in those patients. On the other hand, high levels of apoptosis have been observed in arrhythmogenic right ventricular dysplasia, a condition characterized by myocardial replacement with fibro fatty material [12].

The recent results publicated by Dr Jeff Safitz clearly demonstrate that pts with ARVD are 10fold more susceptible to mechanical stretch and electrical force then normal cardiomyocytes, explaining why those pts are at risk for early and massive apoptosis.

Pathoanatomical and Pathophisiological Basis of the Disease

During embriological development human heart follows ontogenetical transformations and repeating the pattern of the Universe it finally becomes double helix [13,22]. According to Torrent-Guasp's model human heart is a double helicoid structure organized by singular muscular band [13,14,15], (Figure 2).

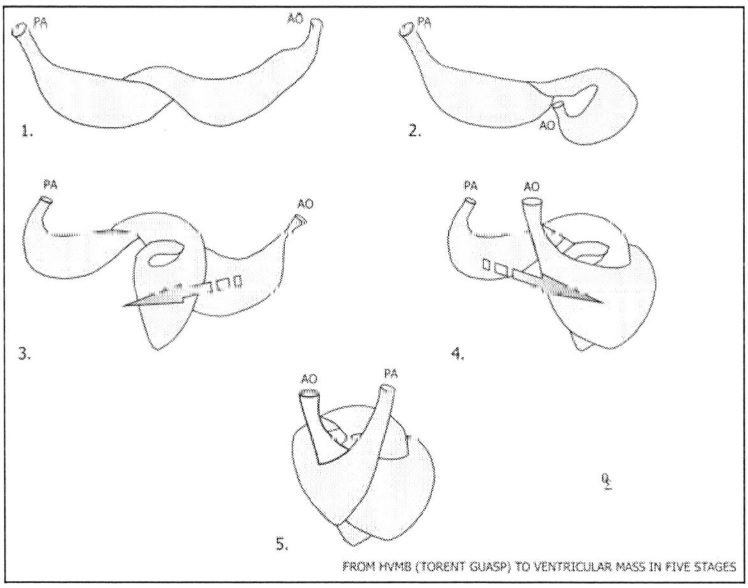

Figure 2. Simplified explaination of heart's development morphological changes.

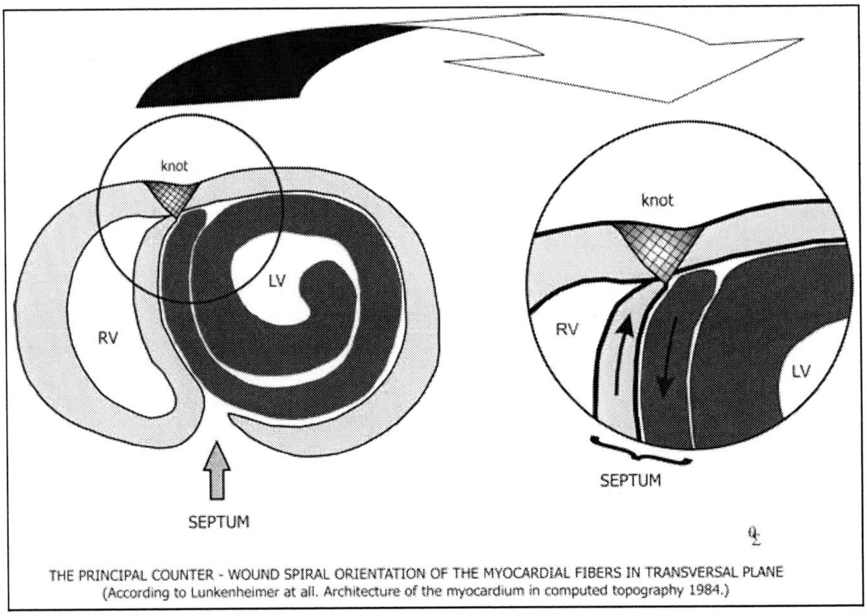

Figure 3. Arrows represent different vectors of force of contraction through LV systole "*vide intra*".

Specific place in the human ventricular muscular band (HVMB) is the knot formed by twisting along the instrinsic axis and folding for up to 180 degreees [17,18]. That central twist of HVMB, or knot, defines two loops: basal, from pulmonary artery root to the central fold and apical loop, from central fold to the aortic root [13,14,16,17], (Figure 2,3).

The parts of basal loop are free right ventricular wall and free left ventricular wall divided by posterior linear border of right ventricular cavity (sulcus inerventricularis posterior). The fibers forming apical loop after the knot make descendent part and with 90 degrees turn and propagate upwards, as ascending part to the root of the aorta (Figure 2).

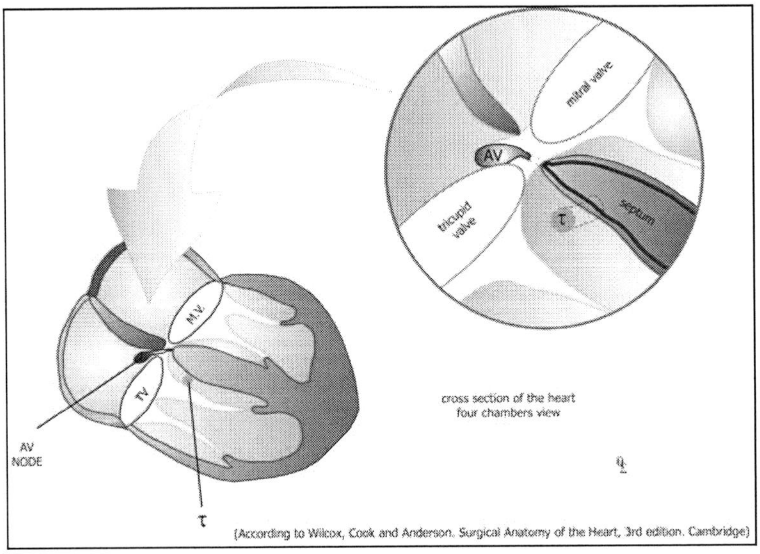

Figure 4. Location of the "τ" point-part a.

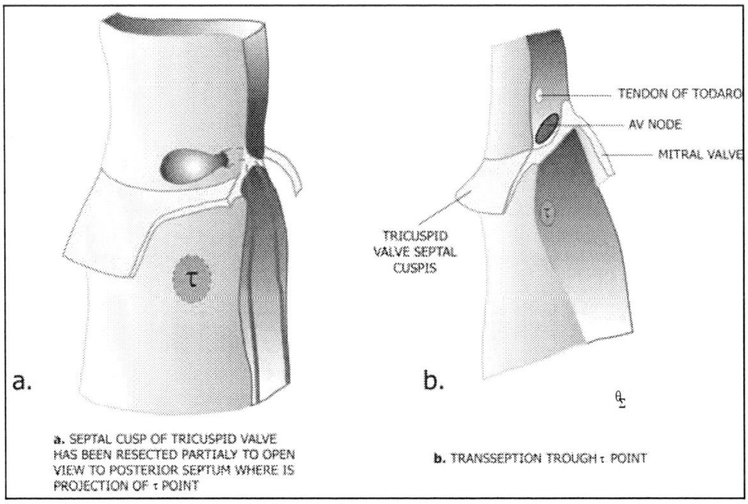

Figure 5. Location of the "τ" point-part b.

During the cardiac cycle the wave of excitation goes along ventricular muscular band and contraction follows the same route [15,18,19]. The cardiac cycle thus, is the consequence of spatial orientation of VMB and net effect of forces developed inside them [18,19]. The heart movements during the normal cardiac cycle, it is our impression, resemble the rhythm of Cuban salsa: ejection, twist-untwist, suction.

One of the first signs in the early stage of ARVD is the abnormal movement of basal part of the interventricular septum, seen by TDI on 2D echo, already described and named "V sign" by Dr Ivana Vranic a few years ago, now transparent to understanding with pathoanatomical interplay of HVMB and early apoptotic process due to mechanical streching in the specific point of septum interventricularis named "τ" point [30,31,32], (Figures 4,5).

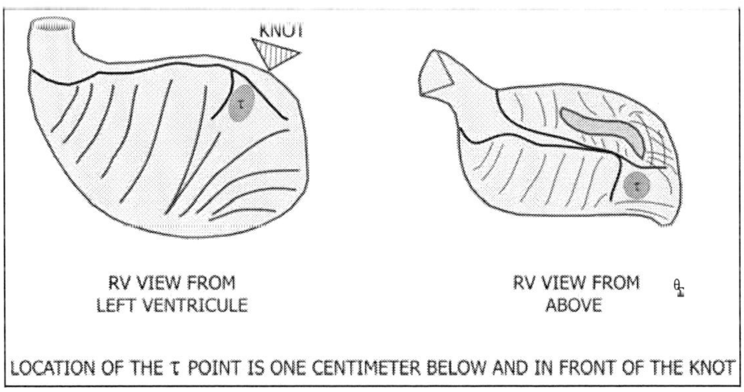

Figure 6. The relationship between "τ" and knot of MVB.

Tau point and knot of MVB are very close to each other and connecting fibers exist from knot to right ventricular band-septal portion as well as to the LV first loop and LV second loop (Fig 6).

Thus the structure of septum is of a special interest concerning impact of statical forces implyed in ARVD. According to Torrent-Guasp model of the heart, both ventricles participate in formation of septum. Right ventricle with anterior and posterior reccurent fibres, a tiny superficial fibers that have vertical direction. Deeper, there is a layer of ascendent segment fibers, that after sinking into the anterior interventicular sulcus, run obliquely and upwads in the destianation of aortic root. Third fiber direction in septum belongs to the descending segment whose orientation is different and at 90 degrees crosses the former layer. This is also clearly visible on the histological preparations of septum (Figure 3,7).

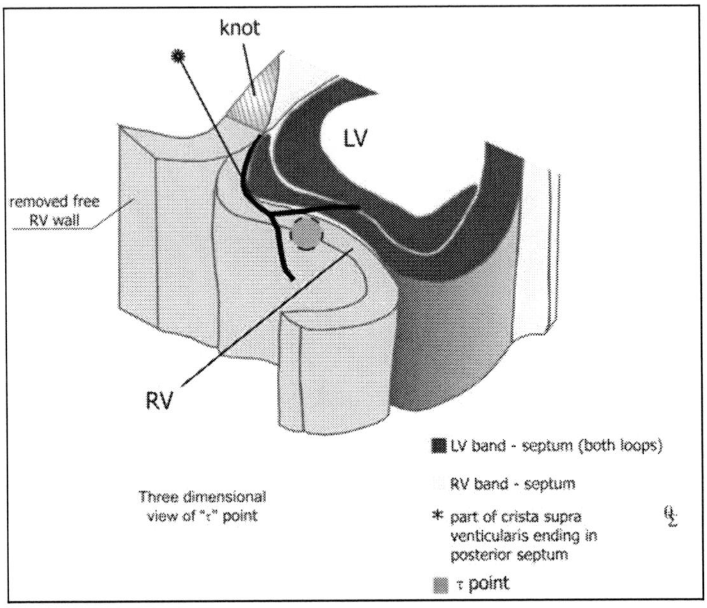

Figure 7. Transsection of IVS at the level of knot.

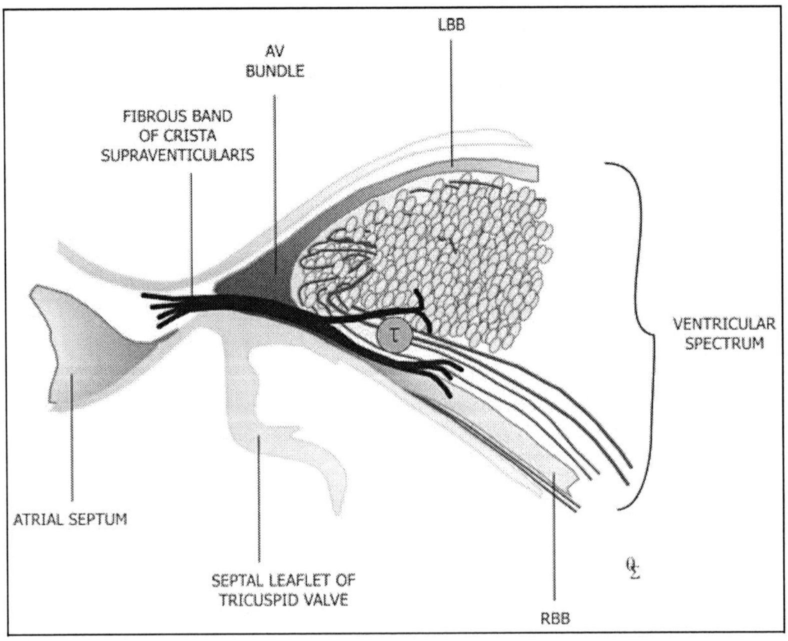

Figure 8. Schematic hystological architecture of interventricular septum with regard to fibrous anchoring of CSV and Tau point.

Note the existence of two patterns of myofibrillar space orientation in ventricular septum: a longitudinal, belonging to the right ventricular band and transversal, belonging to the left ventricular band (Figure 8), [21].

Crista supraventicularis finishes by deep anchoring in posterior septum approximatelly 1 cm bellow the knot divided in two parts: one part ending in the internal loop of LV and the other one in the septal part of exterior LV loop and right ventricle (Figures 7,8).

Tau point is located directly between these two parts exposed to three different tracton forces which stretch along projections in three ortogonal system (Figure 9).

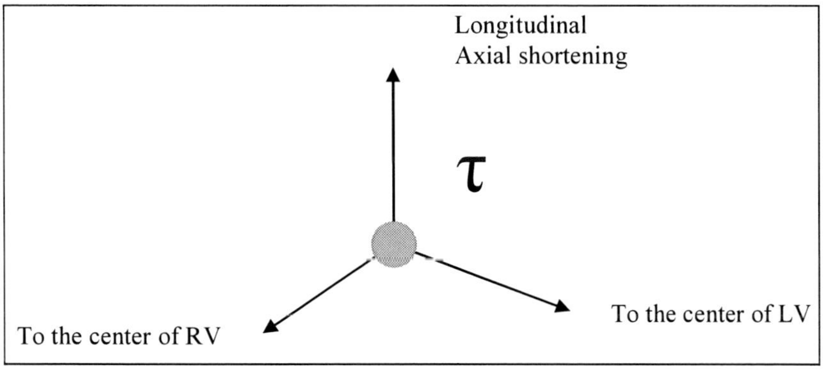

Figure 9. Schematic representation of different traction forces at the "τ" point.

The first force is centripetal, e.i to the centre of LV and is a consequence of the first loop contraction. The second force is a consequence of propagation of electromechanical wave along the muscular band making the two layers of septum to move in opposite directions from the "τ" point. The third force is active in saggital plane, and is a consequence of the ejection phase due to the action of longitudinal forces along the heart axis (Fig.9).

Myocardium at that point undergoes maximum shear stress during the cardiac cycle and in special pathological conditions is first to degenerate.

There is no other point along the myocardial band that undergoes traction of more physical forces, so it represents "locus resistentiae minoris" for adiposis prone patients. At that particular point of the heart, "τ" point, begins the loss of heart "SALSA" rhythm and deterioration seen as sudden jerky movements. At that point, also, begins the fomation of an obstacle to normal electrical conduction and cause for instability and fatal arrhythmias.

Definition

Right ventricular dysplasia/cardiomyopathy is genetically transmitted condition characterized by structural and functional abnormalities that involve mostly the right ventricle and sometimes the left ventricle as well. It is caused by the replacement of myocardial tissue by fat and fibrous tissue. The most striking morphological feature of the disease is massive diffuse or segmental loss of myocardium and replacement with fat and fibrous tissue in the mediomural and epicardial layers of the right ventricular free wall [25].

Clinical forms and genetics. Classification of Right Ventricular Cardiomyopathies

Dr Guy Fontaine [25] has proposed new classification of ARVC during the last SCD Internet symposium held in 2007, wich encompassed folowing similar conditions:

ARVD

Phenotype: This disease is, as it is with most of the other forms of ARVC, an inherited condition transmitted in a dominant form with variable expressions and penetrance in family members (20 to 50%). It is generally discovered during adolescence by signs of ventricular arrhythmias originating in the right ventricle. Sudden death can be the first presenting symptom especially during endurance and competitive sports. It is generally a progressive condition, but the disease may remain stable for decades.

Histology: The epicardial and frequently mediomural layers of RV myocardium are occupied by fat and fibrosis. Some aspects suggest that the pathologic process starts in the mediomural layers mostly extending toward the epicardium, which can be totally made of fat and fibrosis, wrongly suggesting that the disease progresses from epicardium to endocardium. Fibrosis generally borders or embeds surviving fibers. Full thickness of the RV myocardium is necessary to depict the typical topographic features of the lesions. Therefore, histology is the gold standard to ascertain the diagnosis. The frust forms and forms observed at the beginning of the disease, especially those observed in family members, can be difficult to diagnose. Involvement of the left ventricle is frequently observed mostly at the apex, which looks covered by fat. However, some focal zones of fibrosis and fatty tissue can be found all over the full thickness of LV myocardium. This may explain the decrease in the LV function found even in the moderate forms of the disease.

Genotype: Genes identified are coding for Desmoplakin and recently Plakophilin 2 and Desmoglein 2. These genes are parts of the desmosomal structure and fascia adherens, which plays a major role in longitudinal cell-cell adhesion. However, Transforming Growth Factor (TGF Beta3) is a new gene related to the phenotypic presentation of one of these cardiomyopathies. Plakophillin 2 appears currently as the most frequently observed gene (11 to 43% of the series).

Biventricular Dysplasia

Phenotype: Because of the loss of myocardial tissue of the left ventricle, this form frequently leads to congestive heart failure.

Histology: In this form, the same evidence of fatty tissue and fibrosis is observed in both ventricles. However, the disease seems to progress from epicardium to endocardium as opposed to classical ARVD, where fibrosis and fat seems to start in the mediomural layers.

RVD Without Arrhythmia (Quiescent)

Phenotype: There are no obvious arrhythmias as opposed to the previous form. This might be related to the fact that the arrhythmogenic substrate is totally silent or that minor arrhythmias are present, but not severe enough to lead to hospitalization.

Histology: In this form, observed in 3.7% of the general population, the typical histologic pattern of ARVD is observed in the RV free wall. However, the arrhythmogenic substrate is dormant. It is postulated that the occurrence of arrhythmias that may lead to sudden death is either due to the development of critical electrophysiologic parameters leading to sustained re-entry or the result of neutrophiles activation or both.

RVD with Congestive Heart Failure

Phenotype: This can be the result of two different mechanisms. The first is due to major progression of the dysplastic phenomenon, producing more and more myocardium by fat and fibrosis in the right ventricle, and leading to subsequent involvement of the left ventricle by the same disease process. The second is due to a superimposed myocarditis (see below). Because of absence or minor arrhythmias, these cases can mimic Idiopathic dilated cardiomyopathy.

ARVD + Superimposed Myocarditis

Clinical as well as histologic data, may exhibit various forms of myocarditis superimposed on ARVD suggesting a particular susceptibility of dysplastic myocardium to inflammatory phenomena in particular viruses (this concept can be extended to other forms of cardiomyopathies). The presence of coxsackies as well as adenoviruses has been observed in the myocardium of ARVD patients. In most cases myocarditis involves both the right and left ventricle. Both the severity of left ventricular involvement and speed of myocarditis progression, determines the prognosis. Clinical patterns are quite variable.

A. Quiescent

Phenotype: Asymptomatic.

Histology: presence of lymphocytes is common (0.1-5.5%) in the general population. In our opinion it seems nevertheless more frequent in ARVD patients.

B. Hyper Acute

Phenotype: Fever, asthenia, dyspnea, hypotension, fulminant heart failure and death within a few days.

Histology: Diffuse round cells infiltration, polymorphonuclear, eosinophils.

C. Acute

Phenotype: Fever, Chest pain, AV conduction disorder. May last from a few days up to several weeks and is associated with the release of cardiac enzymes (troponine).

Histology: Round cells (lymphocytes). Value of endocardial biopsies that may lead to therapeutic implications (Beta-interferon).

D. Chronic

Phenotype: Moderate clinical signs of heart failure, asthenia, dyspnea, etc.

Histology: Healed myocarditis leaves patchy areas of "replacement" fibrosis. Lymphocytes have disappeared or remain in small quantities.

E. Chronic-active

Phenotype: Moderate clinical signs of heart failure, asthenia, dyspnea, increasing with time, palpitations, syncope, etc.

Histology: Myocarditis, which is frequently multifocal, progresses replacing more and more myocardium by fibrosis and patchy zones of adipocytes. Lymphocytes are present. These multiple forms explain the polymorphism of clinical presentations. We think that superimposed myocarditis is a major cause of the trigger of arrhythmias and sudden death.Therefore the pathology of the hearts of patients who died suddenly have shown more frequently than in the common forms of RVD the evidence of signs of inflammation. Gene mutations explaining viral susceptibility is an open question.

Naxos Disease

This is a very rare disease discovered in the island of Naxos (Greece) in 24 patients from 6 families. The form of transmission is recessive; some other isolated cases have been discovered in the world.

Phenotype: The phenotype is identical to classical ARVD associated with Woolly hair and Keratoderma.

Histology: Typical ARVD association. The association of signs of myocarditis and arrhythmias is frequent, as is sudden death.

Genotype: Plakoglobin truncation is the monogenic factor producing the disease. All patients are homozygous. The asymptomatic heterozygous patients may have Right Ventricular Outflow Tract ventricular tachycardia.

Israelian Desmoplakin Recessive Dysplasia

Phenotype: There is a syndrome found in the non-Jewish population of Israel associated with woolly hair, keratoderma and RVD similar to Naxos disease.

Genotype: Desmoplakin truncation is the monogenic factor producing the disease.

Venetian Desmoplakin Dominant Dysplasia

(Transmission is autosomal dominant)

Phenotype: Seems similar to ARVD.

Histology: Similar to ARVD.

Genotype: Desmoplakine located in series between plakoglobin and desmin, supporting the complex actin-myosin, is responsible for the disease.

Uhl's Anomaly
(A rare anomaly)

Phenotype: Two forms. *Pediatric form*: Newborns (differential diagnosis with Ebstein disease) with congestive heart failure. *Adult form*: Arrhythmias, congestive heart failure or both. This form is frequently confused with ARVD.

Histology: The pathologic examination is pathognomonic and unmistakable. There is total absence of myocardium on the RV free wall consisting only of epicardium and endocardium separated by a thin layer of adipocytes occupied by coronary vessels, which could exhibit abnormal proliferation of the media. Thus, the wall is, properly speaking, transparent.

ARVD Mimicking Uhl's Anomaly

Phenotype: One case with huge RV (Dr G Fontaine). Extremely thin RV free wall mimicking Uhl's anomaly (all imaging techniques).

Histology: After heart transplant for terminal heart failure, a thin layer of myocardium was present. The wall was translucent but not transparent. This is therefore different from typical Uhl's anomaly

Biventricular Spongy Dysplasia

Phenotype: Slowly progressing congestive heart failure. One case from Portugal (Dr G Fontaine). No other case in the literature.

Histology: Total disappearance of myocardium in RV with thick endocardium and epicardium. LV dissociated by interstitial fat with minor fibrosis, suggesting apoptosis.

Catecholaminergic VTs

Phenotype: Episodes of Polymorphic VTs triggered by effort or psychological stress. High risk of sudden death.

Histology: Two presentations: *With structural heart disease:* Histology similar to classical ARVD. *Without structural heart disease.*

Genotype: Mutation of the gene coding for RyR2 Ryanodine receptor on Sarcoplasmic reticulum playing a role in the regulation of intracellular calcium. The overload of calcium can explain the particular morphology of ventricular arrhythmias. This is different from ARVD arrhythmias, which are mostly the result of slow intramyocardial conduction and reentry.

Brugada Syndrome (BS)
(Some patients only)

Phenotype: Nocturnal sudden death, dizziness, "vasovagal syncope". In some cases this syndrome shows an overlapping pattern with ARVD. Nevertheless, effectiveness of Isoprenaline in the BS is in sharp contrast with ARVD, where it is used to induce ventricular arrhythmias. Therefore, it seems appropriate to include in the database only those BS ECG patients who meet the new ARVD criteria.

Histology: Pathology of some cases of BS who died suddenly showed, in 38% of them, structural heart disease, some with signs of inflammation/fibrosis andothers with a typical histologic pattern of ARVD.

Genotype: Multiple mutations in SCN5A that now appears as a cofactor rather than the unique cause of the disease.

Right Ventricular Outflow Tract (RVOT)

(About 50% of patients)

Phenotype: Extrasystoles, runs of repetitive short runs of ventricular tachycardia. Imaging techniques have identified a structural heart disease.

Histology: A typical pattern of dysplasia localized to the infundibular area has been reported (including small vessels disease).

Septal Ventricular Outflow Tract (SVOT)

Ventricular extrasystoles progressing to VT have been observed in intraseptal exploration by using a special needle probe inserted inside the RV septum during surgery and showing highly fragmented potentials.

Left Ventricular Outflow Tract (LVOT)

Extrasystoles and VTs have been recently identified. Structural heart disease has not been reported yet.

Fat Dissociation Syndrome (FDS)

Phenotype: No symptoms, presence of hypersignal of fat at MRI examination (false positive diagnosis for ARVD). The risk of sudden death is very low.

Histology: Presence of fatty tissue in the right ventricular myocardium has been known by pathologists for a long time. However, its quantitative assessment is recent. In addition, fat in the RV appears to be specific to the human species. This is observed in up to 60% of the general population. It has not been observed in the RV of eight non-Bonobo monkeys. Therefore, FDS seems to be the result of a mutation that has occurred specifically in the human species. Basically, there is no fibrosis in FDS, which seems less dangerous than ARVD.

Clinical Picture

ARVD manifests as a wide spectrum of clinical presentations [23], including mechanical myocardial dysfunction and various arrhythmias, generally of right ventricular origin, such as isolated extrasystoles, nonsustained or sustained ventricular tachycardia (VT), and ventricular fibrillation responsible for SD. Atrial arrhythmias are sometimes present because of dilated right atrium.

Diagnosis

Diagnosis of ARVD is based on the presence of major and minor criteria encompassing structural, electrocardiographic, arrhythmic, and genetic factors [26]. Among these criteria inverted T waves beyond V1 are a sign of diagnostic value that should attract attention, particularly in young patient with a normal heart at physical examination. However, these criteria are about to be reconsidered on more objective grounds.

The recognition of mild, fruste, or localized forms of the disease remains a clinical challenge. It is difficult to diagnose ARVD in patients with minimal right ventricular abnormalities by echocardiographic or contrast angiographic examination. Magnetic resonance imaging is a promising technique in showing right ventricular anatomy and function as well as in characterizing the composition of the right ventricular wall, especially with regard to the presence of adipose tissue.

Pitfalls in Diagnosing ARVD

Arrhythmogenic right ventricular dysplasia is a genetic disorder followed by peculiar RV involvement and its structural and functional abnormalities (due to the replacement of myocardium by fatty and fibrous tissues) and electrical instability that precipitates ventricular arrhythmias and sudden death [25,26]. However, all non-invasive and invasive methods of evaluating RV structure and function have inherent limitations, which are due to the complex anatomy of RV. Evaluation of the RV can present awesome experience since of its very complicated geometry and fact of being separated into three parts: inflow, outflow and belonging body which is crescentic and truncated. Not to mention the right ventricular free wall which also has a variable trabecular pattern that in combination with its retrosternal position limits precise measurement of cavity size and wall thickness. Nevertheless, tricuspid anterior plane systolic excursion (TAPSE) has been shown to correlate with its overall function (in adults), particularly in systole, as assessed by ejection fraction, which can be objectively estimated by radionuclide ventriculography (done in a standard way). The recognition of mild, *fruste*, or localized forms of the disease remains a clinical challenge. It is difficult to diagnose ARVD in patients with minimal right ventricular abnormalities by echo or contrast angiography examination. So far only V sign has been attributed as pathognomonic in ARVD but no other signs have been reported yet. Standardized diagnostic criteria have been proposed by the ISFC, however this condition may be overlooked by the insufficiency of its signs at the early stage of disease.

Relevance of right Ventricular Function

The right ventricle is a structurally and functionally complex chamber whose importance has been neglected previously. However, it maintains haemodynamic stability by propelling systemic venous blood returning from the right atrium through the pulmonary vascular bed.

Therefore, right ventricular dysfunction is relevant in a variety of conditions such as: chronic lung disease, primary pulmonary vascular disease, pulmonary thrombo-embolic disease, myocardial infarction, congenital heart disease and cardiopulmonary transplantation. Right ventricular diastolic function is first to be affected in those conditions with relative preservation of systolic function. Nevertheless, in ARVD patients diastolic function may be pseudonormalized (due to the phenomenon of ventricular interdependence) in the clinically silent form of the disease and having only slightly impaired systolic function of a right ventricle.

Echocardiography in Diagnosing ARVD

In the former sugessted protocol for ARVC search by echo, it was highlighted that thorough and systematic examination of both ventricles should be performed and particularly because of the fact that the disease process can be localised also in the left ventricle. The procedure must be reproducible and relevant in the context of a clinical setting. Therefore, the suggested protocol concentrated on the sites of disease predilection, namely the RV apex, inflow and outflow tracts- the so-called "triangle of dysplasia". The degree of RV dilatation can be described in relation to the left ventricle (LV) with RV enlargement described as follows: *mild*: RV enlarged but a 2D area less than LV area; *moderate*: RV area equals LV area; *severe*: RV larger than LV area [27].

Dimensions of right Ventricle Region of Interest

Foale et al studied normal adult right ventricles to determine the reproducibility of various tomographic planes and to obtain measurements of normal cavity sizes. From this study the most easily obtained and reproducible measurements were ascertained and are suggested as part of the standard examination. Because the inflow tract (RVIT), ventricular body, and outflow tract (RVOT) are three distinct regions of the right ventricle that are orientated in different axis, two measurements of each region should be obtained from separate views: RVIT1 and RVIT3, RVOT1 and RVOT3, and RVSAX (short-axis) and RVLAX (long-axis)

Typically the echocardiogram is performed with the subject in the left lateral decubitus position. At least three sinus beats of each view should be recorded during quiet respiration or at end expiration. If the patient is in atrial fibrillation at least 5 beats should be recorded.

For each view, the gain and compression should be optimized so that the best echocardiographic image of the endocardial borders is obtained. The selection of harmonics or fundamental frequency should depend upon which yields the best definition of structures. The depth should be selected that allows visualization of all of the structures of interest. All images should have an ECG tracing and clear calibration markings. If visualization of the RV is inadequate, an intravenous contras agent can be administered to obtain better RV border delineation.

The RV shape is complex and its inflow, body and outflow portions cannot all be visualized from one view. Thus imaging of the chamber is necessary from several views. The echocardiographic examination should be performed according to a standard procedure (Table I):

Table I. Echocardiographic Examination: Methods

1)	Parasternal long axis
2)	Parasternal long axis to visualize the tricuspid valve (RV inflow view)
3)	Parasternal short axis (multiple levels including the base of heart to visualize RVOT)
4)	Apical four-chamber
5)	Apical two-chamber (separately of left ventricle and right ventricle)
6)	Subcostal long axis
7)	Subcostal short axis of RV inflow and outflow

1) The first echocardiographic window that should be obtained is the **parasternal long axis**. This imaging plane is recorded with the transducer in the third or fourth intercostals space immediate to the left of the sternum. The transducer should be angled so that aortic valve, mitral valve and left ventricle are in their long axis. This view should be performed at a depth that allows visualization of all structures and then at a lower depth focusing on the RV. Structures of interest in this view include:

    - Left ventricle – dimensions and wall motion
    - Left atrium – size
    - Mitral valve – structure and function
    - Aortic valve – structure and function
    - Right ventricle – dimension, morphology and wall motion

    In this view, M-mode of the LV should be obtained at the highest sweep speed. The line of interrogation should be at the leaflet tip and perpendicular to the long axis of the LV. Color Doppler of the MV and AV should be obtained.
2) The second view is the parasternal long axis of the RV which allows visualization of the tricuspid valve (**RV inflow view**). This is obtained by angling the transducer to the right from the parasternal long axis of the LV and rotating the transducer slightly. *The inferoposterior wall of the right ventricular inflow tract under the tricuspid valve is the most important region to be visualized*, because it is a frequently affected region. To evaluate this region the transducer should be angled toward the inferior vena cava or the liver. In ARVD this region may appear as thinned and have diastolic bulging or wall motion abnormalities (hypokinesis, akinesis or dyskinesis). In ARVD subjects the inferoposterior wall motion is generally reduced as compared to healthy subjects. In severe ARVD the only motion in this region is that of the leaflet plane. Color Doppler of the TR jet should also be attempted.
3) The **parasternal short axis** at the aortic valve level is obtained by angling the probe 90° with respect to the parasternal long axis of the LV. This view provides information about the outflow portion of the right ventricle. In many subjects the ratio between the right ventricular outflow tract and the aorta (in systole) will be enlarged. The outflow tract is one of the places where there are saccular dilatations and wall motion abnormalities. The anterior wall, especially in its apical portion, may be commonly affected by fibro-fatty replacement. Therefore, it is important to view the anterior wall of the right ventricle from several short axis views including mid-ventricle and apex. These are obtained by angling or moving the probe more toward the apex while maintaining a tomographic cut

of the LV. These views are important for the analysis of the left ventricle and septal configuration. Color Doppler of pulmonic regurgitation and a peak velocity of the tricuspid regurgitation jet by continuous wave Doppler should be obtained from the short axis views of RV outflow and inflow respectively.

4) The **apical four-chamber** view provides considerable information including the relative sizes of the right and the left ventricle. The four-chamber view is defined as a view which maximizes the LV long axis and the tricuspid and mitral annular dimensions. In this view, the full excursion of the mitral and tricuspid valves should be seen. From this view, the morphology and the motion of the left ventricle and right ventricle are assessed. In order to permit visualization of the trabecular pattern of the RV, an image should be obtained by moving the transducer toward the midline and magnifying the RV. In the apical four chamber view, color Doppler of mitral regurgitation and tricuspid regurgitation should be recorded. Also pulse wave Doppler at the leaflet tips of the mitral and tricuspid valves should be recorded at the fastest sweep speed in order to assess diastolic function. Pulse wave Doppler or a pulmonary vein should be recorded when feasible. Lastly, the continuous wave Doppler of the tricuspid regurgitation jet should be recorded in order to calculate the peak RV systolic pressure.
5) Since the inferoposterior wall of the right ventricle is commonly involved in ARVD, it is important to visualize this region from as many views as possible the **apical RV two-chamber** view. Starting from the apical four-chamber, the transducer is positioned over the RV apex and then angled and rotated to visualize the inferoposterior wall of the RV and its apex. These walls are assessed for wall motion and the myocardial trabecular pattern.
6) The echocardiographic analysis continues with the study of the **subcostal long-axis view**. This view is obtained with the transducer moved to a subxyphoid position and directed superiorly and leftward. The view is aligned so that the orientation of the LV an RV are similar to that obtained in the apical four chamber view. From this subcostal long-axis view one can obtain information about the RV size and motion of its free wall and apex. The transducer is then angled upward to visualize the shape and motion of the RVOT and to assess for saccular dilatation and wall motion abnormalities.
7) Finally the transducer is rotated into the **subcostal short axis view**. From this projection both the inflow tract and the outflow tract of the right ventricle are assessed. Again in this view key findings of ARVD include alteration of motion such as diastolic bulging or wall motion abnormalities of the inflow tract and enlargement, and saccular dilatation of the outflow tract.

   The compilation of these views will allow for calculation of:

- Cardiac chamber dimensions (including left ventricle, left atrium, right atrium and right ventricle)
- Right ventricular areas and volumes (RV volume will be calculated by the previously validated biplane area-length method)
- Right ventricular function

  - ♦ Systolic: calculated by "descent of the base" method, endocardial area change method and volume change
  - ♦ Diastolic: E/A wave, deceleration time, dP/dt.

- Right ventricular wall thickness
- Severity of tricuspid valve regurgitation
- Estimation of the right ventricular systolic pressure
- Right ventricular regional function
- Presence and location of RV aneurysms

New Echocardiographic Perspectives in Early Diagnozing SCD Prone Patients

In previous few years Dr Ivana Vranic reported of V sign [22,29], (Pictures 1,2) as early patognomonic sign in ARVD patients. As for V sign to be searched for we use pulsed wave Doppler tissue imaging in the hope to observe an abnormal posterior septal wall motion. The pulsed wave Doppler sample volume (size 4) is usually placed on the right ventricular side at the basal interventricular septum in the apical 4-chamber view, as well as in the long axis parasternal view and in the short axis on the mitral valve level. Special attention is paid to the Doppler velocity to avoid aliasing (Nyquist limit 15cm/s) and aligning the Doppler beam to the interventricular septum to optimize measurements which we obtain during end expiration. Based on the septal wall motion velocity pattern, peak myocardial velocities are measured in pre-ejection (peak PE), in systole (peak S), in early diastole (peak E) and in late diastole (peak A). Values for all echocardiographic parameters are however, averaged over five cardiac cycles.

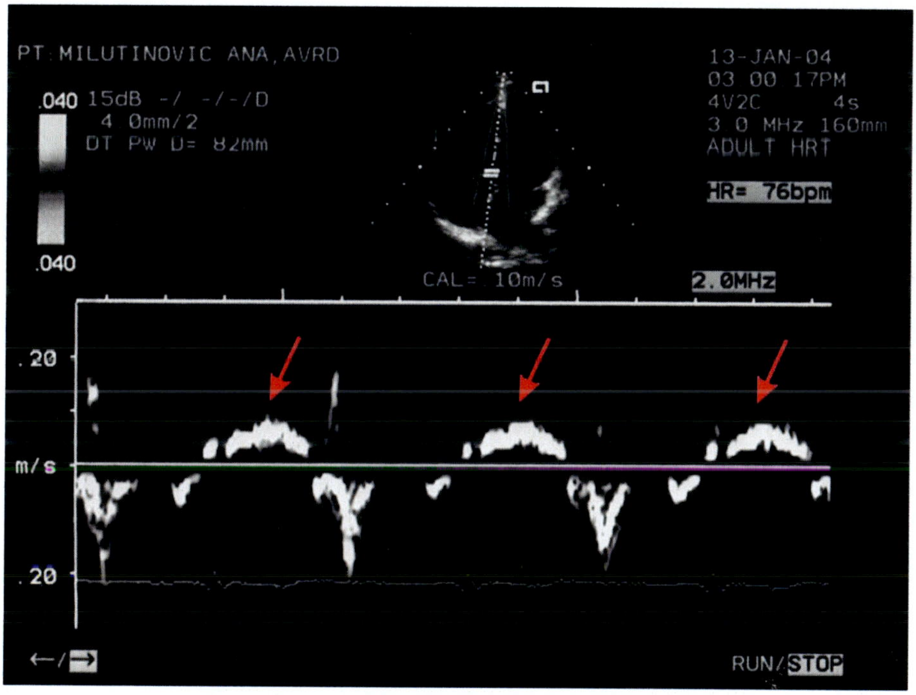

Picture 1. ARVD pt. Red arrow depicits V sign postsystolic shortening.

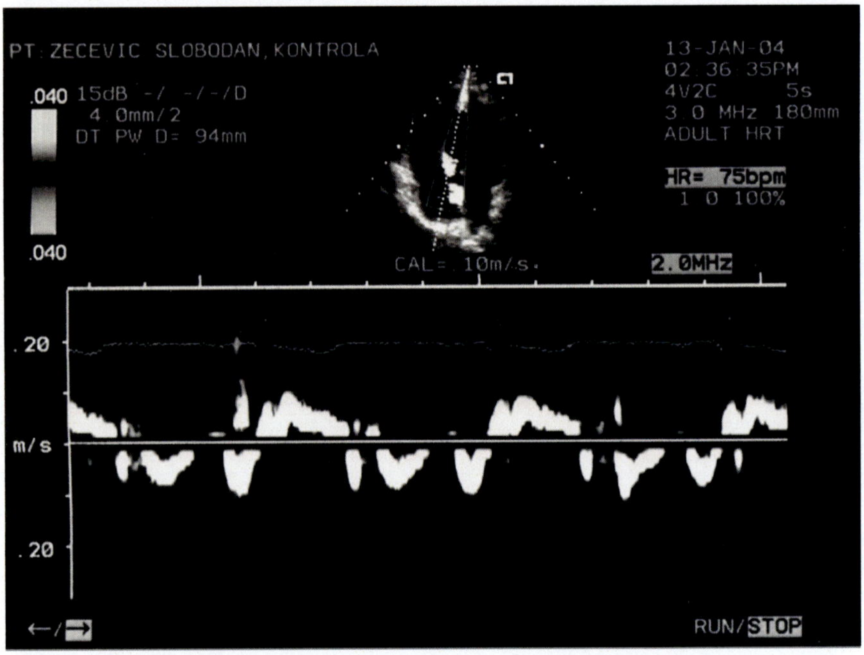

Picture 2. Normal individual. Postsystolic lenthening- no V sign.

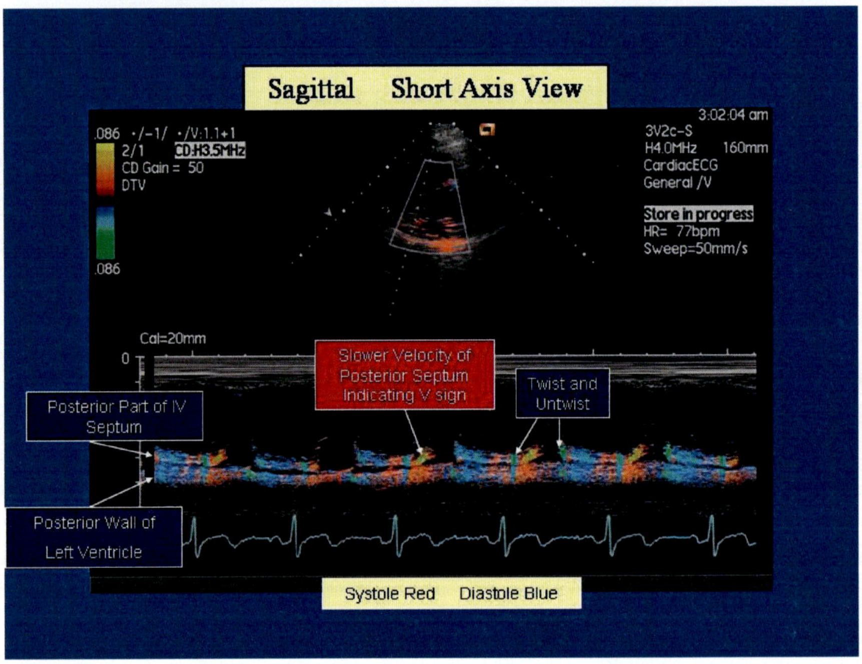

Picture 3. ARVD pt. Note the existence of V sign.

It is much easier though, with color coded M mode TDI (Pictures 3,4,5,6,7,8) to objectivize the difference between normal subject and a patient with ARVD (or any other clinical form above mentioned). Tau point clearly indicates the region affected with early apoptosis due to any discovered defect in cell to cell athesion proteins that loose contact as a consequence of different forces applied to the locus minoris resistentiae in the double helicoid structure of the heart.

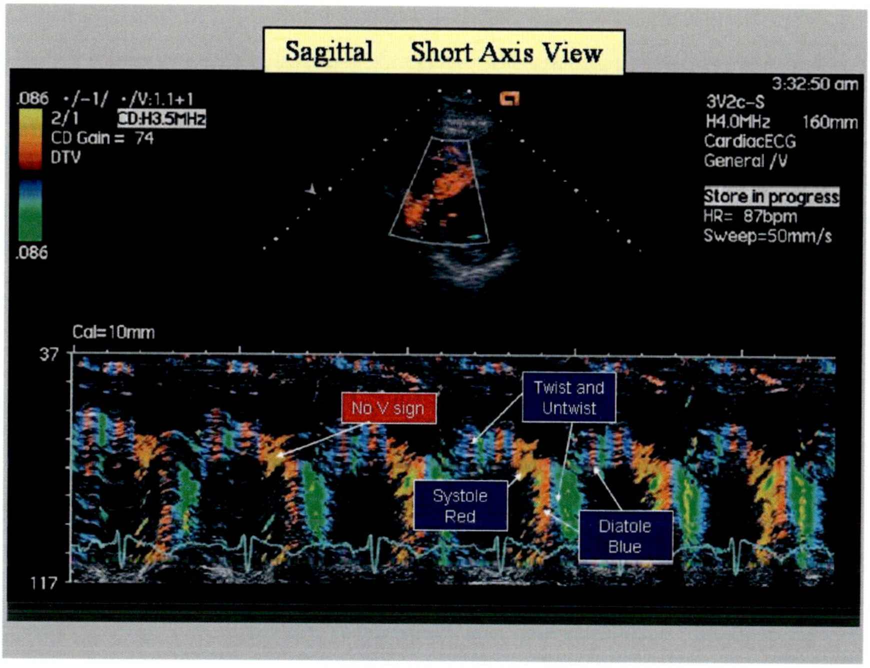

Picture 4. Normal individual-no V sign.

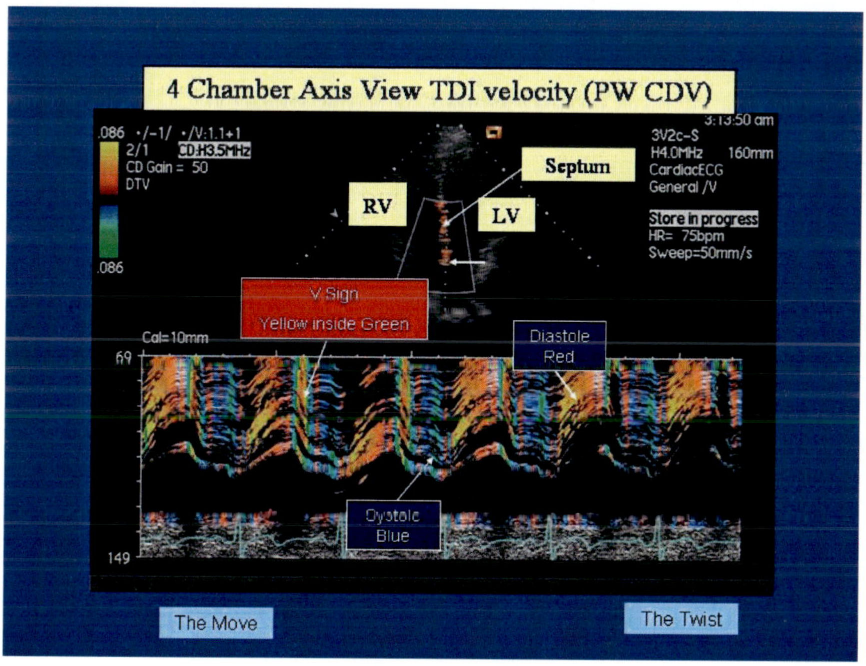

Picture 5. ARVD pt. Note the existence of V sign.

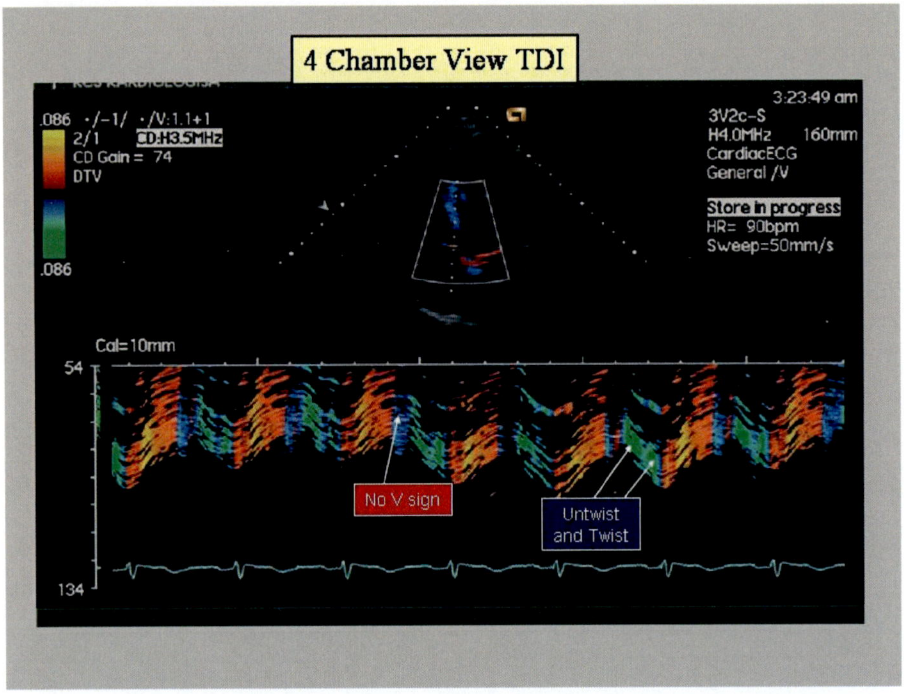

Picture 6. Normal individual-no V sign.

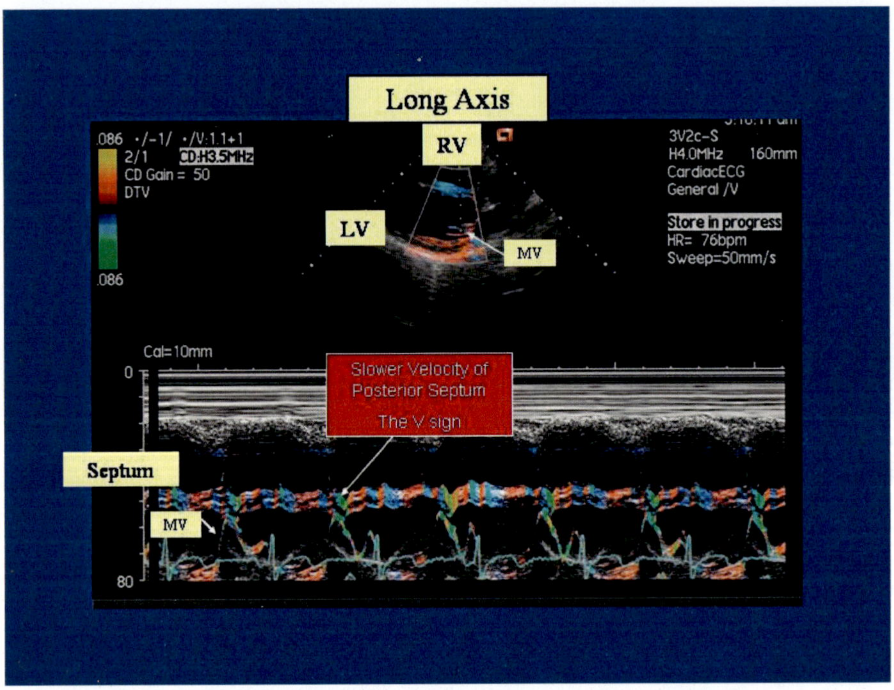

Picture 7. ARVD pt. Note the existence of V sign.

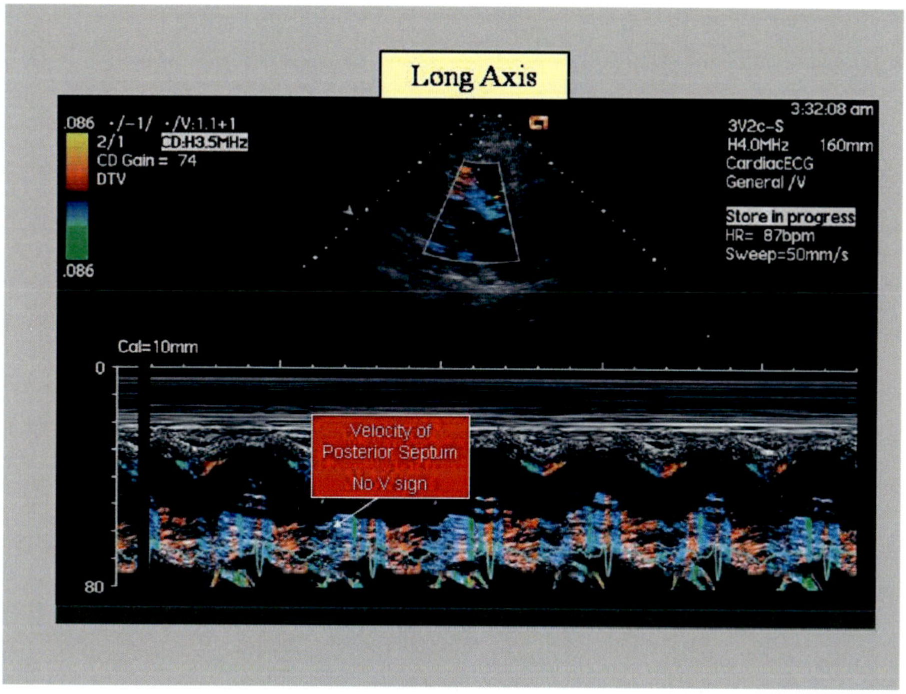

Picture 8. Normal individual-no V sign.

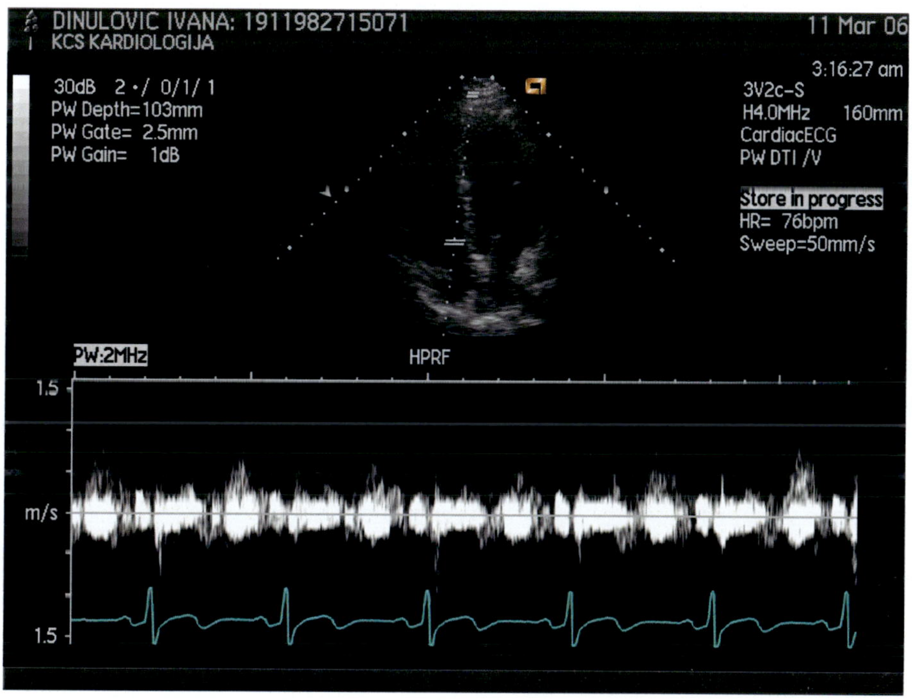

Picture 9. Characteristic appearance of E/A ratio changeable interplay.

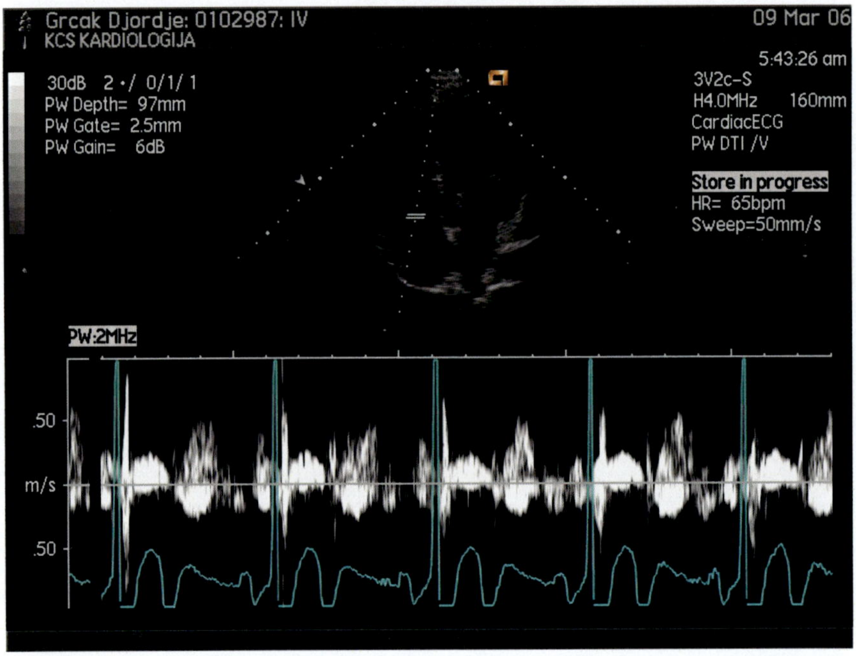

Picture 10. Normal transtricuspid flow-slight changes in E amplitude due to respiratory changes.

However, in our 10 years experience with patients with ARVD, a second sign in close relation to the existence of Tau point has been discovered and named "T sign" [30,31,32,35]. This sign is also pathognomonic of ARVD in relation to registered changes in motion of the septal cusp of tricuspid valve at the early stage of the disease. The explaination for this lies in the affected region of the Tau point where the loss of support for the posterior part of cusp exists. In search for this T sign echo examination is performed in similar fashion. 2D echo is always performed in apical four chamber view with technique of pulsed Doppler tissue imaging. The pulsed wave Doppler sample volume (size 4) is to be placed on the right ventricular side at the basal part of septal cusp and special attention paid to aligning the Doppler beam to the interventricular septum to optimize measurements which are obtained during end expiration. Consequently transtricuspid flow profile is being recorded and values of all echocardiographic parameters are averaged over five cardiac cycles to avoid respiratory changes. 2D echo examination is to be performed in each patient in apical 4-chamber view, parasternal long axis view and parasternal short axis view on the mitral valve area level.

Significant change in E/A velocity due to complex volume oscillations in right heart as a consequence of septal cusp lack of support in the posterior basal part due to existence of Tau point in pts prone to SCD. E wave velocity measures 0.5; 0.7; 0.6; 0.4; 0.5; 0.8. A wave measures 0.3; 0.2; 0.4; 0.4; 0.5; 0.1. It means the more blood is held in the right atrium the more has to be pushed out in the next consecutive beat (Picture 9).

Conversely, in normal subjects there is only respiratory pressure volume changes in emptying RV (Picture 10). It is therefore possible, if no other arrhythmia exists to spot this sophisticated interdependent relationship that is clearly visible in ARVD or any other form SCD risk patients even in the very early phase of the disease process, long before any morphological changes in the heart may occur.

ECG Newly Observed Signs

Among research attempts in discovering new diagnostic signs in ARVD patients Dr Guy Fontaine has reported of late potentials derived epsilon waves in diferent localization on ECG and named them prepsilon, topsilon, bipsilon, tripsilon, and giant epsilon during last Cardiostim conference. This idea is not easily aplicable because of technical limitations and quality of ECG machine but it is of significant importance in the clinical practice.

Vectorcardiography in Diagnosing ARVD

However, in evaluating ECG tracings vectorcardiography is more susceptible to delicate changes and is more superior than late potentials (signal averaged electrocardiograms) in detecting electricaly non conductive areas of myocardium. In that sense Dr Ivana Vranic has reported of specific early changes due to Tau point. The explaination of this lies in the electrical propagation through HVMB and vector sequence by time changeble. It is now subject of ongoing trial in checking its wide aplicability.

Discussion

The discovery of the ventricular myocardial band by Dr Francisco Torrent Guasp reconciled the form and function of ventricular myocardium, giving explaination for electrical and mechanical events in human heart. It has been clearly demonstrated by fast Fourier analyses of ventricular MUGA scans, that muscular contractile activity, during the cardiac cycle, progresses (in a peristaltoid manner), along successive VMB segments. Since the excitation necessarily precedes contraction, the most logical pattern of ventricular electrical activation should follow both spatially and temporarily, previously described sequence of its mechanical action. V sign is therefore easy to explain because crista supraventricularis is driven by three orthogonaly opposed forces as embaded in inferioposterior septal part being ephemerally behind the time in the contraction. The observation of septal posterior displacement by 2D echo may be in accordance with localized cell to cell adhesion protein distortion suspected in this condition, or localized apoptosis demonstrated in the posteroseptal part of crista supraventricularis by Dr Thomas N. James. On the basis of anatomic study of human and other mammalian hearts, it has been suggested that it is crucial to the understanding of right ventricular failure to consider the normal functions of the crista supraventricularis. As long as the crista supraventricularis remains intact, left ventricular systole can tether even the damaged right ventricular free wall sufficiently to empty the right ventricle into the pulmonary artery. An intact crista supraventricularis is also necessary for normal function of the tricuspid valve, both by its purse-string action on the tricuspid orifice and by providing essential support for the anterior leaflet of the tricuspid valve. For its optimal mechanical effectiveness in coordinating and facilitating hemodynamic efficiency of the right ventricle with that of the left ventricle (including most of the interventricular septum), the anatomic configuration of the apoptotic tissue (septal band of the crista supraventricularis) in the upper right side of the crest of the interventricular septum explains some probable contractile advantages [28]. Although the connection of the septal band with the rest of the crista supraventricularis is thin when seen in cross section, it is actually a broad sheet extending from an area posterior to the membranous interventricular septum to a region well anterior to the normal location of the Hiss bundle. Furthermore, the bottom of the septal band tissue seen in cross section has a pronglike configuration, suggesting a firm anchor deep within the mass of interventricular septal myocardium.

Conclusion

Because right ventricular function may be impaired either by primary right sided heart disease, or secondary to left sided cardiomyopathy or valvular heart disease, it is obvious that RV function should be evaluated with caution. In practice, clinicians largely rely on non-invasive imaging methods for assessment of RV function. Two dimensional echocardiography is the mainstay for analysis of RV function, but recently alternative techniques have been proposed, including tissue Doppler imaging (TDI) techniques, three dimensional echocardiography, magnetic resonance imaging (MRI), and even invasive assessment of pressure-volume loops. Also, vectorcardiography gives clear cut potential in analyzing RV function and even eary diagnosis for the risk of SCD due to inhereted disorders that affect desmosomes, such as ARVD as most common one.

Valid WHO criteria during last the 12 years failed to detect disease at its early stage and recommended diagnostic methods were shown to have low sensitivity for majority of patients even in its overt phase (because of lack of scoring system) [33,34]. Investigation of this population is further complicated by disease rarity and lack of large databases. New research published data give priority to vectorcardiography and ultrasound.

A possible explanation for this lies in the existence of specific place in the heart exposed to most physical forces during cardiac cycle. Nevertheless, this place is *locus minoris rezistenitae* during contraction and relaxation of the heart. It is presently the focus of an ongoing clinical study regarding two aforementioned methods in detecting early stage of ARVD/C. It is also registered by WIPO as SOPHIE methodology (suggesting wisdom to detect). Soon enough we can expect this technique to be incorporated in new medical equipment (for stratification of risk for SCD).

References

[1] Myerburg RJ, Castellanos A. Cardiac arest and sudden death. In: Zipes DP, Libby P, Bonow RO and Braunwald E, ed. *Braunwald's Heart Disease: A Textbook of Cardiovascular Medicine*. 7th edn. Elsevier Saunders Company, Philadelphia, PA, 2004:865-908.

[2] Priori SG, Aliot E, Blomstrom-Lundqvist C et al. Task force on sudden cardiac death of the European Society of Cardiology. *Eur Heart J* 2001; 22: 1374-1450.

[3] Escobedo LG, Zack MM. Comparison of sudden and nonsudden coronary deaths in the United States. *Circulation* 1996; 93: 2033-36.

[4] Arntz HR, Willich SN et al. Diurnal, weekly and seasonal variation of sudden death. Population based analysis of 24 061 consecutive cases. *Eur Heart J* 2000; 21:315-20.

[5] Holmberg M, Holmberg S, Herlitz J. Incidence, duration and survival of ventricular fibrilation in out-of-hospital cardiac arrest patients in Sweden. *Resuscitation* 2000; 44:7-17.

[6] Rampazzo A., Nava A., Danieli G.A., Buja G. et al. The gene for arrhythmogenic right ventricular cardiomyopathy maps to chromosome 14q23-q24. *Hum Moll Gen* 1994; Vol 3(6): 959-62.

[7] Saffitz E. Jeffrey. 2005. Dependence of Electrical Coupling on Mechanical Coupling in Cardiac Myocytes. *Ann.N.Y.Sci.*2005; 1047: 336.-44.

[8] Fatkin, D. and R.M.Graham. Molecular mechanisms of inherited cardiomyopathies. *Physiol. Rev.* 2002; 82: 945-80.

[9] McKoy, G.N. Protonotarios, A. Crosby, et al. Identification of a deletion of plakoglobin in arrhythmogenic right ventricular cardiomyopathy with palmoplantar keratoderma and wooly hair-Naxos disease. *Lancet* 2000; 355: 2119-24.

[10]Fisher SA, Langille LB, Srivastava D. Apoptosis during cardiovascular development. *Circulation Research* 2000; November 10: 856-64.

[11]Perlman H, Maillard L, Krasinski K et al. Evidence for the rapid onset of apoptosis in medial smooth muscle cells after baloon injury. *Circulation* 1997; 95:981-7.

[12]Ashkenazi A, Dixit V. Death receptors: signalling and modulation. *Science* 1998; 281: 1305-8.

[13]Torrent-Guasp F, Buckberg GD,Clemente C,Cox JL et al The structure and function of the helical heart and its buttress wrapping.I.The normal macroscopic structure of the heart. *Semin Thorac Cardiovasc Surg* 2001;13(4):301-19

[14]Torrent-Guasp F, Kocica MJ, Corno A, Komeda M et al.Systolic ventricular filling. *Eur J Cardiothorac Surg* 2004;25(3):376-86

[15]Lunkenheimer PP, Redmann K, Florek J, Fassancht U .et al The forces generated within the musculature of the left ventricular wall. *Heart* 2004;90:200-7

[16]Streeter DD,Torrent -Guasp F.Geodesic paths in the left ventricle of the mammalian heart. *Circuulation* 1973,48 (Suppl. 4).4-14.

[17]Greenbaum RA, Ho SY, GibsonDG ,Becker AE, Anderson RH.Left ventricular fibre architecture in man. *British Heart Journal* 1981; 45:248-63

[18]Buckberg GD, Clemente C, Cox JL, Coghlan HC, Castella M, Torrent-Guasp F et al.The structure and the function of the helical heart and its buttress wrapping IV.Concepts of dynamic function from the nirmal macroscopic helical structure. *Semin Thoracic Cardiovasc Surg* 2001; 13(4):342-57

[19]Torrent- Guasp F, Ballerter M, Buckberg GD et al.Spatial orientation of the ventricular muscle band: physiologic contribution and surgical implicamions. *J Thorac Cardiovasc Surg* 2001;122(2):389-92

[20]Marino B, Corno AF. Spiral pattern: universe, normal heart, and complex congenital defects. *J Thorac Cardiovasc Surg* 2003;126(4):1225-6.

[21]Wilcox,Cook and Anderson. *Surgical Anatomy of the Heart*, Cambridge 2003.

[22]Ivana Vranic. Un nouveau signe echocardiographique pour identifier la DVDA. *Cardinale* Tome XVI No 2 Fevrier 2004; p 22-4.

[23]McKenna WJ, Thiene G, et al. Diagnosis of arrhythmogenic right ventricular dysplasia/cardiomyopathy. Task Force of the Working Group Myocardial and Pericardial Disease of the European Society of Cardiology and of the Scientific Council on

Cardiomyopathies of the International Society and Federation of Cardiology. *Br Heart J.* 1994 Mar; 71(3):215-8.

[24]Thiene G, Nava A et al. Right ventricular cardiomyopathy and sudden death in young people. *N Engl J Med.* 1988 Jan 21;318(3):129-33.

[25]Fontaine G, Fontaliran F, Frank R. Arrhythmogenic right ventricular cardiomyopathies: clinical forms and main differential diagnoses. *Circulation.* 1998 Apr 28;97(16):1532-5.

[26]Corrado D, Fontaine G et al. Arrhythmogenic right ventricular dysplasia/cardiomyopathy: need for an international registry. Study Group on Arrhythmogenic Right Ventricular Dysplasia/Cardiomyopathy of the Working Groups on Myocardial and Pericardial Disease and Arrhythmias of the European Society of Cardiology and of the Scientific Council on Cardiomyopathies of the World Heart Federation. *Circulation.* 2000 Mar 21;101(11):E101-6.

[27]Yoerger DM, Marcus F, Sherrill D, et al. For the Multidisciplinary Study of Right Ventricular Dysplasia. Echocardiographic findings in patients meeting task force criteria for arrhythmogenic right ventricular dysplasia: new insights from the Multidisciplinary Study of Right Ventricular Dysplasia. *J Am Coll Cardiol* 2005;45:860 –5.

[28]Ivana I Vranic. Assessment of right ventricular function in ARVC/D patients by 2D ECHO. Abstracts of EUROECHO 7 December 3-6, 2003. *Eur J Echocard* 2003; Vol 4 Suppl 1, p S74

[29]Ivana I Vranic. Pathognomonic sign of ARVC/D by Echo? Abstracts of EUROECHO 7 December 3-6, 2003. *Eur J Echocard* 2003; Vol 4 Suppl 1, p S74

[30]Ivana I Vranic, M Ristic, T Simic. Specific and sensitive enough to reveal the fruste forms of arrhythmogenic right ventricular dysplasia. *J Am Soc Echocardiog*, May 2004; Vol 17 No 5: 524.

[31]Ivana I Vranic, M Ristic, et al.. Septal cusp irregular motion of tricuspid valve in ARVD patients. *Echocardiog*, May 2004; Vol 21 No 4: 358.

[32]Ivana I Vranic, T Simic. Contribution of the crista supraventricularis function in development of heart failure in ARVD patients. *Eur J Echocardiog*, Dec 2004; Vol 5 Suppl 1:177S.

[33]Ivana I Vranic, M Matic. Sudden cardiac death in young athletes- is it preventable? *Europace*, June 2005; Vol 7 -Suppl 1: 85.

[34]Ivana I Vranic, Mihailo Matic. Arrhythmogenic right ventricular dysplasia non qualifying for criteria of WHF but echo positive. *Eur J Echocardiog*, Dec 2005; Vol 6 Suppl 1:S26.

[35]Ivana I Vranic. Another pathognomonic sign in arrhythmogenic right ventricular dysplasia vizualized by pulsed wave doppler in septal cusp of tricuspid valve. *J Am Soc Echocardiog*, May 2006; Vol 19 No 5: 632.

Index

A

B

C

D

E

F

G

H

I

J

N

O

P

Q

R

S

T

U